FROM
PATIENT TO PAYMENT

Insurance Procedures for the Medical Office

SIXTH EDITION

Cynthia Newby, CPC

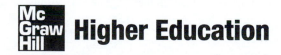 **Higher Education**

Boston   Burr Ridge, IL   Dubuque, IA   New York   San Francisco   St. Louis
Bangkok   Bogotá   Caracas   Kuala Lumpur   Lisbon   London   Madrid   Mexico City
Milan   Montreal   New Delhi   Santiago   Seoul   Singapore   Sydney   Taipei   Toronto

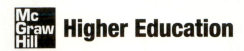

Higher Education

FROM PATIENT TO PAYMENT: INSURANCE PROCEDURES FOR THE MEDICAL OFFICE

Published by McGraw-Hill, a business unit of The McGraw-Hill Companies, Inc., 1221 Avenue of the Americas, New York, NY, 10020. Copyright © 2010 by The McGraw-Hill Companies, Inc. All rights reserved. Previous editions © 1993, 1998, 2002, 2005, and 2008. No part of this publication may be reproduced or distributed in any form or by any means, or stored in a database or retrieval system, without the prior written consent of The McGraw-Hill Companies, Inc., including, but not limited to, in any network or other electronic storage or transmission, or broadcast for distance learning.

Some ancillaries, including electronic and print components, may not be available to customers outside the United States.

This book is printed on acid-free paper.

2 3 4 5 6 7 8 9 0 QPD/QPD 0 9

ISBN   978-0-07-340201-7

MHID   0-07-340201-X

Vice president/Editor in chief: *Elizabeth Haefele*
Vice president/Director of marketing: *John E. Biernat*
Sponsoring editor: *Natalie J. Ruffatto*
Director of development, Allied Health; Patricia Hesse
Developmental editor: *Bonnie Hemrick*
Executive marketing manager: *Roxan Kinsey*
Lead media producer: *Damian Moshak*
Media producer: *Marc Mattson*
Director, Editing/Design/Production: *Jess Ann Kosic*
Project manager: *Marlena Pechan*

Senior production supervisor: *Janean A. Utley*
Designer: *Marianna Kinigakis*
Media project manager: *Mark A. S. Dierker*
Cover design: *Jessica M. Lazar*
Typeface: *11.5/13 Minion*
Compositor: *Aptara, Inc.*
Printer: *Quebecor World Dubuque Inc.*
Cover credit: © *Veer/Corbis Photography*

Library of Congress Cataloging-in-Publication Data

Newby, Cynthia.
    From patient to payment : insurance procedures for the medical office / Cynthia Newby. —6th ed.
        p. cm.
    Rev. ed. of: Glencoe from patient to payment. 3rd ed. c2002.
    Includes index.
    ISBN-13: 978-0-07-340201-7 (alk. paper)
    ISBN-10: 0-07-340201-X (alk. paper)
    1. Medical offices—Management. 2. Medical fees. 3. Health insurance. I. Newby, Cynthia.
Glencoe from patient to payment. II. Title.
R728.5.C64 2010
610.68—dc22

2008052998

The Internet addresses listed in the text were accurate at the time of publication. The inclusion of a Web site does not indicate an endorsement by the authors or McGraw-Hill, and McGraw-Hill does not guarantee the accuracy of the information presented at these sites.

Codeveloped by McGraw-Hill Higher Education and Chestnut Hill Enterprises, Inc. chestnuthl@aol.com

The Medisoft Student Data files, illustrations, instructions, and exercises in *From Patient to Payment: Insurance Procedures for the Medical Office* are compatible with the Medisoft™ Advanced Version 14 Patient Accounting software available at the time of publication. Adaptations may be necessary for use with subsequent versions of the software. Text changes will be made in reprints when possible. Medisoft Advanced Version 14 software must be available to access the Medisoft Student Data files. It can be obtained by contacting your McGraw-Hill sales representative.

All brand or product names are trademarks or registered trademarks of their respective companies.

CPT five-digit codes, nomenclature, and other data are copyright 2008 American Medical Association. All rights reserved. No fee schedules, basic unit, relative values, or related listings are included in the CPT. The AMA assume no liability for the data contained herein.

CPT codes are based on CPT 2009.

ICD-9-CM codes are based on ICD-9-CM 2009.

All names, situations, and anecdotes are fictitious. They do not represent any person, event, or medical record.

www.mhhe.com

Brief Contents

Contents

CHAPTER 16   Medisoft Claim Simulations   286

Guide to the Interactive Simulated CMS-1500 Form   316

Glossary   322

Index   335

Preface

Welcome to the sixth edition of *From Patient to Payment*. This text/workbook is designed for introductory medical insurance courses. Its practical, focused approach provides students with the basics of preparing correct health care claims.

Your Career in Medical Insurance, Billing, and Reimbursement

Medical billing is one of the 10 fastest-growing allied health occupations. This employment growth is the result of the increased medical needs of an aging population, advances in technology, and the growing number of health practitioners.

Medical insurance specialists play important roles in the financial well-being of every health care business. Billing for services in health care is more complicated than in other industries. Government and private payers vary in payment for the same services, and healthcare providers deliver services to beneficiaries of several insurance companies at any one time. Medical insurance specialists must be familiar with the rules and guidelines of each health care plan in order to submit the proper documentation so that the office receives maximum appropriate reimbursement for services provided. Without an effective administrative staff, a medical office would have no cash flow!

Medical billing is a challenging, interesting career, where you are compensated according to your level of skills and how effectively you put them to use. Individuals who have a firm understanding of the medical billing process will find themselves well prepared to enter this ever-changing field.

Overview

Whether your course of study is medical assisting, medical insurance and billing, or health information technology, this text/workbook gives you the background, knowledge and skills needed to successfully handle the medical billing process. It covers procedures as well as basic medical coding guidelines for verifying the diagnosis and procedure codes used to report patients' conditions on health care claims. It also covers the important topic of HIPAA. In today's health care environment, claims cannot be simply correct. Claims, as well as the process used to create them, must also comply with the rules imposed by federal and state law and by government and private payer health care program requirements.

The sixth edition of *From Patient to Payment* is based on a ten-step medical billing process, illustrated on the inside front cover of your text, that organizes the topics for you. This sequence includes:

Step 1   Preregister patients
Step 2   Establish financial responsibility for visits
Step 3   Check in patients
Step 4   Check out patients
Step 5   Review coding compliance
Step 6   Check billing compliance
Step 7   Prepare and transmit claims
Step 8   Monitor payer adjudication
Step 9   Generate patient statements
Step 10 Follow up patient payments and handle collections

The chapters of the text are organized to follow this process:

- Chapters 1 and 2 introduce the major types of medical insurance, payers, and regulators; the medical insurance specialist's functions, ethical responsibilities, and certification; the medical billing process; and HIPAA Privacy, Security, and Electronic Health Care Transactions/Code Sets rules.
- Chapters 3 and 4 build skills in correct coding procedures, use of coding references, and compliance with proper linkage guidelines.
- Chapters 5, 6, and 7 cover payment methods, calculating reimbursement, how to bill compliantly, and preparing, transmitting, and following up claims using the CMS-1500 (08/05) paper claim and the HIPAA electronic claim. Also covered is the collections process.
- Chapters 8 through 13 provide descriptions of the major third-party private and government-sponsored payers' procedures and regulations. Each chapter contains specific filing guidelines. Chapter 14 focuses on dental insurance and billing.
- Chapter 15 provides necessary background in hospital billing, coding, and payment methods.

After studying this text, you can enhance your qualifications for employment by studying *Computers in the Medical Office,* which develops skills in the use of Medisoft™, a popular medical billing and accounting software program, that can easily be transferred to any software program on the job. These skills can then be cemented through *Case Studies for the Medical Office,* an excellent "internship in a box." *Case Studies for the Medical Office* contains a simulation covering two weeks of work in a medical office using Medisoft.

What Every Instructor Needs to Know

What's New in the Sixth Edition?

Chapter 1

- Updated illustrations for Medisoft Version 14, the billing software program available for use with the program

Chapter 2

- The National Plan and Provider Enumeration System (NPPES), a repository for NPIs, introduced as a key resource for complete claim completion
- HIPAA website updated

Chapter 3

- ICD-9-CM codes and concepts updated to 2009

Chapter 4

- CPT/HCPCS codes updated to 2009
- Coverage of FDA pending symbol in CPT
- Decision tree for new versus established patients

Chapter 5

- Updated statistics for insurance coverage

Chapter 6

- 2008 NUCC CMS-1500 (version 4.0) instructions, including new condition codes that can be reported and updated instructions for NPI

Chapter 7

- Real-time claims adjudication (RTCA) concept/procedures added

Chapter 8

- Managed care statistics and trends updated

Chapter 9

- New type of Medicare payers, A/B MACs, introduced
- Physician Quality Reporting Initiative (PQRI) explained
- Instruction on the newly mandated (March 2009) ABN form that replaces the old ABN and eliminates the NEMB

Chapter 9

- CMS-1500 instructions updated for mandatory NPI

Chapter 10

- Content updated
- Medicaid claim form completion instructions for CMS-1500 updated per NUCC

Chapter 11

- Introduces new program TRICARE Prime Remote
- TRICARE claim form completion instructions for CMS-1500 updated per NUCC

Chapter 12

- Workers' Compensation claim form completion instructions for the CMS-1500 updated per NUCC

Chapter 13

- Content and terminology updated

Chapter 14

- Dental claims updated for NPI

Chapter 15

- New Important Message from Medicare illustrated
- Present on admission (POA) reporting for hospital claims
- "Never events"—patients' hospital-acquired conditions (HACs) that Medicare and most major payers will not cover
- Explanation of MS-DRGs as the basis for the new inpatient prospective payments

Chapter 16

The claim case studies have been revised for completion with Medisoft Advanced Version 14. A new installation program has been created for downloading and installing the Medisoft Student Data files directly from the OLC to students' computers.

Medisoft Advanced Version 14

Medisoft Advanced Version 14 is available to adopters who wish to use this popular billing program for claim completion in Chapter 16. In addition to the new instructions for use of Medisoft Version 14, the illustrations of medical billing program software screens have been updated.

New Interactive Simulated CMS-1500 Form

Students have the option to use the new interactive simulated CMS-1500 form to complete claim case studies.

Learning and Teaching Supplements
For the Instructor

The *Medical Insurance Coding Workbook for Physician Practices and Facilities, 2009–2010 edition* (0-07-3402044)

Since medical insurance specialists verify diagnosis and procedure codes and use them to report physicians' services, a fundamental understanding of coding principles and guidelines is the baseline for correct claims. The *Medical Insurance Coding Workbook* provides practice and instruction in coding and compliance skills. The coding workbook reinforces and enhances skill development by applying the coding principles introduced in *From Patient to Payment 6e* and extending knowledge through additional coding guidelines, examples, and compliance tips. It offers over 75 case studies to simulate more real-world application. Also included are inpatient scenarios for coding that require compliance with the *ICD-9-CM Official Guidelines for Coding and Reporting* sequencing rules.

Instructor's Medisoft ™ Advanced Version 14 Software

This full working version allows a school to place the live software on the laboratory or classroom computers (only one copy needs to be sent per campus location). In addition to the software, the following equipment and supplies are needed for the Medisoft claim simulations in Chapter 16:

- Medisoft Student Data files (a base of case study information created for use with the claim cases studies in Chapter 16), available for download from the Online Learning Center, www.mhhe.com/fp2p6e
- PC with 500 MHz or greater processor speed
- 256 MB RAM
- 500 MB available hard disk space (if saving data to a hard drive)
- CD-ROM 2x or faster disk drive
- Windows Vista Business 32-bit version (Medisoft 14 will not work on the 64-bit system), Windows XP Professional, or Windows 2000 Professional
- Medisoft™ Advanced Version 14 Patient Accounting
- External storage device for storing backup copies of the working database
- Printer
- Active Internet connection to access the OLC

Instructor's Interactive Simulated CMS-1500 Form

The simulated form is a PDF file that can be used with Adobe Reader to create and print CMS-1500 forms. Available for download at the Online Learning Center, the form provides an easy-to-use alternative to filling in claim forms by hand. Instructors may choose to have students experiment with the form while completing the claim case studies in Chapter 6 and Chapters 8 through 12.

Instructor's Manual, which is posted to the Instructor Resources on the Online Learning Center, www.mhhe.com/fp2p6e, includes:

- course overview
- information on ordering and installing Medisoft™ Advanced Version 14 software
- chapter-by-chapter lesson plans
- software troubleshooting tips
- end-of-chapter solutions
- correlation tables: SCANS, AAMA Role Delineation Study Areas of Competence, and AMT Registered Medical Assistant Certification Exam Topics

If you elect to use Chapter 16: Medisoft Claim Simulations, you can rely on the manual for important information to help your students work through the Medisoft exercises.

Online Learning Center (OLC), www.mhhe.com/fp2p6e, Instructor Resources include:

- instructor's PowerPoint® presentation of Chapters 1–15
- electronic testing program featuring McGraw-Hill's EZ Test. This flexible and easy-to-use program allows instructors to create tests from book specific items. It accommodates a wide range of question types and instructors may add their own questions. Multiple versions of the test can be created and any test can be exported for use with course management systems such as WebCT, Blackboard, or PageOut.
- Instructor's Manual in Word and PDF format
- links to professional associations
- Medisoft™ Advanced Version 14 installation instructions
- Medisoft tips and frequently asked questions
- Medisoft solutions backup file (Chapter16_solutions.mbk) for instructor use
- PageOut link

For the Student
Student-at-Home Medisoft™ Advanced Version 14 Software
This version is an option for distance education or students who want to practice with the software at home.

Medisoft Student Data
The Student Data files provide the patient database to complete the Medisoft™ Advanced Version 14 claim case studies in Chapter 16. The files, as well as instructions for downloading them, are available at the text's Online Learning Center (OLC) under the heading "Medisoft v14 Data Files."

Online Learning Center (OLC), www.mhhe.com/fp2p6e, includes additional chapter quizzes and other review activities.

Many tools to help you learn have been integrated into your text.

Chapter Features

Learning Outcomes—gives you an overview of the key concepts and organization.

Key Terms—lists the important vocabulary terms alphabetically to build your insurance terminology. Key terms are printed in bold-faced type and defined when introduced in the text.

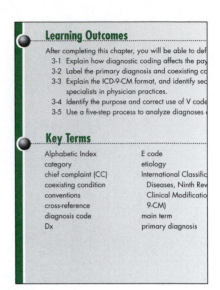

Learning Outcomes

After completing this chapter, you will be able to def

3-1 Explain how diagnostic coding affects the pay

3-2 Label the primary diagnosis and coexisting co

3-3 Explain the ICD-9-CM format, and identify sec
    specialists in physician practices.

3-4 Identify the purpose and correct use of V code

3-5 Use a five-step process to analyze diagnoses

Key Terms

Alphabetic Index	E code
category	etiology
chief complaint (CC)	International Classific
coexisting condition	Diseases, Ninth Rev
conventions	Clinical Modificatio
cross-reference	9-CM)
diagnosis code	main term
Dx	primary diagnosis

Why This Chapter Is Important to You

The information in this chapter will enable you to:
• Use an important reference book, the ICD-9-CM.
• Expand your understanding of why errors in diagnos
  and payment cycle.
• Learn one of the most important steps in completing h

What Do You Think?

To diagnose a patient's condition, the physician follows
making based on the patient's statements, an examinati
information. When the diagnosis is made, the medical
to the insurance carrier through codes on the health car
coding have on the medical office?

Why This Chapter Is Important to You—explains how the information in the chapter relates to the job of a medical insurance specialist.

What Do You Think?—describes a situation or discussion point for you to consider as you study the chapter.

HIPAA and Compliance Tips—connect you to the real world of insurance billing to build your understanding of the correct privacy, security, and code sets to use. These tips also give you hints on the best ways to complete health care claims and on correctly handling situations that may arise in the medical office.

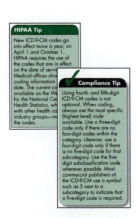

HIPAA Tip

New ICD-9-CM codes go into effect twice a year, on April 1 and October 1. HIPAA requires the use of the codes that are in effect on the date of servi Medical offices sho coding information date. The current co available on the We for the National Ce Health Statistics, wh with other health ca industry groups—m the codes.

✓ **Compliance Tip**

Using fourth- and fifth-digit ICD-9-CM codes is not optional. When coding, always use the most specific (highest level) code available. Use a three-digit code only if there are no four-digit codes within the category. Likewise, use a four-digit code only if there is no five-digit code for that subcategory. Use the five-digit subclassification code wherever possible. Most commercial publishers of the ICD-9-CM use a symbol such as 5 next to a subcategory to indicate that a five-digit code is required.

Professional Focus—related facts about current computer technology, legislation, changing regulations, and career applications.

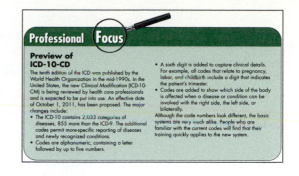

FYI—"For Your Information" boxes with interesting bits of information about topics in the main text.

Explore the Internet—the URLs of useful websites for medical insurance specialists.

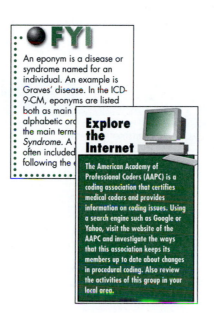

Chapter Review

Chapter Summary—provides a useful review of the chapter's concepts and provides a summary of each learning outcome.

Check Your Understanding—test your knowledge of the chapter's concepts and terms with various types of exercises.

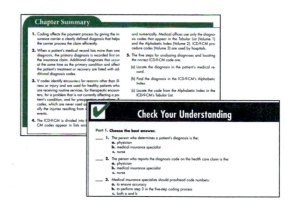

Case Studies—throughout the chapter, Case Studies ask you to apply the knowledge gained by studying the chapter for correct answers.

Claim Case Studies

The claim case studies in Chapter 16 let you practice your knowledge of correct claim preparation using Medisoft software.

Glossary

The most important insurance, billing, and coding definitions are found in the back of the text for each reference.

Online Learning Center (OLC)

www.mhhe.com/fp2p6e
The OLC provides additional learning and teaching tools.

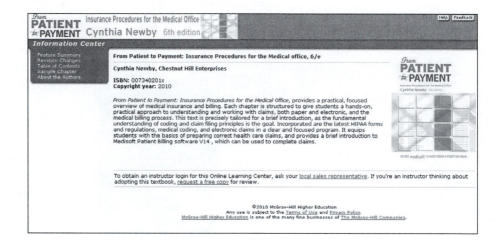

Acknowledgments

A number of people made significant contributions to the sixth edition of *From Patient to Payment*. For insightful reviews, criticisms, helpful suggestions, and information, we would like to acknowledge the following:

From Patient to Payment Reviewers for Sixth Edition

Christa Bartlett, CMA-CPC
University of Alaska Fairbanks

Karen Bean, BS, MS
Blinn College

Amy L. Blochowaik, MBA, ACS, AIAA, AIRC, ALHC, ARA, FLHC, FLMI, HCSA, HIA, MHP, PCS, SILA-F
Northeast Wisconsin Technical College

Deborah K. Cresap, MS
West Virginia Northern Community College

Sheri L. Kraft Haugen
Wisconsin Indianhead Technical College

Pamela Jeffcoat, CMA, MA
Renton Technical College

Tammy Savage, R.N.
Douglas Education Center

Maggie M. Scott, MPH, RHIT
Victor Valley College

Jan Vermiglio-Smith, RN, MS, PhD
Central Arizona College–Allied Health Program

Teresa A. Welch
Spoon River College

Virginia Williams, MS, Associate Professor
Kaskaskia College

Nichole Yerger, MS, RN
PACE Institute

Fifth Edition Reviewers

Roxane Abbott
Sarasota County Technical Institute

Deborah Eid
Apollo College

Carol Hinricher
University of Montana College of Technology

Cecilia Jacob
Tennessee Tech at Memphis

Beverly D. Joe
National Park Community College

Michael Meyer, DO, CCS, CPC
FMU, DeVry Online, South University Online

Latonya Polite
Sanz School

Lori L. Rager, CMA
Eagle Gate College

David Rice
Career College of Northern Nevada

Maggie M. Scott
Victor Valley Community College

FROM
PATIENT TO PAYMENT

Insurance Procedures for the Medical Office

From Patient to Payment: Becoming a Medical Insurance Specialist

Learning Outcomes

After completing this chapter, you will be able to define the key terms and:

1-1 Explain the main differences between indemnity plans and managed care plans.

1-2 Define the various types of insurance coverage.

1-3 Describe the medical office billing workflow.

1-4 List the ten primary responsibilities of a medical insurance specialist.

1-5 Compare medical ethics and etiquette.

1-6 Discuss effects of health care claim errors on medical office routines.

Key Terms

assignment of benefits	fee-for-service	noncovered (excluded)
benefits	health care claim	services
coinsurance	health plan	patient information form
copayment	indemnity plan	payer
deductible	indirect payment	policyholder
dependent	insurance carrier	preauthorization
diagnoses	managed care	preexisting condition
direct payment	managed care organization	premium
electronic claim	(MCO)	procedures
encounter form	medical coder	provider
ethics	medical insurance	remittance advice (RA)
etiquette	medical insurance specialist	
explanation of benefits (EOB)	medically necessary	

Why This Chapter Is Important to You

The information in this chapter will enable you to:

- Understand the medical office billing and reimbursement process.
- Understand the role of a medical insurance specialist in a medical office.
- Understand the importance of working efficiently and accurately in a medical office.
- Begin to gain the skills that will make you a valuable member of a medical office staff.

What Do You Think?

The health care field is constantly changing. Technology offers new medical equipment and drugs to improve care. The demand for medical services is rising, and so is the cost. Most physicians are part of small or large group practices or clinics rather than practicing alone. Electronic versions of medical records are increasingly important. Patients have many choices in health care coverage and must select from a wide range of medical insurance options and prices. Thus, today's medical office staff often communicates with many insurance companies that have many different rules and policies regarding insurance claims. In what ways can the medical insurance specialist keep up-to-date on these issues?

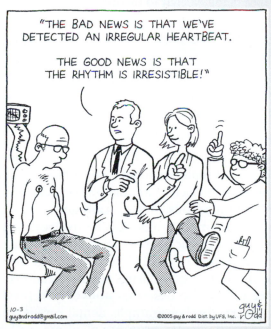

Everyone, no matter how healthy, needs medical care at some time. People need preventive care, such as routine checkups and vaccinations, to stay healthy. They also need treatment for sicknesses, accidents, and injuries. A person who receives medical care owes a charge for the medical services and supplies that are involved. To be able to afford the charges, many people in the United States have **medical insurance,** which is an agreement between a person, who is called the **policyholder,** and a **health plan.** Health plans, also known as **insurance carriers** or **payers,** are organizations that offer financial protection in case of illness or accidental injury. Medical insurance helps pay for the policyholder's medical treatment.

Insurance Basics

A person who buys medical insurance pays a **premium** to a health plan. In exchange for the premium, the health plan agrees to pay amounts, called **benefits**, for medical services. Medical services include the care supplied by **providers**—hospitals, physicians, and other medical staff members and facilities.

The health plan issues the policyholder an insurance policy that contains a list of covered medical services that is called a schedule of benefits. Benefits commonly include payment of medically necessary medical treatments received by policyholders and their dependents. The Health Insurance Association of America defines the insurance term **medically necessary** as "medical treatment that is appropriate and rendered in accordance with generally accepted standards of medical practice." In general, the procedure must meet these conditions to be considered necessary:

- Procedures or services match the patient's illness.
- Procedures are not elective (that is, they are required to treat a condition, rather than being elected to be done by the patient).
- Procedures are not experimental. The procedures must be approved by the appropriate federal regulatory agency, such as the Food and Drug Administration.
- Procedures are furnished at an appropriate level. Simple diagnoses need simple procedures; complex or time-consuming procedures are reserved for complex conditions

Typical covered medical services include surgical, primary care, emergency care, and specialists' services. Other medically related expenses, such as hospital-based services, are usually included. Many health plans also cover preventive medical services, such as annual physical examinations, pediatric and adolescent immunizations, prenatal care, and routine cancer screening procedures such as mammograms. Policies list treatments that are covered at different rates and medical services that are not covered. For example, a plan may pay 80 percent of most physically related treatments but a smaller percentage of the charges for drugs and medications.

The medical insurance policy also describes **noncovered (excluded) services**—what it does not pay for. For example, dental care is generally not included. (However, separate dental insurance plans are available for purchase.) Also, if a new policyholder has a medical condition that was diagnosed before the policy was written—known as a **preexisting condition**—a health plan may not cover medical services for its treatment.

Indemnity Plans

In the last century, most medical insurance policies in the United States were **indemnity plans.** Under an indemnity plan, the medical costs policyholders incur when they receive treatment for accidents and illnesses are paid by the insurance carrier. If a policyholder or a covered **dependent** (a spouse, child, or other relative specified in the insurance policy) gets sick, the health plan pays most of the bill. Benefits are determined on a **fee-for-service** basis. In other words, benefits are based on the fees physicians charge for the services.

Under an indemnity plan, the policy lists the services that are paid for and the amounts that are paid. The benefit may be for all or part of the charges. In many cases, the policyholder owes a percentage of the fees, usually called **coinsurance.** For example, the schedule of benefits in a medical insurance policy may say that it pays 80 percent of the fees for surgery performed in a hospital and that the policyholder must pay 20 percent. Under this contract, if the policyholder has surgery in the hospital and the bill is $2,000, the health plan pays 80 percent of $2,000, or $1,600. The policyholder is responsible for the coinsurance—the other 20 percent, or $400 in this example.

Managed Care Plans

Under indemnity plans, it is difficult for insurance carriers to control costs because there have been few restrictions on providers' charges, especially for new technology, drugs, and procedures. To counter this trend, the concept of **managed care** was introduced. Managed care is a way of supervising medical care with the goal of ensuring that patients get needed services in the most appropriate, cost-effective setting.

To accomplish managed care goals, the financing and management of health care are combined with the delivery of services. **Managed care organizations (MCOs)** establish links among provider, patient, and payer. Instead of only the patient's having a policy with the health plan, under managed care both the patient and the provider have agreements with the MCO. The patient agrees to the payments for the services, and the provider agrees to accept the fees the MCO offers for services. This arrangement gives the managed care plan more control over the services the provider performs and the fees the plan pays.

Managed care is the leading type of health plan, and many different kinds of managed care programs are available. These are covered in detail in Chapter 5. In some cases, patients pay fixed premiums at regular time periods, such as monthly. A patient may also pay a **copayment**—a small fixed fee, such as $10, for each office visit. In some plans, this "copay" is a percentage of the amount the provider receives. In either case, the copayment must always be paid by the patient at the time of service.

Cost Containment

Most health plans, including indemnity plans, now have cost-containment practices to help control costs. For example, patients may be required to choose from a specific group of physicians and hospitals for all medical care. A visit to a specialists may require a referral from the patient's primary care physician. A second physician's opinion may be required before surgery can be reimbursed. Also, many services that previously involved overnight hospital stays are now covered only if done during daytime hospital visits, with patients recuperating at home.

Preauthorization is another example of a cost-containment practice. If preauthorization is required, the health plan must approve a procedure before it is done in order for the procedure to be covered. For example, many nonemergency services must be approved before patients are admitted to the hospital. Also, shorter hospital stays are encouraged, and weekend hospital admissions for Monday services may not be permitted.

COMMON TYPES OF MEDICAL INSURANCE

Some patients seen in a medical office are covered by private insurance. Others qualify for programs sponsored by state or federal governments.

Private Insurance

Private health plans offer a variety of types of medical insurance coverage. Most people enrolled in private insurance are covered under group contracts—policies that cover people who work for the same employer or belong to the same organization. Examples include private companies, professional associations, labor unions, and schools. Other plans are offered as individual contracts, which are policies purchased by people who do not qualify as members of a group.

Some employers have established themselves as self-insured health plans. Rather than paying a premium to an insurance carrier, the organization assumes the risk of paying directly for medical services, establishes contracts with local physician practices, and sets up a fund with which it pays for claims. The organization itself establishes the benefit levels and the plan types it will offer.

People may also have medical coverage through their liability insurance and automobile insurance. For example, people injured in automobile accidents may be insured through the medical benefit of their or another party's automobile policy. Coverage varies by state.

Government Plans

The most common government plans in effect in the United States are:

- *Medicare*—Medicare is a federal health plan that covers most citizens aged sixty-five and over, people with disabilities, end-stage renal disease (ESRD), and dependent widows.
- *Medicaid*—Low-income people who cannot afford medical care are covered by Medicaid, which is cosponsored by federal and state governments. (Medicaid is a state-run program; there are matching federal dollars available for states that satisfy certain requirements, such as providing prenatal care and child vaccinations.) Qualifications and benefits vary by state.
- *Workers' Compensation*—People with job-related illnesses or injuries are covered under workers' compensation insurance

through their employer. Workers' compensation benefits vary according to state law.

- *TRICARE (formerly CHAMPUS)*—This program covers expenses for dependents of active-duty members of the uniformed services and for retired military personnel. It also covers dependents of military personnel who were killed while on active duty.
- *CHAMPVA*—The Civilian Health and Medical Program of the Department of Veterans Affairs is for veterans with permanent service-related disabilities and their dependents. It also covers surviving spouses and dependent children of veterans who died from service-related disabilities.

THE MEDICAL OFFICE BILLING WORKFLOW

In most cases, a person covered by a health plan receives insurance benefits by filing a **health care claim.** This claim identifies the policyholder (and the patient, if this person is not the policyholder) and tells the health plan which medical services were performed and why. Most medical offices file claims for their patients. The billing workflow for a patient's health care is as follows:

1. The patient presents for an appointment.
2. Medical services are provided to the patient.
3. The health plan is billed for the appointment.
4. The health plan responds to the claim.
5. The patient is billed as appropriate.

The patient presents for an appointment.

After making an appointment, the patient arrives at the medical office reception area and completes (or updates) initial forms. A new patient who comes to a medical office usually fills out a **patient information form,** also known as a registration form. Returning patients are asked to check and update their patient information forms. Most medical offices make sure that patients' forms are updated at least every twelve months. As shown in Figure 1-1, page 8, the patient information form provides the demographic data—personal, employment, and medical insurance information—needed to file a claim.

Patient information forms usually ask for the patient's signature or for a parent's or guardian's signature if the patient is a minor. As part of the form or separately, the patient usually signs an **assignment of benefits.** The assignment of benefits is a statement that tells the health plan to pay benefits directly to the physician. If the patient does not sign the assignment of benefits, the insurance benefit check goes to the policyholder, who must then pay the provider. Another signature permits the provider to give the health plan information needed to help process the claim. Although providers have a right to do this under federal law without a patient's signature (explained in Chapter 2), most medical offices have patients sign this line.

CENTRAL PRACTICE CENTER
1122 E. University Drive
Mesa, AZ 85204
602-969-4237

Patient				
Last Name	First Name	MI	Sex __ M __ F	Date of Birth / /
Address	City	State		Zip
Home Ph # ( )	Marital Status		Student Status	
SS#	Allergies:			
Employment Status	Employer Name	Work Ph # ( )		Primary Insurance ID#
Employer Address	City	State		Zip
Referred By		Ph # of Referral ( )		

Responsible Party (Complete this section if the person responsible for the bill is not the patient)

Last Name	First Name	MI	Sex __ M __ F	Date of Birth / /
Address	City	State Zip		SS#
Relation to Patient __ Spouse __ Parent __ Other	Employer Name		Work Phone # ( )	
Spouse, or Parent (if minor):			Home Phone # ( )	

Insurance (If you have multiple coverage, supply information from both carriers)

Primary Carrier Name	Secondary Carrier Name
Name of the Insured (Name on ID Card)	Name of the Insured (Name on ID Card)
Patient's relationship to the insured __ Self __ Spouse __ Child	Patient's relationship to the insured __ Self __ Spouse __ Child
Insured ID #	Insured ID #
Group # or Company Name	Group # or Company Name
Insurance Address	Insurance Address
Phone #	Copay $	Phone #	Copay $

Other Information

Is patient's condition related to:
__ Employment __ Auto Accident (if yes, state in which accident occurred: ___) __ Other Accident

Date of Accident: / / Date of First Symptom of Illness: / /

Reason for visit:

Financial Agreement and Authorization for Treatment

I authorize treatment and agree to pay all fees and charges for the person named above. I agree to pay all charges shown by statements, promptly upon their presentation, unless credit arrangements are agreed upon in writing.

I authorize payment directly to CENTRAL PRACTICE CENTER insurance benefits otherwise payable to me. I hereby authorize the release of any medical information necessary in order to process a claim for payment in my behalf.

Signed: _____ Date: _____

Figure 1-1 Patient Information Form

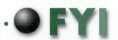
If the patient has insurance coverage, the medical office staff verifies the patient's eligibility by communicating with the health plan to:

- Check that the patient will be covered for services being provided.
- Find out the terms and conditions of the insurance coverage, such as whether a copayment is required.

The medical insurance specialist files the patient information form in the financial section of the patient's medical record. Patients' financial records include insurance and billing information. The patient's medical record is a file that also includes the patient's medical history, a record of treatment and progress, and other communications.

Medical services are provided to the patient.

In many cases, the physician examines the patient, evaluates the patient's condition, and treats the patient. At times, the patient's care is handled by a nonphysician practitioner (NPP), such as a nurse or physician assistant.

The complaint and symptom(s) are documented in the patient's medical record. Also stated are the **diagnoses**—the physician's opinion of the nature of the patient's illness or injury—and the **procedures,** which are the services, tests, and treatments provided, including any medicines prescribed.

The provider then fills out some type of **encounter form.** This form has spaces for the diagnosis, the medical services, the fees for the day's visit, and the provider's signature. An example is shown in Figure 1-2, page 10. Although the encounter form may be as simple as a receipt, usually it is a specially designed form. In some offices, it may be called a superbill or charge ticket. Encounter forms list procedures typically performed in a particular medical office.

The health plan is billed for the appointment.

In most cases, the patient's encounter will be reported to the health plan using a standardized claim. (This claim is described in detail in Chapter 6.) The claim is completed using information from the patient information form, the patient's medical record, and the encounter form.

The charges for the day's visit are totaled from the encounter form. These charges are the basis for completing the health care claim. Any payments due from the patient at the time of service are collected and noted on the claim, which is transmitted to the health plan.

Medical billing programs are typically used to prepare health care claims. Billing programs streamline the important process of creating and following up on claims sent to health plans and bills sent to patients. The completed claim is recorded in the billing program's insurance log, a running list of insurance claims that have been sent to all carriers. The health care claim is then sent to the health plan in one of two ways. Most claims are sent as an **electronic claim,** transmitted by transferring information from a computer in the provider's office to a health plan's computer. The other claims—paper claims—are printed and mailed to the payer.

CENTRAL PRACTICE CENTER
1122 E. University Drive
Mesa, AZ 85204
602-969-4237

PATIENT NAME				APPT. DATE/TIME			

PATIENT NO.				DX			
				1.			
				2.			
				3.			
				4.			

DESCRIPTION	√	CPT	FEE	DESCRIPTION	√	CPT	FEE
EXAMINATION				**PROCEDURES**			
New Patient				Diagnostic Anoscopy		46600	
Problem Focused		99201		ECG Complete		93000	
Expanded Problem Focused		99202		I&D, Abscess		10060	
Detailed		99203		Pap Smear		88150	
Comprehensive		99204		Removal of Cerumen		69210	
Comprehensive/Complex		99205		Removal 1 Lesion		17000	
Established Patient				Removal 2-14 Lesions		17003	
Minimum		99211		Removal 15+ Lesions		17004	
Problem Focused		99212		Rhythm ECG w/Report		93040	
Expanded Problem Focused		99213		Rhythm ECG w/Tracing		93041	
Detailed		99214		Sigmoidoscopy, diag.		45330	
Comprehensive/Complex		99215					
				LABORATORY			
PREVENTIVE VISIT				Bacteria Culture		87081	
New Patient				Fungal Culture		87101	
Age 12-17		99384		Glucose Finger Stick		82948	
Age 18-39		99385		Lipid Panel		80061	
Age 40-64		99386		Specimen Handling		99000	
Age 65+		99387		Stool/Occult Blood		82270	
Established Patient				Tine Test		85008	
Age 12-17		99394		Tuberculin PPD		86580	
Age 18-39		99395		Urinalysis		81000	
Age 40-64		99396		Venipuncture		36415	
Age 65+		99397					
				INJECTION/IMMUN.			
CONSULTATION: OFFICE/ER				DT Immun		90702	
Requested By:				Hepatitis A Immun		90632	
Problem Focused		99241		Hepatitis B Immun		90746	
Expanded Problem Focused		99242		Influenza Immun		90660	
Detailed		99243		Pneumovax		90732	
Comprehensive		99244					
Comprehensive/Complex		99245					
				TOTAL FEES			

Figure 1-2 Encounter Form

Anthem Blue Cross Blue Shield
900 West Market Street
Phoenix, AZ 84209
Date prepared: 6/22/2010

Patient's name	Dates of service from - thru	POS	Proc	Qty	Charge amount	Eligible amount	Patient liability	Amt paid provider
Claim number 0347914								
Daiute, Angelo X	06/17/10 - 06/17/10	11	36415	1	$11.00	$11.00	$00.00	$11.00
Daiute, Angelo X	06/17/10 - 06/17/10	11	80050	1	$98.00	$98.00	$00.00	$98.00
Daiute, Angelo X	06/17/10 - 06/17/10	11	81000	1	$12.00	$12.00	$00.00	$12.00
Daiute, Angelo X	06/17/10 - 06/17/10	11	93000	1	$51.00	$51.00	$00.00	$51.00
Daiute, Angelo X	06/17/10 - 06/17/10	11	99386	1	$123.00	$123.00	$00.00	$123.00

Figure 1-3 Sample Physician Remittance Advice

The health plan responds to the claim.

At the health plan's office, the claim is received and processed by the claims department. After verifying basic information and patient eligibility, the diagnosis and procedures are reviewed to be sure the treatment was medically necessary.

To use an extreme example, a claim may indicate that the patient had a broken arm and that the procedure was removal of the tonsils. Since removing the tonsils is not a medically necessary treatment for a broken arm, the claim would be denied. If the patient were instead treated with a cast for the broken arm, the treatment would suit the diagnosis and would be considered medically necessary.

The claims department compares the services to the schedule of benefits in the patient's policy and determines the amount of benefit to be paid on the claim. Many plans include a **deductible,** an amount the policyholder must pay (usually annually) before insurance benefits are paid. Only medical services that are covered in the schedule of benefits count toward the deductible.

For example, suppose Glenda Williams's plan has a $250 annual deductible. This means that her insurance company does not pay any benefits until she has spent $250 for services covered by her policy. If her medical bills total $400, she must pay the first $250. The insurance carrier will pay part or all of the remaining $150 according to the schedule of benefits in her policy.

Once the amount of benefit is determined, the insurance company issues a check. At the same time, it issues an **explanation of benefits (EOB)** or **remittance advice (RA)**. As shown in Figure 1-3, the RA/EOB shows how the amount of benefit was determined. The insurance carrier may send payment to the physician or to the policyholder. If payment goes directly to the physician, it is called a **direct payment**. If it goes to the policyholder, it is an **indirect payment**. In either case, the patient receives a document that explains the payment, as shown in Figure 1-4, page 12.

CUSTOMER'S EXPLANATION OF BENEFITS

1324   0664402

THIS IS NOT A BILL. RETAIN FOR YOUR RECORDS.

CUSTOMER'S NAME: SUSAN BILTON
ID NUMBER: 140385526
PATIENT'S NAME: SUSAN BILTON

COVERAGE: BCBS OF NJ

CONSUMER DIVISION

CLAIM NUMBER: 7970920006160000
CLAIM RECEIVED: 04/02/2010
CLAIM FINALIZED: 04/08/2010
CHECK NUMBER: 0005890315

MEDICAL SURGICAL/MAJOR MEDICAL CLAIM SUMMARY

CHARGES FOR THIS CLAIM ....$ 1,224.00
AMOUNT OF CUSTOMER BALANCE REMAINING.............$ 367.20
BENEFITS PAID TO SUSAN BILTON ....$ 856.80

DO NOT SUBMIT A SEPARATE MAJOR MEDICAL CLAIM FORM
THIS CLAIM HAS BEEN PROCESSED UNDER YOUR MEDICAL-SURGICAL AND MAJOR MEDICAL CONTRACTS

PATIENT'S NAME: SUSAN BILTON   IDENTIFICATION NUMBER: 140385526   CLAIM NUMBER: 7970920006160000

PROVIDER NAME		1	2	3	4	5	6	7	8	9
TYPE OF SERVICE - PLACE OF SERVICE	DATE OF SERVICE FROM TO	CHARGE AMOUNT	OTHER INS PAYMENT	NOT COVERED AMOUNT	ELIGIBLE AMOUNT	DEDUC- TIBLE	COINS/ CO-PAY	BENEFIT AMOUNT	CUSTOMER BALANCE	MSG CODES
ANESTHESIA CONSLTNTS CENTRL JERSEY										
ANESTHESIA-INPATIENT	03/13/10 03/13/10	1224.00			1224.00		367.20	856.80		
MAJOR MEDICAL		1224.00						0.00	367.20	
TOTALS		1224.00			1224.00		367.20	856.80	367.20	
MESSAGES										

CRP02B (1-97)

* SUSAN HAS SATISFIED $1,000.00 OF HER DEDUCTIBLE FOR THE PERIOD 01-01-10 TO 12-31-10. (0O55)

Figure 1-4 Sample Patient Explanation of Benefits

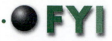
The patient is billed as appropriate.

When the RA/EOB arrives, it must be reviewed and checked. The amount paid is posted (that is, entered) in the medical billing program. If the patient has more than one insurance plan, the cycle is repeated, and the claim and payment information are sent to the second payer. The billing program is used to determine whether the patient owes an additional payment on the account. If so, this amount is billed to the patient. An example of a bill sent to a patient is shown in Figure 1-5.

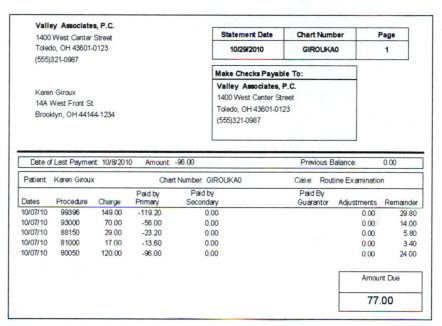

Figure 1-5 Sample Patient Invoice

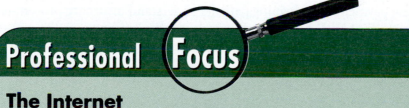

Professional Focus

The Internet and Medical Insurance

The World Wide Web is a valuable source of information about many topics of interest to medical insurance specialists. For example, many insurance carriers have websites that post updates to their claims submission procedures. Professional organizations, such as the American Medical Association, offer information and opinions on timely medical topics.

Each chapter of this text contains an Explore the Internet box that suggests a website that may be of use to you. Visit these sites, and begin to build a reference library of resources that will help you in your future role as a medical insurance specialist.

THE RESPONSIBILITIES OF A MEDICAL INSURANCE SPECIALIST

Explore the Internet

Using a search engine such as Google or Yahoo, explore the job statistics gathered by the Bureau of Labor Statistics. At the Bureau's home page, choose Keyword Search of BLS web pages, and enter a job title of interest to you. Two possible choices for your search are (1) medical assistants and (2) health information technicians. In particular, review the job outlook information.

It is clear that teamwork is essential in the medical office. The **medical insurance specialist** works with the professional staff of physicians and nonphysician practitioners as well as with other administrative personnel. An overall focus is smoothing the way for payments from health plans and from patients. The work includes much more than entering data in a billing program to complete a health care claim. It requires knowledge of the billing and reimbursement process and the ability to work with a variety of complex insurance plans.

In addition to physicians' practices, medical insurance specialists work in clinics, for hospitals or nursing homes, and in other health care settings such as insurance companies as claims examiners, provider relations representatives, or benefits analysts. Positions are also available in government and public health agencies. Employment with companies that offer billing or consulting services to health care providers is an option, as is self-employment as a claims assistance professional who helps consumers with medical insurance problems or as a billing service for providers.

In small physician practices, medical insurance specialists handle a variety of billing and collections tasks. In larger medical practices, duties may be more specialized. Billing, insurance, and collections duties may be separated, or a medical insurance specialist may work exclusively with claims sent to just one of many payers, such as Medicare or workers' compensation. The administrative functions in larger groups or networks are usually headed by a practice manager, office manager, or administrator to whom the administrative staff, such as medical transcriptionists, receptionists, accounting personnel, and medical insurance specialists, report.

Job Duties: The Medical Billing Process

The physicians and, often, the practice manager determine the medical insurance specialist's job duties. Although parts of the job may vary, most medical insurance specialists perform similar tasks. Examples include gathering patient information and signatures, filing health care claims, reviewing payments, and helping patients understand insurance procedures. These medical billing and reimbursement tasks, as shown in Figure 1-6, require knowledge of the office workflow relating to claims and skills in

Step 1 Preregister patients
Step 2 Establish financial responsibility for visits
Step 3 Check in patients
Step 4 Check out patients
Step 5 Review coding compliance
Step 6 Check billing compliance
Step 7 Prepare and transmit claims
Step 8 Monitor payer adjudication
Step 9 Generate patient statements
Step 10 Follow up patient payments and handle collections

Figure 1-6 Medical Billing Process

using the medical billing program, accurately entering data, and carefully proofreading data.

Tasks at the Time of Service

1. Preregister patients.

The billing and reimbursement process really begins before patients arrive at the office.

Tasks related to this area of responsibility include scheduling appointments and gathering basic patients' demographic and insurance information.

2. Establish financial responsibility for the visit.

Medical insurance specialists check insurance coverage and eligibility for benefits. They also check preauthorization requirements and any other payer rules. Duties also include asking patients for appropriate signatures authorizing assignment of benefits, and scanning or photocopying insurance cards.

3. Check in patients.

During the check-in process, medical insurance specialists ask patients for appropriate signatures authorizing assignment of benefits, and scan or photocopy insurance cards. Copayments are collected, and the patient's previous financial record is reviewed for current balances.

4. Check out patients.

After the encounter, diagnoses, treatments, and charges must be located on the encounter forms in patients' medical records in order to total the patient's charges. If the patient owes a balance from previous visits, this amount may also be collected during the visit, subject to state laws. If balances are not collected at this time, arrangements for payment are made. Payments may be made by cash, check, or credit or debit card. When a payment is made, a receipt is given to the patient. Patients' follow-up visits are also scheduled.

Tasks to Prepare Claims

5. Review coding compliance.

Medical insurance specialists double-check the links between diagnoses and procedures to be sure of the medical necessity for the services. The correct codes for the diagnoses and procedures must be used on claims. The patient's primary illness is assigned a code from the *International Classification of Diseases*, Ninth Revision, *Clinical Modification* (ICD-9-CM) (see Chapter 3). For example:

The ICD code for Alzheimer disease is 331.0.
The ICD code for influenza with bronchitis or with a cold is 487.1.

Similarly, each procedure the physician performs is assigned a code that stands for the particular service, treatment, or test. This code is selected from the *Current Procedural Terminology* (CPT) (see Chapter 4). For example:

99460 is the CPT code for the physician's examination of a newborn infant. 27130 is the code for a total hip replacement operation.

In some medical practices, the physicians assign these codes; in others, a **medical coder** or the medical insurance specialist handles this task.

6. Check billing compliance.

A second part of claim preparation is to verify that the billing meets the payer's conditions for correct claims. Each charge for a visit is related to a specific procedure code. Although a separate fee is associated with each code, each code is not necessarily billable. Whether it can be billed depends on the payer's rules. Some payers include particular codes in the payment for another code. Medical insurance specialists apply their knowledge of payer guidelines to analyze what can be billed on health care claims.

7. Prepare and transmit claims.

A key task is preparing accurate, timely health care claims. Most practices prepare claims for their patients. Claims communicate information about a patient's diagnosis, procedures, and charges to a payer. Correct claims help the office receive payment on time.

Tasks to Help Collect the Maximum Appropriate Payment

8. Monitor payer adjudication.

Payers review health care claims by following a process known as adjudication. This term means that the payer puts the claim through a series of steps designed to judge whether it should be paid. What the payer decides about the claim—to pay it in full, to pay some of it, or to deny it—is reported back to the provider on the RA/EOB sent with the payment. The medical insurance specialist reviews each payment and explanation by comparing the claim with the payment.

9. Generate patient statements.

Payers' payments are posted to the appropriate patients' accounts. In many cases, patients will be billed for charges that were not fully paid by their medical insurance plans. The amount paid by all payers (the primary insurance and any other insurance) plus the amount to be billed to the patient should equal the expected fee. Bills that list the dates and services provided, any payments made by the patient and the payer, and the balances now due are mailed to patients.

10. Follow up patient payments, and handle collections.

Patient payments are regularly analyzed for overdue bills. A collection process is often started when patient payments are later than permitted under the practice's financial policy. Patient medical records and financial records are filed and retained according to the medical practice's policy. Federal and state laws govern which documents are kept and for how long.

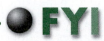

FYI

Some services performed by physicians do not take place in medical offices but rather in other locations, such as hospitals. When a patient is admitted to a hospital, the medical insurance specialist is responsible for gathering complete and correct information. Hospitals may send reports to the physician's office. These reports are used to complete health care claims.

Helping Patients

Another key area of responsibility in the medical office is helping patients by answering their questions about insurance reimbursement and the health care claim process. Patients also need assistance when problems with payers arise.

Requirements for Success

A number of skills and attributes are required for successful mastery of the tasks of a medical insurance specialist.

Skills

- *Knowledge of medical terminology, anatomy, physiology, and medical coding:* Medical insurance specialists must analyze physicians' descriptions of patients' conditions and treatments and relate these descriptions to the systems of diagnosis and procedure codes used in the health care industry.

- *Communication skills:* The job of a medical insurance specialist requires excellent communications skills, both oral and written. For example, patients often need explanations of insurance benefits or clarification of instructions such as referrals. Courteous, helpful answers to questions strongly influence patients' desire to continue to use the practices' services. Memos, letters, the telephone, and e-mail are used to research and follow up on changes in health plans' billing rules. These skills also are needed to send claim attachments that explain special conditions or treatments to obtain maximum reimbursement from payers, and to create and send effective collection letters.

- *Attention to detail:* Many aspects of the job involve paying close attention to detail, such as correctly completing health care claims, filing patients' medical records, recording preauthorization numbers, calculating the correct payments, and posting payments for services.

- *Flexibility:* Working in a changing environment requires the ability to adapt to new procedures, handle varying kinds of problems and interactions during a busy day, and work successfully with different types of people with various cultural backgrounds.

- *Information technology (IT) skills:* Most medical practices use computers to handle billing and to process claims. Many also plan to use computers to keep patients' medical records. General computer literacy, including a working knowledge of (1) the Microsoft Windows operating system, (2) a word-processing program, (3) a medical billing program, and (4) Internet-based research, is essential. Data entry skills are also necessary. Many human errors occur during data entry, such as pressing the wrong key on the keyboard. Other errors are a result of a lack of computer literacy—not knowing how to use a program to accomplish tasks. For this reason, proper training in data-entry techniques so that errors are caught, as well as knowing how to use computer programs, are both essential for medical insurance specialists.

- *Honesty and integrity:* Medical insurance specialists work with patients' medical records and with finances. It is essential to maintain the confidentiality of patient information and communications, as well as to act with integrity when handling these tasks.

- *Ability to work as a team member:* Patient service is a team effort. To do their part, medical insurance specialists are cooperative and focus on the best interests of patients and the practice.

Attributes

A number of attributes are also very important for success as a medical insurance specialist. Most have to do with the quality of professionalism, which is key to getting and keeping employment. These factors include:

- Appearance: a neat, clean, professional appearance increases confidence in your skills and abilities. Being well-groomed, with clean hair, nails, and clothing, presents a businesslike demeanor to patients and other staff members.
- Attendance: Being on time for work demonstrates that you are reliable and dependable.
- Initiative: Being able to start a course of action and stay on task is an important quality to demonstrate.
- Courtesy: Treating patients and fellow workers with dignity and respect is an interpersonal quality that helps build good professional relationships at work.

Ethics and Etiquette in the Medical Office

Licensed medical staff members and other employees working in physicians' practices share responsibility for observing a code of ethics and for following correct etiquette.

Ethics

Medical **ethics** are standards of behavior requiring truthfulness, honesty, and integrity. Ethics guide the behavior of physicians, who have the training, the primary responsibility, and the legal right to diagnose and treat human illnesses and injuries. All medical office employees and those working in health-related professions share responsibility for observing the ethical code.

Each professional organization has a code of ethics that is to be followed by its members. In general, this code states that information about patients, other employees, and confidential business matters should not be discussed with anyone not directly concerned with them. Behavior should be consistent with the values of the profession. For example, it is unethical for an employee to take money or gifts from a company in exchange for giving them business. Study Figures 1-7 and 1-8, page 20, as examples of codes of ethics that relate to the role of medical insurance specialists.

Etiquette

Professional **etiquette** is also important for medical insurance specialists. Correct behavior in the office is generally covered in the practice's employee policy and procedure manual. For example, guidelines establish which types of incoming calls must go immediately to a physician or to a nurse or assistant, and which require a message to be taken.

THE EFFECTS OF HEALTH CARE CLAIM ERRORS

Efficient and accurate completion of the health care claim process helps a medical office run smoothly. The job of the medical insurance specialist is important because most medical office income comes from insurance payments. Errors in filing claims slow the reimbursement process and

AHIMA Code of Ethics

Ethical Principles: The following ethical principles are based on the core values of the American Health Information Management Association and apply to all health information management professionals.

HIM professionals:

I. Advocate, uphold, and defend the individual's right to privacy and the doctrine of confidentiality in the use and disclosure of information.

II. Put service and the health and welfare of persons before self-interest and conduct themselves in the practice of the profession so as to bring honor to themselves, their peers, and to the health information management profession.

III. Preserve, protect, and secure personal health information in any form or medium and hold in the highest regard the contents of the records and other information of a confidential nature, taking into account the applicable statutes and regulations.

IV. Refuse to participate in or conceal unethical practices or procedures.

V. Advance health information management knowledge and practice through continuing education, research, publications, and presentations.

VI. Recruit and mentor students, peers, and colleagues to develop and strengthen professional work force.

VII. Represent the profession accurately to the public.

VIII. Perform honorably health information management association responsibilities, either appointed or elected, and preserve the confidentiality of any privileged information made known in any official capacity.

IX. State truthfully and accurately their credentials, professional education, and experiences.

X. Facilitate interdisciplinary collaboration in situations supporting health information practice.

XI. Respect the inherent dignity and worth of every person.

Figure 1-7 AHIMA Code of Ethics

Reprinted with permission from the American Health Information Management Association.

interfere with other work. Some examples of problems that can arise from filing inaccurate claims are the following:

Lower Payments and Denied Claim

A typographical error or incorrect code will communicate the wrong diagnosis or treatment to the payer. This can result in a lower benefit payment or in denial of the claim.

Delays in Payments

If the health plan must request additional information, payment will be delayed. The payer's claims department can correct an error, but it takes time, so issuing the benefit payment will take longer.

Disruption of Other Work

When a medical insurance specialist has to correct a claim form or fill out a request for a review, the time spent means that new claims for other patients have to wait. Correcting information may also require the assistance of the physician or other members of the office staff, who then must interrupt their activities.

Patients' Questions and Complaints

If a patient has already paid for services, errors in the claim process can slow reimbursement. The medical insurance specialist or another member of the office staff may have to interrupt activities to handle inquiries and complaints.

American Academy of Professional Coders

Code of Ethical Standards

- Members of the American Academy of Professional Coders shall be dedicated to providing the highest standard of professional coding and billing services to employers, clients and patients. Behavior of AAPC members must be exemplary.

- AAPC members shall maintain the highest standard of personal and professional conduct. Members shall respect the rights of patients, clients, employers and all other colleagues.

- Members shall use only legal and ethical means in all professional dealings, and shall refuse to cooperate with or condone by silence, the actions of those who engage in fraudulent, deceptive or illegal acts.

- Members shall respect the laws and regulations of the land, and uphold the mission statement of the AAPC.

AAPC Mission Statement

Establish and maintain ethical and educational standards for professional coders.

Provide a national certification and credentialing process.

Support the national and local membership by providing educational products and opportunities to network.

Increase and promote national recognition and awareness of procedural and diagnostic coding.

- Members shall pursue excellence through continuing education in all areas applicable to their profession.

- Members shall strive to maintain and enhance the dignity, status, competence and standards of coding for professional services.

- Members shall not exploit professional relationships with patients, employees, clients or employers for personal gain.

- Above all else, we will commit to recognizing the intrinsic worth of each member.

This code of Ethical Standards for members of the American Academy of Professional Coders strives to promote and maintain the highest standard of professional service and conduct among its members. Adherence to these standards assures public confidence in the integrity and service of professional coders who are members of the American Academy of Professional Coders.

Figure 1-8 Code of Ethical Standards, American Academy of Professional Coders
Copyright © 2008 American Academy of Professional Coders. Reprinted with permission.

Chapter Summary

1. A health plan pays for patients' medical services according to the policy's schedule of benefits. Most health plans require payment of premiums. Some plans pay a percentage of the charge, while others require just a copayment. Indemnity plans pay benefits on a fee-for-service basis. Under managed care plans, which are the most popular plans, providers' fees are set in advance. Most health plans now have some cost-containment features.

2. Common kinds of private medical insurance include group insurance, individual insurance, self-insured health plans, liability insurance, and automobile insurance. Government programs include Medicare, Medicaid, workers' compensation, TRICARE, and CHAMPVA.

3. These are five steps in the health care billing workflow:

   (a) *The patient presents for an appointment*—The patient completes or updates the patient information form and indicates whether to assign benefits. Insurance coverage is verified.

   (b) *Medical services are provided to the patient*—The health care professional examines the patient, evaluates the patient's condition, treats the patient, documents the patient's condition and the procedures provided, and completes the encounter form.

   (c) *The health plan is billed for the appointment*—A health care claim is prepared and transmitted to the health plan.

   (d) *The health plan responds to the claim*—The health plan processes the claim, makes appropriate payment, and provides an explanation of benefits/ remittance advice that explains how the payment was determined.

   (e) *The patient is billed as appropriate*—The health plan's payment is checked for accuracy and recorded. If additional payments are due from another insurance plan, another claim is prepared. If a balance is due from the patient, a bill is prepared and mailed to the patient.

4. The ten main duties performed by the medical insurance specialist are:

   1. Preregister patients.

   2. Establish financial responsibility for the visit.

   3. Check in patients.

   4. Check out patients.

   5. Review coding compliance.

   6. Check billing compliance.

   7. Prepare and transmit claims.

   8. Monitor payer adjudication.

   9. Generate patient statements.

   10. Follow up patient payments and handle collections.

5. Insurance claim errors slow the reimbursement process and interfere with other work in the medical office. Effects of errors include lower payments and denied claims, delays in payments, disruption of other work, and increased questions and complaints by patients.

Part 1. Put the five steps in the medical office billing work flow in the correct order.

    a. Physician examines the patient, evaluates the patient's condition, treats the patient, and completes the patient's encounter form.

    b. Patient completes or updates the patient information form.

    c. Health plan processes the claim, makes appropriate payment, and provides a remittance advice.

    d. Medical insurance specialist records payment, reviews the accompanying remittance advice for accuracy, and determines whether the patient owes an additional payment.

    e. Medical insurance specialist completes the health care claim and transmits it to the health plan.

Part 2. Choose the best answer.

_____ **1.** The amount an insurance carrier will pay for a covered medical service is the:
    a. benefit
    b. premium
    c. claim

_____ **2.** Under an indemnity plan, benefits are determined on what basis?
    a. fee-for-service
    b. cost-containment
    c. either a or b

_____ **3.** Under a managed care plan, fixed fees for medical procedures and services are set by the:
    a. health care provider
    b. managed care organization
    c. patient

_____ **4.** The patient information form gives information about:
    a. the patient
    b. the insurance company
    c. both a and b

_____ **5.** The file that contains the patient's medical and insurance information is the:
    a. encounter form
    b. patient's medical record
    c. code

_____ **6.** Which of the following represent the amount of money a patient must pay before the health plan will pay for services? List all that apply.
    a. benefit
    b. premium
    c. deductible

_____ **7.** The medical billing program is used to record:
    a. claims sent
    b. health plan payments
    c. both a and b

_____ **8.** When treatment is appropriate for the patient's diagnosis, it is said to be:
    a. medically necessary
    b. deductible
    c. direct

_____ **9.** The assignment of benefits allows the health plan to:
    a. pay the physician for services
    b. withhold payments for services
    c. pay the patient for services

____**10.** Coding means:
   a. writing prescriptions so patients cannot read them
   b. assigning proper numbers to identify the diagnoses and procedures on claims
   c. using a billing program for the patient's progress notes

Part 3. Write "T" or "F" in the blank to indicate whether you think the statement is true or false.

____ **1.** The job of the medical insurance specialist is not important in a medical office.

____ **2.** The job description of a medical insurance specialist is determined by the physicians and the practice manager.

____ **3.** The encounter form lists the diagnosis, medical services, and fees for a patient's visit.

____ **4.** The medical insurance specialist files the patient information form in the patient's medical record.

____ **5.** The only duty a medical insurance specialist has is to transmit health care claims to insurance carriers.

____ **6.** The physician, the medical insurance specialist, or a medical coder finds the correct codes for diagnosis and treatment.

____ **7.** Once the health care claim is transmitted to the payer, the job of the medical insurance specialist is finished.

____ **8.** If a patient calls with a question about insurance, the call should be directed to the physician.

____ **9.** The term *remittance advice* means that the medical insurance specialist explains insurance problems to the patient.

____**10.** If there seems to be a mistake in the amount of money paid by an insurance carrier, the medical insurance specialist should request a review.

Part 4. Match the following insurance programs to the patients who qualify for them. Note that some letters are used more than one time.

   A. TRICARE   **B.** CHAMPVA
   C. Medicare   **D.** Medicaid
   E. workers' compensation   **F.** individual insurance
   G. group insurance

____ **1.** Tom Kahler is seventy-three years old.

____ **2.** Linda Belize hurt her back lifting a case of motor oil in the warehouse at work.

____ **3.** Amy Jenks is the five-year-old daughter of a U.S. Army sergeant stationed in Korea.

____ **4.** Rachel Marinaccio is a vice president of First Bank, where she participates in the company's health insurance plan.

____ **5.** Cynthia Weiner's husband died of complications from paralysis that resulted from stepping on a land mine when he was a U.S. Marine during the Vietnam War.

____ **6.** Jill Ludwig receives state welfare benefits.

____ **7.** Captain Cheryl Kupper is retired from the U.S. Navy.

____ **8.** Emelina Valdez subscribes to health insurance through the same agent who carries her automobile and homeowner's insurance.

____ **9.** Kenji Ito has a permanent disability that is not related to service in the armed forces and is not a work-related injury.

____**10.** Thurman Jackson is covered by his wife's insurance through the Automobile Dealers' Association.

HIPAA and the Legal Medical Record

Learning Outcomes

After completing this chapter, you will be able to define the key terms and:

2-1 Discuss the importance of medical record documentation in the billing and payment process.

2-2 Define the facts that are included in patients' protected health information (PHI).

2-3 Discuss the purpose of the HIPAA Privacy Rule, the HIPAA Security Rule, and the HIPAA Electronic Health Care Transactions and Code Sets standards.

2-4 Describe which PHI can be released without patients' authorization.

2-5 Discuss patients' authorizations to use or disclose PHI.

2-6 Describe the purpose of a retention schedule.

2-7 Discuss how to guard against potentially fraudulent situations.

Key Terms

Acknowledgment of Receipt of Notice of Privacy Practices

authorization

clearinghouse

compliance plan

documentation

electronic health records (EHR)

fraud

Health Insurance Portability and Accountability Act (HIPAA)

HIPAA Electronic Health Care Transactions and Code Sets (TCS)

HIPAA Privacy Rule

HIPAA Security Rule

medical records

minimum necessary standard

National Plan and Provider Enumeration System (NPPES)

National Provider Identifier (NPI)

Notice of Privacy Practices (NPP)

Office of Civil Rights (OCR)

protected health information (PHI)

retention schedule

subpoena

subpoena *duces tecum*

treatment, payment, and operations (TPO)

Why This Chapter Is Important to You

The information in this chapter will enable you to:

- Understand the importance of keeping medical records private and secure.
- Feel confident about how to respond when someone requests information about a patient.
- Know how to protect yourself, the physician, and other staff members from potentially fraudulent situations.

What Do You Think?

The work of physicians involves many legal issues, such as possible accusations of false billing or of incorrectly disclosing a patient's private information. The work of the medical insurance specialist also involves many legal considerations. Not only must patients' protected health information be respected and kept confidential, but physicians must also be guarded from potentially fraudulent situations. For example, a patient may attempt to persuade the medical insurance specialist to change a fact on a claim in order to receive benefits falsely. In your opinion, is it ever appropriate for a medical insurance specialist to alter a claim?

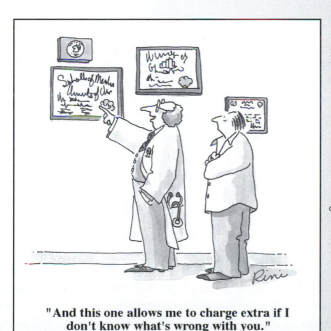

"And this one allows me to charge extra if I don't know what's wrong with you."

MEDICAL RECORDS

Patients' **medical records** contain all facts, findings, and observations about their health history. The medical record also contains all communications with and about the patient. The medical record in the medical office begins with a patient's first contact and continues through all treatments and services. The record provides continuity and communication among physicians and other health care professionals who are involved in a patient's care. Patient medical records are also used in research and for education.

Patient medical records are legal documents. Physicians own the physical record (although patients own the information about themselves), and properly documented patient care is part of a physician's defense against accusations that patients were not treated correctly. Medical records should clearly state who performed what service and describe why, where, when, and how it was done. Physicians document the rationale behind their treatment decisions. This rationale is the basis for the concept of medical necessity—a clinically logical link between a patient's condition and the treatment provided. For example, when a test or drug is ordered for a patient, the physician documents the diagnosis or condition that is being confirmed or ruled out.

Although they do not make entries in patient medical records, medical insurance specialists work with the records in the billing and payment process. The documentation of diagnoses and procedures is used as proof of billed services. An unwritten law of medical insurance is that if it was not documented, it was not done, and if it was not done, it cannot be billed. Payers also use documentation to decide whether reported services should be reimbursed. The record must clearly document where, why, when, and how each service occurred.

> ✓ **Compliance Tip**
>
> The connection between documentation and billing bears repeating: If a service is not documented, it was not done, and if it was not done, it cannot be billed.

DOCUMENTATION STANDARDS

In medical record **documentation,** a patient's health status is recorded in chronological order using a systematic, logical, and consistent method. A patient's health history, examinations, tests, and results of treatments are all documented. Because of the importance of patients' medical records, the leading health care industry groups set standards for documentation. Standardization helps make medical records more efficient and improves the quality of patient care. Since medical insurance specialists help organize and maintain patient medical records, it is important to be aware of the following standards and to encourage their use:

- *Records Must Be Clear*—Medical records should be complete and accurate. If the records are handwritten, the entries should be legible to others, made in black ink (not pencil), and dated.
- *Entries Must Be Signed and Dated*—Whether digitally entered by the provider, handwritten, or transcribed, each entry must have the signature or initials and title of the responsible provider and the date.
- *Changes Must Be Clearly Made*—An incorrect entry is marked with a single line through the words to be changed; the correct

information is entered after it, so that the previous copy can be read. Corrections are also dated and signed by the person making the change. No part of a record should be otherwise altered or removed, deleted, or destroyed

Example

Correct	Incorrect	Guideline
85 5/7/2007 this 80-year old *jrb*	85 this 80-year old	Corrections should be clear, signed, and dated.

- *No Blank Spaces May Be Left Between Entries*—Entries are made chronologically, without spaces between them, to prevent out-of-order entries.
- *Each Patient Should Have a Single Record*—Each patient should have one medical record, often called a unit record. (Note, however, that practices should be sure to have a separate file in a patient's medical record when workers' compensation claims are involved; see Chapter 12.)
- *Records Should Use Consistent Vocabulary and Format*—All entries should reflect standard, accepted medical vocabulary and abbreviations. All medical records in a practice should be consistently labeled and have logical sections.
- *Diagnostic Information Must Be Easy to Locate*—Past and present diagnoses should be placed so that they are easy to locate by each physician who uses the medical record.
- *Practitioners' Entries Must Be Made Promptly*—Entries should be made in a timely manner and filed in a consistent chronological order, either ascending or descending.

Documentation Formats

Medical insurance specialists work with various formats that are used to organize patients' medical records. The most common format used in general medical practices is called a *problem-oriented medical record* (POMR). The problem-oriented medical record contains a general section with data from the initial patient examination and assessment. When the patient makes subsequent visits, the reasons for those encounters are listed separately in a problem list, each with its own notes. For example, the patient's record might have a general section followed by sections labeled "skin disorder" and "right eye scleral abrasion" with notes about these conditions.

Progress notes for each problem are in the SOAP format, beginning with the problem and then four points: *Subjective, Objective, Assessment,* and *Plan*:

S—The *subjective* information is based on the patient's descriptions of symptoms along with other comments.

O—The *objective* information includes the physical examinations and laboratory reports or tests.

A—The *assessment,* also called the impression or conclusion, is the physician's diagnosis, or interpretation of the subjective and objective information.

P—The *plan,* also called treatment, advice, or recommendations, includes the necessary patient monitoring, follow-up, procedures, and instructions to the patient.

Documentation Content

Providers follow generally recognized guidelines to document encounters. The initial examinations and assessments (see Figure 2-1) show the treatment plan for the patient. Progress reports document the patient's progress

James E. Ribielli
5/19/2010

CHIEF COMPLAINT: This 79-year-old male presents with sudden and extreme weakness. He got up from a seated position and became light-headed.

PAST MEDICAL HISTORY: History of congestive heart failure. On multiple medications, including Cardizem, Enalapril 5 mg qd, and Lasix 40 mg qd.

PHYSICAL EXAMINATION: No postural change in blood pressure. BP, 114/61 with a pulse of 49, sitting; BP, 111/56 with a pulse 50, standing. Patient denies being light-headed at this time.

HEENT: Unremarkable.

NECK: Supple without jugular or venous distension.

LUNGS: Clear to auscultation and percussion.

HEART: S1 and S2 normal; no systolic or diastolic murmurs; no S3, S4. No dysrhythmia.

ABDOMEN: Soft without organomegaly, mass, or bruit.

EXTREMITIES: Unremarkable. Pulses strong and equal.

LABORATORY DATA: Hemoglobin, 12.3. White count, 10.800. Normal electrolytes. ECG shows sinus bradycardia.

DIAGNOSIS: Weakness on the basis of sinus bradycardia, probably Cardizem induced.

TREATMENT: Patient told to change positions slowly when moving from sitting to standing, and from lying to standing.

John R. Ramirez, MD

Figure 2-1 Example of Physical Examination Documentation

Jennifer Delgado
8/14/2010

SUBJECTIVE: The patient has had epilepsy since she was 10. She takes her medication as prescribed; denies side effects. She reports no convulsions or new symptoms. She is a full-time student at Riverside Community College.

OBJECTIVE: Phenobarbital 90 mg twice a day as prescribed since 1994. The motor and sensory examination results are normal.

ASSESSMENT: Well-controlled epilepsy.

PLAN: Patient advised to continue medication regimen. Schedule for follow-up in 6 months.

Jared R. Wandaowsky, MD

Figure 2-2 Example of a Progress Note

and response to the treatment plan (see Figure 2-2). Discharge summaries are prepared during the patient's final visit for a particular treatment plan. If either the patient or the physician ends the relationship, the physician must still maintain the patient's medical record. The physician also sends the patient a letter that documents the situation and provides for continuity of care with the next provider.

Every patient visit should be documented with the following information:

- The patient's name.
- The encounter date and reason.
- Appropriate history and physical examination.
- Review of all tests that were ordered.
- The diagnosis.
- The plan of care, or notes on treatments that were given.
- The instructions or recommendations that were given to the patient.
- The signature of the provider who saw the patient.

In addition to this encounter information, a patient's medical record must contain:

- Biographical and personal information, including the patient's full name, Social Security number, date of birth, full address, marital status, home and work telephone numbers, and employer information as applicable.
- Duplicates of all documents that communicate with the patient, including letters, telephone calls, faxes, and e-mail messages; the

patient's responses; and a note of the time, date, topic, and physician's response to each communication from the patient.

- Duplicates of prescriptions and instructions given to the patient, including refills.
- Any original documents that the patient has signed, such as an authorization to release information (see page 37, Figure 2.5) and an advance directive.
- Medical allergies and reactions, or the lack of them.
- Up-to-date immunization record and history if appropriate, such as for a child.
- Previous and current diagnoses, test results, health risks, and progress.
- Copies of referral or consultation letters.
- Hospital admissions and release documents.
- A record of any missed or canceled appointments.
- Any requests for information about the patient (from a health plan or an attorney, for example), and a detailed log of to whom information was released.

The patient medical record also includes the identification number assigned by the practice to the patient. Billing and insurance information is usually stored separately from the medical record.

Electronic Health Records

Because of the advantages, health care leaders in business and government are pressing for laws to require the switch to **electronic health records (EHR).** An electronic health record is a running collection of health information that provides immediate electronic access by authorized users. The federal government has set the goal of using electronic records for all patients by 2014. Although few small physician practices have electronic patient records now, due to the cost, this is expected to change rapidly.

In most practices, billing records are handled with a billing program, but most of the clinical recordkeeping is on paper. Providers' notes are usually written on the patients' records or transcribed from dictation and placed in the record, where they are signed and dated by the responsible provider. Lab test results are printed; X-rays, ECGs , and other routine test results are included.

In electronic health records, documents may be created in a variety of ways, but they are ultimately viewed on a computer screen. For example, a practice may use various medical history-taking templates for gathering and recording consistent history and physical (H&P) information from patients. The computer-based templates range in focus from abdominal pain to depression, with from ten to twenty questions each. Clinical staff members enter patient responses directly into patient records using computers in the exam rooms. Responsible providers then sign the entries using technology for electronic signatures that verifies the identity of the signer.

PROTECTED HEALTH INFORMATION AND MEDICAL RECORDS

Health is a personal and private matter. The health information that patients share with physicians could change their lives or cause them to lose jobs or friends. Nevertheless, medical information must be recorded in medical records and communicated to others in the course of treatment and payment. To ensure that health information is protected from misuse, a federal law, the **Health Insurance Portability and Accountability Act,** or **HIPAA** (pronounced hip-uh), regulates how electronic patient information is stored and shared.

HIPAA has three rules that are important in medical offices:

1. *HIPAA Privacy Rule*—The privacy requirements cover patients' health information.
2. *HIPAA Security Rule*—The security requirements state the administrative, technical, and physical safeguards that are required to protect patients' health information.
3. *HIPAA Electronic Transaction and Code Sets Standards*—These standards require every provider who does business electronically to use the same health care transactions, code sets, and identifiers.

HIPAA Privacy Rule

The **HIPAA Privacy Rule** must be followed by health plans, health care clearinghouses, and health care providers as well as by the outside businesses that work with them, such as medical billing companies and accounting firms.

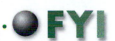

A **clearinghouse** is a company that helps medical offices and health plans exchange claim data in correct formats. Clearinghouses, for instance, are able to accept paper claims from a physician and transform them into electronic claims that are HIPAA compliant.

Protected Health Information

The Privacy Rule establishes the definition of each patient's **protected health information (PHI).** PHI is any individually identifiable health information that is transmitted or maintained by electronic media, such as sent over the Internet or stored in the office's computer files. Under this definition, a physician's report of the number of people treated who have diabetes is not PHI, but the names of the patients are protected. PHI includes many facts about people, such as names, addresses, birth dates, employers, telephone numbers, Social Security numbers, and health plan beneficiary numbers, any of which could be used to identify them.

Privacy Practices

The Privacy Rule also sets out the things that medical offices must do to properly handle patients' PHI:

- The practice must adopt privacy practices that are appropriate for its health care services.
- The practice must notify patients about their privacy rights and how their information may be used or disclosed.
- Office employees must be trained so that they understand the privacy practices.

- A staff member must be appointed as the office's privacy official, and this person must be responsible for seeing that privacy practices are adopted and followed.
- Patients' records containing individually identifiable health information must be maintained and stored so that they are not readily available to those who do not need them.

Notice of and Acknowledgment of Receipt of Notice of Privacy Practices

To comply with the Privacy Rule, medical offices, as well as other providers and health plans, must give each patient an explanation of privacy practices at the patient's first contact or encounter. To satisfy this requirement, a medical office gives the patients a copy of the office's **Notice of Privacy Practices** (see Figure 2-3). The notice explains how patients' PHI may be used and describes the patients' rights. The office must also ask each patient to review this notice and sign an **Acknowledgment of Receipt of Notice of Privacy Practices,** showing that he or she has read and understood the document (see Figure 2-4, page 35).

Professional Focus

Office for Civil Rights

Patients who observe privacy problems in their providers' offices can complain either to the medical office or to the Department of Health and Human Services (HHS). Complaints must be put in writing—on paper or electronically—and sent to the **Office for Civil Rights (OCR),** which is part of HHS, usually within 180 days. The office must cooperate with an HHS investigation and give HHS access to its facilities, books, records, and systems, including relevant protected health information.

Sharing Protected Health Information

The Privacy Rule recognizes that medical offices and payers must be able to exchange PHI in the normal course of business. The rule says that there are three everyday situations in which PHI can be released *without* the patient's permission: **treatment, payment, and operations (TPO).**

- *Treatment* means providing and coordinating the patient's medical care. Physicians and other medical staff members can discuss patients' cases in the office and with other physicians. Laboratory or X-ray technicians may call to obtain clarification of unreadable

Central Practice Center

NOTICE OF PRIVACY PRACTICES

THIS NOTICE DESCRIBES HOW MEDICAL INFORMATION ABOUT YOU MAY BE USED AND DISCLOSED AND HOW YOU CAN GET ACCESS TO THIS INFORMATION. PLEASE REVIEW IT CAREFULLY.

WHY ARE YOU GETTING THIS NOTICE?

Central Practice Center is required by federal and state law to maintain the privacy of your health information. The use and disclosure of your health information is governed by regulations under the Health Insurance Portability and Accountability Act of 1996 (HIPAA) and the requirements of applicable state law. For health information covered by HIPAA, we are required to provide you with this Notice and will abide by this Notice with respect to such health information. If you have questions about this Notice, please contact our Privacy Officer at 877-555-1313. We will ask you to sign an "acknowledgment" indicating that you have been provided with this notice.

WHAT HEALTH INFORMATION IS PROTECTED?

We are committed to protecting the privacy of information we gather about you while providing health-related services. Some examples of protected health information are:

- Information indicating that you are a patient receiving treatment or other health-related services from our physicians or staff;
- Information about your health condition (such as a disease you may have);
- Information about health care products or services you have received or may receive in the future (such as an operation); or
- Information about your health care benefits under an insurance plan (such as whether a prescription is covered);

when combined with:

- Demographic information (such as your name, address, or insurance status);
- Unique numbers that may identify you (such as your Social Security number, your phone number, or your driver's license number); and
- Other types of information that may identify who you are.

SUMMARY OF THIS NOTICE

This summary includes references to paragraphs throughout this notice that you may read for additional information.

1. Written Authorization Requirement

We may use your health information or share it with others in order to treat your condition, obtain payment for that treatment, and run our business operations. We generally need your written authorization for other uses and disclosures of your health information, unless an exception described in this Notice applies.

2. Authorizing Transfer of Your Records

You may request that we transfer your records to another person or organization by completing a written authorization form. This form will specify what information is being released, to whom, and for what purpose. The authorization will have an expiration date.

3. Canceling Your Written Authorization

If you provide us with written authorization, you may revoke, or cancel, it at any time, except to the extent that we have already relied upon it. To revoke a written authorization, please write to the doctor's office where you initially gave your authorization.

4. Exceptions to Written Authorization Requirement

There are some situations in which we do not need your written authorization before using your health information or sharing it with others. They include:

Treatment, Payment and Operations
As mentioned above, we may use your health information or share it with others in order to treat your condition, obtain payment for that treatment, and run our business operations.

Family and Friends
If you do not object, we will share information about your health with family and friends involved in your care.

Figure 2-3 Example of a Notice of Privacy Practices

Research
Although we will generally try to obtain your written authorization before using your health information for research purposes, there may be certain situations in which we are not required to obtain your written authorization.

De-Identified Information
We may use or disclose your health information if we have removed any information that might identify you. When all identifying information is removed, we say that the health information is "completely de-identified." We may also use and disclose "partially de-identified" information if the person who will receive it agrees in writing to protect your privacy when using the information.

Incidental Disclosures
We may inadvertently use or disclose your health information despite having taken all reasonable precautions to protect the privacy and confidentiality of your health information.

Emergencies or Public Need
We may use or disclose your health information in an emergency or for important public health needs. For example, we may share your information with public health officials at the State or city health departments who are authorized to investigate and control the spread of diseases.

5. How to Access Your Health Information

You generally have the right to inspect and get copies of your health information.

6. How to Correct Your Health Information

You have the right to request that we amend your health information if you believe it is inaccurate or incomplete.

7. How to Identify Others Who Have Received Your Health Information

You have the right to receive an "accounting of disclosures." This is a report that identifies certain persons or organizations to which we have disclosed your health information. All disclosures are made according to the protections described in this Notice of Privacy Practices. Many routine disclosures we make (for treatment, payment, or business operations, among others) will not be included in this report. However, it will identify any non-routine disclosures of your information.

8. How to Request Additional Privacy Protections

You have the right to request further restrictions on the way we use your health information or share it with others. However, we are not required to agree to the restriction you request. If we do agree with your request, we will be bound by our agreement.

9. How to Request Alternative Communications

You have the right to request that we contact you in a way that is more confidential for you, such as at home instead of at work. We will try to accommodate all reasonable requests.

10. How Someone May Act On Your Behalf

You have the right to name a personal representative who may act on your behalf to control the privacy of your health information. Parents and guardians will generally have the right to control the privacy of health information about minors unless the minors are permitted by law to act on their own behalf.

11. How to Learn about Special Protections for HIV, Alcohol and Substance Abuse, Mental Health and Genetic Information

Special privacy protections apply to HIV-related information, alcohol and substance abuse treatment information, mental health information, psychotherapy notes and genetic information.

12. How to Obtain A Copy of This Notice

If you have not already received one, you have the right to a paper copy of this notice. You may request a paper copy at any time, even if you have previously agreed to receive this notice electronically. You can request a copy of the privacy notice directly from your doctor's office. You may also obtain a copy of this notice from our website or by requesting a copy at your next visit.

13. How to Obtain A Copy of Revised Notice

We may change our privacy practices from time to time. If we do, we will revise this notice so you will have an accurate summary of our practices. You will be able to obtain your own copy of the revised notice by accessing our website or by calling your doctor's office. You may also ask for one at the time of your next visit. The effective date of the notice is noted in the top right corner of each page. We are required to abide by the terms of the notice that is currently in effect.

14. How To File A Complaint

If you believe your privacy rights have been violated, you may file a complaint with us or with the federal Office of Civil Rights. To file a complaint with us, please contact our Privacy Officer.

No one will retaliate or take action against you for filing a complaint.

Figure 2-3 Example of a Notice of Privacy Practices (*cont.*)

Acknowledgment of Receipt of Notice of Privacy Practices

I understand that the providers of Central Practice Center may share my health information for treatment, billing and healthcare operations. I have been given a copy of the organization's notice of privacy practices that describes how my health information is used and shared. I understand that Central Practice Center has the right to change this notice at any time. I may obtain a current copy by contacting the practice's office or by visiting the website at www.xxx.com.

My signature below constitutes my acknowledgment that I have been provided with a copy of the notice of privacy practices.

_____
Signature of Patient or Legal Representative   Date

If signed by legal representative,
relationship to patient:_____

Figure 2-4 Example of an Acknowledgment of Receipt of Notice of Privacy Practices

---

HIPAA Tip

PHI and Electronic Transmission

Medical insurance specialists receive training in handling electronically transmitted information using the practice's computer system and the Internet. HIPAA allows the use of e-mail, but the e-mail system needs to be designed for secure transmission of confidential information.

---

requests. This information can be provided by the physician or another medical staff member.

- *Payment* refers to the exchange of information with health plans. Medical office staff members can take the required information from patients' records and prepare health care claims that are transmitted to health plans.
- *Operations* are the general business management functions needed to run the office.

Minimum Necessary Standard

When using protected health information, a medical office must try to limit the information shared to the minimum amount of PHI necessary to accomplish the intended purpose. The **minimum necessary standard** means taking reasonable safeguards to protect PHI from incidental disclosure. For example, a medical insurance specialist would not disclose a patient's history of cancer on a workers' compensation claim for a sprained ankle. Only the information the recipient needs to know is given.

Authorizations

For use or disclosure of PHI other than for treatment, payment, or operations (TPO), the patient must sign an **authorization** to release the information. For example, information about alcohol and drug abuse may not be released without a specific authorization from the patient.

The authorization document must be in plain language and include the following:

- A description of the information to be used or disclosed.
- The name or other specific identification of the person(s) authorized to use or disclose the information.
- The name of the person(s) or group of people to whom the covered entity may make the disclosure.
- A description of the purpose of each requested use or disclosure.
- An expiration date.
- Signature of the individual (or authorized representative) and date.

A sample authorization form is shown in Figure 2-5.

Patients have the right to an accounting of disclosures of their PHI other than for treatment, payment, or operations purposes. The medical office keeps a disclosure log for each patient so that authorized disclosures can be listed. When accidental disclosure of a patient's PHI occurs, it should also be documented in the individual's medical record, since it did not fall into a permitted disclosure purpose for TPO and the individual did not authorize it. An example is sending a consultation report to the wrong physician's office.

Exceptions to the Privacy Rule

There are a number of exceptions to the Privacy Rule. All these types of disclosures must also be logged, and release information must be available to the patient who requests it.

- *Release Under Court Order*—If the patient's PHI is required as evidence by a court of law, the provider may release it without the patient's approval upon judicial order. In the case of a lawsuit, a

Case Study

Medical information must be kept confidential, even in a moral dilemma. For example, a woman with a sexually transmitted disease identified John as one of her sexual partners. John came into the office and began receiving treatment with an antibiotic. One day, John's wife Marsha received billing notices and called to ask whether there had been a billing error. Near tears and frightened, Marsha pleaded, "Why is he seeing the doctor? Can't you tell me what's wrong with my husband?" The medical insurance specialist was caught in a moral dilemma. It appeared that John had not told Marsha about his disease despite the fact that she most likely would be infected.

A medical insurance specialist is not allowed to release John's protected health information even in a case like this. In responding to Marsha, the correct thing to say is "I cannot disclose patient information. Why don't you discuss the bill with your husband?"

Patient Name: _____

Health Record Number: _____

Date of Birth: _____

1. I authorize the use or disclosure of the above named individual's health information as described below.

2. The following individual(s) or organization(s) are authorized to make the disclosure: _____

3. The type of information to be used or disclosed is as follows (check the appropriate boxes and include other information where indicated)
- ❑ problem list
- ❑ medication list
- ❑ list of allergies
- ❑ immunization records
- ❑ most recent history
- ❑ most recent discharge summary
- ❑ lab results (please describe the dates or types of lab tests you would like disclosed): _____
- ❑ x-ray and imaging reports (please describe the dates or types of x-rays or images you would like disclosed): _____
- ❑ consultation reports from (please supply doctors' names): _____
- ❑ entire record
- ❑ other (please describe): _____

4. I understand that the information in my health record may include information relating to sexually transmitted disease, acquired immunodeficiency syndrome (AIDS), or human immunodeficiency virus (HIV). It may also include information about behavioral or mental health services, and treatment for alcohol and drug abuse.

5. The information identified above may be used by or disclosed to the following individuals or organization(s):

Name: _____

Address: _____

Name: _____

Address: _____

6. This information for which I'm authorizing disclosure will be used for the following purpose:
- ❑ my personal records
- ❑ sharing with other health care providers as needed/other (please describe): _____

7. I understand that I have a right to revoke this authorization at any time. I understand that if I revoke this authorization, I must do so in writing and present my written revocation to the health information management department. I understand that the revocation will not apply to information that has already been released in response to this authorization. I understand that the revocation will not apply to my insurance company when the law provides my insurer with the right to contest a claim under my policy.

8. This authorization will expire (insert date or event): _____

If I fail to specify an expiration date or event, this authorization will expire six months from the date on which it was signed.

9. I understand that once the above information is disclosed, it may be redisclosed by the recipient and the information may not be protected by federal privacy laws or regulations.

10. I understand authorizing the use or disclosure of the information identified above is voluntary. I need not sign this form to ensure healthcare treatment.

Signature of patient or legal representative: _____ Date: _____

If signed by legal representative, relationship to patient

Signature of witness: _____ Date: _____

Distribution of copies: Original to provider; copy to patient; copy to accompany use or disclosure

Note: This sample form was developed by the American Health Information Management Association for discussion purposes. It should not be used without review by the issuing organization's legal counsel to ensure compliance with other federal and state laws and regulations.

What specific information can be released

To whom

For what purpose

Figure 2-5 Example of an Authorization to Use or Disclose Health Information

court sometimes decides that a physician or medical practice staff member must provide testimony. The court issues a **subpoena,** an order of the court directing a party to appear and testify. If the court requires the witness to bring certain evidence, such as a patient's medical record, it issues a **subpoena** *duces tecum,* which directs the party to appear, to testify, and to bring specified documents or items.

- *Workers' Compensation Cases*—State law may provide for release of records to employers in workers' compensation cases (see Chapter 12). The law may also authorize release to the state workers' compensation administration board and to the insurance company that handles these claims for the state.

- *Statutory Reports*—State laws require the release of some specific types of information to state health or social services departments. For example, physicians must make such statutory reports for patients' births and deaths and for cases of abuse. Because of the danger of harm to patients or others, communicable diseases such as tuberculosis, hepatitis, and rabies must usually be reported.

- *HIV and AIDS*—A special category of communicable disease control is applied to patients with diagnoses of human immunodeficiency virus (HIV) infection and acquired immunodeficiency syndrome (AIDS). Every state requires AIDS cases to be reported. Most states also require reporting of the HIV infection that causes the syndrome. However, state law varies concerning whether only the fact of a case is to be reported or if the patient's name must also be reported. The medical office's guidelines will reflect the state laws and must be strictly observed, as all these regulations should be, to protect patients' privacy and to comply with the regulations.

- *Research Data*—PHI may be made available to researchers approved by the practice. For example, if a physician is conducting clinical research on a type of diabetes, the practice may share information from appropriate records for analysis. When the researcher issues reports or studies based on the information, specific patients' names may not be identified.

- *De-identified Health Information*—There are no restrictions on the use or disclosure of "de-identified" health information— information that does not identify an individual.

HIPAA Security Rule

The **HIPAA Security Rule** requires medical offices to establish safeguards to protect PHI. The security rule specifies how to secure protected health information on computer networks, the Internet, and storage disks such as CDs. A number of techniques, such as passwords, keep stored PHI accessible only to those who need to use it. Computer users must enter user IDs and passwords to be able to use the files to which they have been granted access rights.

For example, receptionists may view the names of patients coming to the office on one day, but they should not see those patients' medical records. However, the nurse or physician needs to view the patient records. Receptionists are given an individual computer password that lets them view the day's schedule but denies entry to patient records. The physicians and nurses possess computer passwords that allow them to see all patient records.

The practice also maintains activity logs indicating who has accessed—or has tried to access—information. The need to use passwords prevents unauthorized users from gaining access to information on a computer or network.

HIPAA Electronic Health Care Transactions and Code Sets

The **HIPAA Electronic Health Care Transactions and Code Sets (TCS)** standards are rules that make it possible for physicians and health plans to exchange electronic data using the standard format and standard codes. Under this rule, three types of standards have been set:

1. Electronic formats.
2. Codes.
3. Identifiers.

Electronic Formats

The HIPAA transactions standards apply to the data that are regularly sent back and forth between providers and health plans. Examples of formats are electronic forms to verify insurance coverage and electronic claims. Each standard is labeled with both a number and a name. Either the number or the name may be used to refer to the particular electronic document format. For example, the number X12 837 stands for health care claims. The complete list of transaction standards is shown in Table 2-1.

Table 2-1 HIPAA Electronic Transaction Standards

Number	Name
X12 837	Health care claims or equivalent encounter information as well as coordination of benefits (COB)—an exchange of information between payers when a patient is covered by more than one medical insurance plan
X12 276/277	Health care claim status inquiry/response
X12 270/271	Eligibility for a health plan inquiry/response
X12 278	Referral authorization inquiry/response
X12 835	Health care payment and remittance advice
X12 820	Health plan premium payments
X12 834	Health plan enrollment and disenrollment

Code Sets

There are also standard sets of codes for diseases; treatments and procedures; and supplies or other items used to perform these actions. These standards are listed in Table 2-2.

Table 2-2 HIPAA Standard Code Sets

Purpose	Standard	*From Patient to Payment* Chapter
Codes for diseases, injuries, impairments, and other health-related problems	*International Classification of Diseases,* Ninth Edition, *Clinical Modification* (ICD-9-CM), Volumes 1 and 2	**Chapter 3**
Codes for procedures or other actions taken to prevent, diagnose, treat, or manage diseases, injuries, and impairments	Physicians' Services: *Current Procedural Terminology* (CPT) Inpatient Hospital Services: *International Classification of Diseases,* Ninth Edition, *Clinical Modification,* Volume 3: *Procedures*	**Chapter 4 and Chapter 15**
Codes for other medical services	Healthcare Common Procedures Coding System (HCPCS)	**Chapter 4**
Codes for dental services	*Current Dental Terminology* (CDT-4)	**Chapter 14**

Identifiers

Identifiers are numbers of predetermined length and structure, such as a person's Social Security number. They are important for billing because the unique numbers can be used in electronic transactions. Two identifiers—for employers and for providers—have been set up by the federal government, and two—for patients and for health plans—are to be established in the future.

- The employer identifier is used to identify the patient's employer on claims. The Employer Identification Number (EIN) issued by the Internal Revenue Service is the HIPAA standard.
- The **National Provider Identifier (NPI)** is the standard unique health identifier for health care providers to use in filing health care claims and other transactions. The NPI replaces other identifying numbers that had been in use, such as the UPIN for Medicare. The NPI is ten positions long, with nine numbers and a check digit. The numbers are assigned to individuals, such as physicians and nurses, and also to organizations, such as hospitals, pharmacies, and clinics. If a physician is in a group practice, both the individual doctor and the group have NPIs.
- CMS is maintaining the NPIs as they are assigned in the **NPPES (National Plan and Provider Enumerator System),** a national database of all assigned numbers.

RECORD RETENTION

Each medical office develops a **retention schedule** to control how long patient information is stored. The retention schedule is based on state law and, if the office sees Medicare or Medicaid patients, on federal regulations. The guidelines cover what information should be kept, for how long, and in what storage medium, such as paper, microfilm, or computer files. If records are to be destroyed at some point after retention, the means of disposal is also covered in the guidelines.

Medical records have a high degree of credibility because the law assumes that patients state only true information to their physicians. A medical office's financial records can be audited for up to seven years from a patient's last visit and for a longer period if embezzlement of government funds has occurred. Patients' medical records, on the other hand, should be maintained indefinitely if an account is contested or if there is a possibility that a patient's illness may not be resolved.

The physician documents critical patient-physician events in the patient's medical record. For example, a physician who is withdrawing from a case usually states in writing the patient's status and confirms that he or she is not doing further work. If a patient does not follow the treatment plan, the physician should document this in writing with a copy of the letter to the patient. This information is maintained in the patient's file. Depending on the physician's policy, if a patient has not returned for medical care after seven years, the records can be destroyed. Medical offices have written procedures that cover how long records are retained and what method is used to destroy them at the proper time.

> ## HIPAA Tip
>
> Medical insurance specialists must be careful about giving out information over the telephone. Never give out information unless the caller is entitled to it (such as a medical professional who is involved with the patient's care). Take the caller's name, phone number, and company name. Call the company to verify that the caller does work there. If the request is from an insurance carrier representative, ask the caller to send a letter, preferably with the claim in question, stating what facts are needed to process the claim.

AVOIDING FRAUD

Fraud occurs when someone intentionally misrepresents facts to receive a benefit illegally. A person who cooperates in a fraudulent situation is also personally responsible. In a medical office, some of the most common fraudulent situations include:

- Altering the patient's chart to increase the amount reimbursed.
- Upgrading or falsifying medical procedures to increase the amount reimbursed.
- Overbilling primary and secondary insurance carriers while at the same time collecting payment from the patient.

Fraud and HIPAA

HIPAA clearly defines health care fraud as a crime. The act set up the Health Care Fraud and Abuse Control Program to coordinate federal, state, and local law enforcement through investigations, audits, evaluations, and inspections. This program is not limited to Medicare and Medicaid. It covers any plan or program that provides health benefits, such as health insurance policies. When fraud is determined, the law permits fines of up to $10,000 per item or service for which fraudulent payment was received. Criminal penalties—fines and imprisonment—exist for knowingly planning to obtain money or property owned by the health care benefit program. If a patient is seriously hurt because of a fraudulent act, a guilty person can be imprisoned for up to twenty years. Life imprisonment is possible if the violation results in a patient's death.

Knowingly is a key word in fraud cases. Most physicians maintain honest relationships with insurance carriers. Some, however, do not. For example, suppose a physician asks a staff member to code a patient's headaches as a subdural hematoma (pool of blood below the dura mater membrane of the brain) in order to justify billing an expensive procedure. An employee must never falsify medical records. Here is what can happen: The physician might receive the higher payment, but the federal government audits the records of the medical office, finds that the patient's record does not match the insurance claim, and successfully prosecutes the physician and the staff member, finding the staff member responsible.

The Medical Insurance Specialist's Role

✔ Compliance Tip

Only physicians who are in clinical practice can prescribe medications. For example, doctors in research cannot write prescriptions. Furthermore, to dispense narcotic drugs, the physician must register with the Drug Enforcement Administration and receive a permit. In the medical office, all drugs and prescription pads must be locked away. Concerns about the way drugs are stored should be reported to the office manager or the physician.

To avoid accidental involvement in fraud, make sure all insurance information is true. A diagnosis or procedure code must not be added to an insurance claim if the physician has not documented the information in the patient's record. If the medical insurance specialist suspects that something has been mistakenly left out, the physician should be asked to update the record before the information is entered on the claim.

Because of their contracts with physicians, many health plans have the right to audit the physician's billing practices. Sometimes carriers audit selected physicians because they provide extraordinary or very specialized services. Other audits are conducted in cases where fraud or other misrepresentation of services is suspected. The health plan will notify the physician before an audit is conducted, and the types of records that will be audited are specified ahead of time. The role of the medical insurance specialist is to make sure the records are available, complete, and signed by the physician.

Professional Focus

Compliance Plans

Under federal law, the Office of Inspector General (OIG) is responsible for investigating suspected health care fraud. So that physicians can take steps to prevent the submission of erroneous claims or other unlawful conduct, the OIG has issued the Compliance Program for Individual and Small Group Physician Practices. This program outlines the parts of a **compliance plan** that each medical office should write and then communicate to staff members. An effective program has these parts: (1) conducting audits and monitoring how well the medical office follows the applicable rules, (2) implementing compliance and practice standards, (3) appointing a compliance officer on staff, (4) conducting appropriate staff training, (5) responding appropriately to fix problems that are found, (6) making sure that employees can communicate openly if they think there are compliance problems, and (7) enforcing the standards and publicizing the rules in the medical office.

Chapter Summary

1. Patients' medical records, which contain the complete, chronological, and comprehensive documentation of patients' health history and status, are used by providers to communicate and coordinate patients' health care. The records are used by medical insurance specialists to prepare and support insurance claims. If a service is not documented, it should not be billed.

2. Patients' protected health information (PHI) is defined as individually identifiable health information that is transmitted or maintained by electronic media. HIPAA requires medical offices to observe a number of regulations in order to protect the use and disclosure of PHI.

3. The HIPAA Privacy Rule regulates the use and disclosure of PHI. It requires medical offices to have a Notice of Privacy Practices, for example, and also to give patients this notice. The HIPAA Security Rule requires medical offices to establish safeguards to protect the confidentiality, integrity, and availability of health information. The HIPAA Electronic Health Care Transactions and Code Sets establish standards for the exchange of financial and administrative data that require the use of common electronic transaction methods and code sets. The four National Identifiers are for employers, health care providers, health plans, and patients.

4. For use or disclosure for treatment, payment, or operations (TPO), no release is required from the patient.

5. To release PHI for other than TPO, a medical office must have the patient sign an authorization. The authorization document must be in plain language, have a description of the information to be used, indicate who can disclose it and for what purpose, indicate who will receive it, and have an expiration date and the patient's signature.

6. A retention schedule provides guidelines on the items in the patient's medical record that must be retained and on the length of time for retention. Also, the provider must be able to justify the level and nature of treatment when a claim is investigated or challenged.

7. To protect against potential fraud, the medical practice should have a compliance plan in place. Medical insurance specialists must observe the appropriate rules about release of patient information and about correct coding and billing.

Part 1. Write "T" or "F" in the blank to indicate whether you think the statement is true or false.

_____ **1.** Medical office staff members are free to share information about patients with their families and friends.

_____ **2.** Health care fraud is a crime.

_____ **3.** Reporting services that were not performed to improve cash flow is an acceptable practice.

_____ **4.** The medical record must contain documentation that supports a billed service.

_____ **5.** The HIPAA law is different in each state.

_____ **6.** The minimum necessary standard helps to determine what PHI should be shared.

_____ **7.** Under the HIPAA Privacy Rule, patients' protected health information can be released to payers for payment purposes.

_____ **8.** A retention schedule does not apply to clinical records.

_____ **9.** The authorization to use and disclose medical information form authorizes the sharing of all confidential information with the patient's family members.

_____**10.** Information about a patient should never be released over the telephone without being sure that the inquirer is entitled to it.

Part 2. Match each term below with its correct definition.

A. HIPAA Privacy Rule

B. authorization

C. minimum necessary standard

D. fraud

E. clearinghouse

F. Notice of Privacy Practices

G. compliance plan

H. subpoena

I. retention schedule

J. PHI

_____ **1.** Law under HIPAA regulating the use and disclosure of patients' individually identifiable health information that is transmitted or maintained by electronic media.

_____ **2.** An order to appear or produce something in court.

_____ **3.** The principle that individually identifiable health information should be disclosed only to the extent needed to support the purpose of the disclosure.

_____ **4.** A HIPAA-mandated document that presents a medical office's principles and procedures related to the protection of patients' protected health information.

_____ **5.** A company that offers providers, for a fee, the service of receiving electronic or paper claims, checking and preparing them for processing, and transmitting them in proper data format to the correct carriers.

_____ **6.** Document signed by a patient that permits release of medical information under the specific stated conditions.

_____ **7.** A medical practice's written plan that includes auditing and monitoring compliance with government regulations, developing consistent written policies and procedures, providing ongoing staff training and communication, and responding to and correcting errors.

_____ **8.** Wrongdoing or misconduct.

_____ **9.** Any information about a patient that might be used to identify the person, such as name, address, or Social Security number.

_____**10.** An office policy governing the information from patients' medical records that is to be stored, for how long it is to be retained, and the storage medium to be used.

Part 3.

The X-ray report below contains four documentation errors. Identify each, and indicate the guideline that has not been followed.

X-RAY REPORT

Patient name
Salvia, Leonard X.

Examination
Esophagus

Report

jdl
7-20-2010

① The patient experiences no difficulty in swallowing barium. A ~~2~~ cm. tablet was given and

② passes readily down to the distal esophagus. After considerable swallowing, the barium

③ tablet remained in place, indicating a significant area of narrowing, less than 1 cm in

④ diameter, located between this distal esophagus that probably represents a stricture related

⑤ to a small hiatus hernia and possible esophagitis. There are no shelf-like defects or masses

⑥ to correspond to neoplasm. The mid and upper ~~position~~ ^portion^ of the esophagus is unremarkable.   *Jane*

⑦ Conclusion: Small hiatus hernia with an area of stenosis, probably on the basis of

⑧ esophagitis, appears to represent a ~~significant~~ ^major^ lesion.   *jdl*

Check Your Understanding (cont.)

Part 4. Classify each of the following situations as fraudulent (F), acceptable practice (A), or a violation of the HIPAA Privacy Rule (V).

_____ **1.** A medical insurance specialist alters a Medicare patient's claim by coding a service that was not performed.

_____ **2.** The physician tells a nurse about a patient's diagnosis.

_____ **3.** The medical practice's receptionist discusses a patient's diagnosis with a friend.

_____ **4.** A patient tells a physician personal details about an old condition unrelated to the current diagnosis.

_____ **5.** A medical office files a report with the state authority regarding births and deaths among the practice's patients in the past year.

_____ **6.** A medical office handling a workers' compensation case tells the patient's employer about his history of skin cancer.

_____ **7.** A primary care physician sends information to a referred specialist without an authorization.

_____ **8.** A medical insurance specialist supplies information about a patient to the patient's insurance carrier.

_____ **9.** The physician performs five services that were not medically necessary.

_____ **10.** A medical insurance specialist submits a Medicare claim form that bills for noncovered services.

Part 5. Read the cases below and answer the questions.

A. Rosalyn Ramirez is a medical insurance specialist employed by Valley Associates, P.C., a midsized multispecialty practice with an excellent record of complying with HIPAA rules. Rosalyn answered the telephone and heard this question: "This is Jane Mazloum, I'm a patient of Dr. Olgivy. I just listened to a phone message from your office about coming in for a checkup. My husband and I were talking about this. Since this is my first pregnancy and I am working, we really don't want anyone else to know about it yet. Has this information been given to anybody outside the clinic?"

How do you recommend that she respond?

B. Mary Kelley, a patient of the Good Health Clinic, asked Kathleen Culpepper, the medical insurance specialist, to help her out of a tough financial spot. Her medical insurance authorized her to receive four radiation treatments for her condition, one every thirty-five days. Because she was out of town, she did not schedule her appointment for the last treatment until today, which is one week beyond the approved period. The insurance company will not reimburse Mary for this procedure. She asks Kathleen to change the date on the record to last Wednesday so that it will be covered, explaining that no one will be hurt by this change and, anyway, she pays the insurance company plenty.

What type of action is Mary asking Kathleen to do?

How should Kathleen handle Mary's request?

C. Angelo Diaz signed the authorization form below. When his insurance company called for an explanation of a reported procedure that Dr. Handlesman performed to treat a stomach ulcer, George Welofar, the clinic's registered nurse, released copies of his complete file. On reviewing Mr. Diaz's history of treatment for alcohol abuse, the insurance company refused to pay the claim, stating that Mr. Diaz's alcoholism had caused the condition. Mr. Diaz complained to the practice manager about the situation.

Should the information have been released?

Patient Name: _Angelo Diaz_

Health Record Number: _AD100_

Date of Birth: _10-12-1945_

1. I authorize the use or disclosure of the above named individual's health information as described below.

2. The following individual(s) or organization(s) are authorized to make the disclosure: _Dr. L. Handlesman_

3. The type of information to be used or disclosed is as follows (check the appropriate boxes and include other information where indicated)
❏ problem list
❏ medication list
❏ list of allergies
❏ immunization records
☑ most recent history
❏ most recent discharge summary
❏ lab results (please describe the dates or types of lab tests you would like disclosed): _____
☑ x-ray and imaging reports (please describe the dates or types of x-rays or images you would like disclosed): _____
❏ consultation reports from (please supply doctors' names): _____
❏ entire record
☑ other (please describe): _Progress notes_

4. I understand that the information in my health record may include information relating to sexually transmitted disease, acquired immunodeficiency syndrome (AIDS), or human immunodeficiency virus (HIV). It may also include information about behavioral or mental health services, and treatment for alcohol and drug abuse.

5. The information identified above may be used by or disclosed to the following individuals or organization(s):
Name: _Blue Cross & Blue Shield_

Address: _____

Name: _____
Address: _____

6. This information for which I'm authorizing disclosure will be used for the following purpose:
❏ my personal records
❏ sharing with other health care providers as needed/other (please describe): _____

7. I understand that I have a right to revoke this authorization at any time. I understand that if I revoke this authorization, I must do so in writing and present my written revocation to the health information management department. I understand that the revocation will not apply to information that has already been released in response to this authorization. I understand that the revocation will not apply to my insurance company when the law provides my insurer with the right to contest a claim under my policy.

8. This authorization will expire (insert date or event): _____

If I fail to specify an expiration date or event, this authorization will expire six months from the date on which it was signed.

9. I understand that once the above information is disclosed, it may be redisclosed by the recipient and the information may not be protected by federal privacy laws or regulations.

10. I understand authorizing the use or disclosure of the information identified above is voluntary. I need not sign this form to ensure healthcare treatment.

Signature of patient or legal representative: _Angelo Diaz_ Date: _3-1-2010_

If signed by legal representative, relationship to patient

Signature of witness: _____ Date: _____

Distribution of copies: Original to provider; copy to patient; copy to accompany use or disclosure

Note: This sample form was developed by the American Health Information Management Association for discussion purposes. It should not be used without review by the issuing organization's legal counsel to ensure compliance with other federal and state laws and regulations.

3 Diagnostic Coding

Learning Outcomes

After completing this chapter, you will be able to define the key terms and:

3-1 Explain how diagnostic coding affects the payment process.

3-2 Label the primary diagnosis and coexisting conditions.

3-3 Explain the ICD-9-CM format, and identify sections used by medical insurance specialists in physician practices.

3-4 Identify the purpose and correct use of V codes and E codes.

3-5 Use a five-step process to analyze diagnoses and locate the correct ICD-9-CM code.

Key Terms

Alphabetic Index
category
chief complaint (CC)
coexisting condition
conventions
cross-reference
diagnosis code
Dx

E code
etiology
International Classification of
   Diseases, Ninth Revision,
   Clinical Modification (ICD-
   9-CM)
main term
primary diagnosis

subcategory
subclassification
subterm
supplementary term
Tabular List
V code

Why This Chapter Is Important to You

The information in this chapter will enable you to:
- Use an important reference book, the ICD-9-CM.
- Expand your understanding of why errors in diagnostic coding interfere with the billing and payment cycle.
- Learn one of the most important steps in completing health care claims.

What Do You Think?

To diagnose a patient's condition, the physician follows a complex process of decision making based on the patient's statements, an examination, and evaluation of this information. When the diagnosis is made, the medical insurance specialist communicates it to the insurance carrier through codes on the health care claim. What impact does incorrect coding have on the medical office?

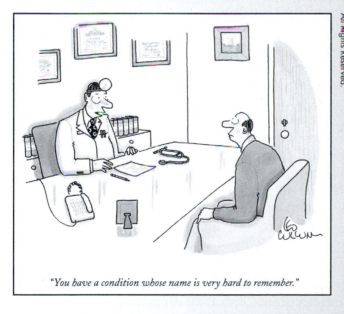

"You have a condition whose name is very hard to remember."

During the course of office encounters (visits) with patients, physicians document their evaluations of patients' conditions in their medical records. For example, in a section called Review of Systems (ROS), the patient's responses to the physician's questions about each body system are recorded. When an examination is conducted, physicians summarize the findings under various headings, such as "neck" or "neurologic" (for the nervous system). Patients' medical records also include treatments, progress notes, follow-up care, laboratory and X-ray reports, and special forms.

When a diagnosis is made by the physician, it is documented in the patient's medical record. The diagnosis, often abbreviated **Dx** in the medical record, describes illnesses or injuries using medical terminology. Medical insurance specialists become familiar with the most common diagnoses of patients seen in their medical offices. For example, in a cardiologist's office, terms such as *hypertension, cardiac infarction, vascular disease, coronary stenosis*, and *angina pectoris* are typical of the medical terminology used to describe a variety of heart conditions. Regardless of the type of medical practice, all diagnoses can be indicated by a coded "language" that is recognized worldwide.

Diagnosis Codes

One of the most important pieces of information on a health care claim is the diagnosis. The code number entered there is based on the physician's opinion of the patient's specific illness(es), sign(s), symptom(s), and complaint(s). This number is the **diagnosis code.**

Coding affects the medical billing and payment process. Diagnosis codes give insurance carriers clearly defined diagnoses to help process claims efficiently. An error in coding conveys to an insurance carrier the wrong reason a patient received medical services. This causes confusion, a delay in processing, and possibly a reduced payment or denial of the claim. An incorrect code may also raise the question of fraudulent billing if the payer decides that, based on the diagnosis, the services provided were not medically necessary.

In some practices, the physician selects the diagnosis codes. In others, a medical coder who has received specialized training in choosing codes handles this task. In still others, medical insurance specialists are expected to assign codes and to stay up to date on new codes.

The ICD-9-CM

The diagnosis codes are found in the **International Classification of Diseases, Ninth Revision, Clinical Modification,** referred to as the **ICD-9-CM.** The ICD-9-CM is a single book or a set of multiple volumes that lists codes according to a system assigned by the World Health Organization of the United Nations. The volumes are distributed by the United States Government Printing Office in Washington, D.C., and by commercial publishers.

The ICD had its beginnings in England in the 1600s. By the late 1800s it was used in the United States for reporting statistics on morbidity (the prevalence of an illness) and mortality (causes of death). Today, computers collect and analyze ICD-9-CM codes used by government health care programs, professional standards review organizations, medical researchers, hospitals, physicians, and other health care providers. Private and public medical insurance carriers also use the codes.

The ICD-9-CM has been revised a number of times. ICD-9, for example, refers to the ninth revision of the ICD. In the title *ICD-9-CM*, the initials *CM* indicate that the edition is a clinical modification. For example, the ICD-9-CM is the clinical modification of the ninth revision of the ICD. Codes in this modification describe various conditions and illnesses with more precision than did earlier codes. Under HIPAA, ICD-9-CM codes must be used to report diagnoses on all claims.

The coding system in the ICD-9-CM contains three-digit **categories** for diseases, injuries, and symptoms. Almost all of these three-digit categories are divided into four-digit code groups called **subcategories.** Many are further divided into five-digit codes called **subclassifications.** In the ICD-9-CM, the fourth and fifth digits are separated from the first three by a period. The purpose of the fourth- and fifth-level diagnosis codes is to permit reporting the most specific diagnosis possible. Figure 3-1 shows an example of several levels of ICD-9-CM codes.

In addition to the categories for diseases, one section of the ICD-9-CM codes begins with the letter *V,* and another section begins with *E.* These letters are followed by up to four digits. The codes that begin with *V* are used for encounters for reasons other than illness or injury. In these situations, patients often do not have a complaint or active diagnosis. For example, a routine annual physical examination is a reason for an office visit without a complaint. Visits for treatments of a diagnosed condition, such as chemotherapy for cancer, also receive codes beginning with *V.* Codes beginning with *E* indicate the external cause of an injury or poisoning. For example, a patient's harmful reaction to the proper dosage of a drug is assigned an E code. Both types of codes are described in more detail later in this chapter.

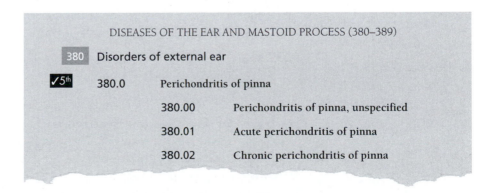

DISEASES OF THE EAR AND MASTOID PROCESS (380–389)

380	Disorders of external ear	
✓5th	380.0	Perichondritis of pinna
	380.00	Perichondritis of pinna, unspecified
	380.01	Acute perichondritis of pinna
	380.02	Chronic perichondritis of pinna

Figure 3-1 Examples of the Three Levels of ICD-9-CM Codes

CODING BASICS FOR PHYSICIAN PRACTICES

✓ Compliance Tip

- If a patient's medical record lists conditions that do not affect treatment during a particular encounter, these conditions are not reported on the claim.
- When a patient has undetermined conditions, indicated by words such as *rule out* or *suspected*, these possible conditions are not reported. Instead, the symptoms are coded and reported.
- If it is hard to determine the primary diagnosis, as in the case of multiple injuries from a motor vehicle accident, usually the diagnosis that supports the medical necessity of the highest-paying procedure is primary.

A health care claim for a patient must show the diagnosis that represents the patient's major health problem *for that particular encounter.* This condition is the **primary diagnosis.** The primary diagnosis must provide the reason for medical services listed on that claim. If a patient has cancer, for example, the disease is probably the patient's major health problem. However, if that patient sees the physician for an ear infection that is not related to the cancer, the primary diagnosis for that particular claim is the ear infection.

At times, there is more than one diagnosis because many patients are treated by a health care provider for more than one illness. Someone with hypertension (high blood pressure), for example, may also have heart disease. A patient with diabetes may seek care for a respiratory infection. The primary diagnosis—the condition that the doctor treated and documented as primary—is listed first on the insurance claim. After that, additional **coexisting conditions** may be listed. Coexisting conditions occur at the same time as the primary diagnosis. If these conditions affect the treatment or recovery from the condition shown as the primary diagnosis, they are reported. For example, a patient with diabetes mellitus often suffers from poor circulation. The diagnosis for this person's office visit to complain of numbness in the fingers and toes would be likely to include the diabetes as a coexisting condition. Sometimes, a diagnosis code contains both the primary and a coexisting condition. For example, code 365.63 means glaucoma associated with vascular disorders.

Examples

The information for identifying a patient's diagnosis and any coexisting conditions is found in the patient's medical record. When the patient goes into the examining room, a medical assistant or nurse may conduct a short interview to find out the patient's **chief complaint** (abbreviated **CC** in the documentation). The chief complaint is the reason the patient seeks medical care on this encounter. Notes about the chief complaint may be entered in the patient's medical record by the medical assistant, nurse, or physician. However, *only* the physician determines the diagnosis.

Suppose Rosa Hernandez, a patient, comes to the office. Notes about the encounter might appear as follows:

CC: Diarrhea X 5 days with strong odor and mucus, abdominal pain and tenderness, no meds.

Dx: Ulcerative colitis.

The notes mean that Ms. Hernandez has had symptoms for five days and has taken no medication. Her chief complaint is noted after the abbreviation *CC.* Her diagnosis, listed after the abbreviation *Dx,* is ulcerative colitis.

Now suppose another patient, Joel Perlman, sees the physician. His record indicates a history of heavy smoking and includes an X-ray report and notes such as these:

CC: Hoarseness, pain during swallowing, dyspnea during exertion.

Dx: Emphysema and laryngitis.

The physician listed emphysema, the major health problem, first. It is Mr. Perlman's primary diagnosis. Laryngitis is a coexisting condition that is being treated.

Finally, a third patient, Janet Chang, has a prior history of breast cancer. For today's visit, her progress notes read:

CC: Laceration of right great toe three days previously, experiencing pain, toe reddened and swollen.

Dx: Complicated open wound of toe.

Ms. Chang's primary diagnosis for this encounter is a complicated open wound of the toe. The cancer is not reported on the health care claim because the physician has not stated that it affects Ms. Chang's recovery time and or the way the wound is treated.

Case Study 3-1

Patient: Hector Garcia

CC: Red swollen lump on thigh noticed four days ago; became painful today.

Dx: Abscess.

What is Hector Garcia's primary diagnosis?

Answer:

_____

Case Study 3-2

Patient: James Jacobson

CC: Left-knee pain, swelling, and weakness. Has had right-knee pain and arthritis in past.

Dx: Left-knee pain and swelling secondary to gouty arthritis.

What is James Jacobson's primary diagnosis?

Answer:

_____

As mentioned earlier, the ICD-9-CM comes in the form of a single book or a set of two or three books. Three sections are available:

Volume 1—Diseases: Tabular List
Volume 2—Diseases: Alphabetic Index
Volume 3—Procedures: Tabular List and Alphabetic Index

Notice that the ICD-9-CM covers two major areas, diseases and procedures. Medical insurance specialists in a medical office use only the diagnosis codes (Volumes 1 and 2) in the ICD-9-CM. The procedures (Volume 3) are used only for hospital tests and treatments. Use of Volume 3 is covered in Chapter 15 of this text.

In the ICD-9-CM, diagnoses are listed two ways, as illustrated in Figure 3-2. One is the **Alphabetic Index,** which lists diagnoses in alphabetic order

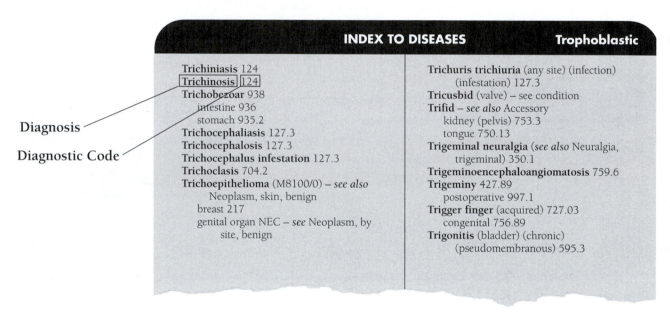

Alphabetic Index

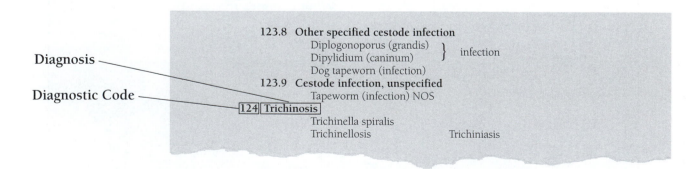

Tabular List

Figure 3-2 ICD-9-CM Alphabetic Index and Tabular List

with their corresponding diagnosis codes. The other is the **Tabular List,** which provides diagnosis codes in numerical order with additional instructions.

Both the Alphabetic Index and the Tabular List are used to find the right code. The Alphabetic Index does not contain all the necessary information, so it is never used alone. After a code is located in the Alphabetic Index, it is looked up in the Tabular List. Notes in this list may suggest or require the use of additional codes. Alternatively, notes may indicate that a condition should be coded differently because of exclusion from a category.

Alphabetic Index

The Alphabetic Index has three sections:

- Section 1 is the index to diseases and injuries, which are the diagnosis codes used most often. This section also contains special tables for indexing the codes for hypertension and neoplasms (tumors).
- Section 2 is a table of drugs and chemicals in alphabetical order, with corresponding codes related to poisoning and external causes.
- Section 3 is an alphabetical index of all external causes of injuries and poisonings, not just those resulting from drugs or chemicals.

The Alphabetic Index is organized by **main terms** in boldfaced type according to condition, as shown in Figure 3-3. A main term may be followed by a series of terms in parentheses called **supplementary terms.** The supplementary terms help define the main term but have no effect on the selection of the code. Because of this fact, they are referred to as "nonessential" supplementary terms. A **subterm** is indented underneath the main term in regular type. Subterms do affect the selection of appropriate diagnosis codes. They describe essential differences in body sites, **etiology** (the cause of disease), or clinical type. Often, a main term or subterm in the Alphabetic Index includes a **cross-reference** that indicates where else to look for additional supplementary terms, anatomical sites, or main terms.

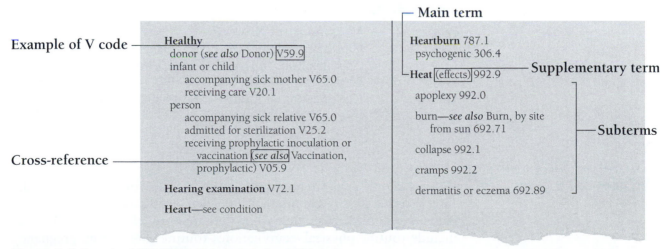

Figure 3-3 Sample of ICD-9-CM Alphabetic Index with Labels

Tabular List

The Tabular List in the ICD-9-CM presents diagnosis codes in numerical order. Many illnesses are classified according to body system, so a particular group of diseases can be found by checking the table of contents, as shown in Table 3-1.

Table 3-1 ICD-9-CM Tabular List Table of Contents

Chapter	Categories
1 Infectious and Parasitic Diseases	001–139
2 Neoplasms	140–239
3 Endocrine, Nutritional, and Metabolic Diseases and Immunity Disorders	240–279
4 Diseases of the Blood and Blood-Forming Organs	280–289
5 Mental Disorders	290–319
6 Diseases of the Central Nervous System and Sense Organs	320–389
7 Diseases of the Circulatory System	390–459
8 Diseases of the Respiratory System	460–519
9 Diseases of the Digestive System	520–579
10 Diseases of the Genitourinary System	580–629
11 Complications of Pregnancy, Childbirth, and the Puerperium	630–677
12 Diseases of the Skin and Subcutaneous Tissue	680–709
13 Diseases of the Musculoskeletal System and Connective Tissue	710–739
14 Congenital Anomalies	740–759
15 Certain Conditions Originating in the Perinatal Period	760–779
16 Symptoms, Signs, and Ill-Defined Conditions	780–799
17 Injury and Poisoning	800–999

Supplementary Classifications

V Codes	Supplementary Classification of Factors Influencing Health Status and Contact with Health Services	V01–V83
E Codes	Supplementary Classification of External Causes of Injury and Poisoning	E800–E999

Appendices

A	Morphology of Neoplasms
B	Glossary of Mental Disorders (deleted in 2004)
C	Classifications of Drugs by American Hospital Formulary Service List Number and Their ICD-9-CM Equivalents
D	Classification of Industrial Accidents According to Agency
E	List of Three-Digit Categories

V Codes and E Codes

V codes and E codes are found in numerical order following the Tabular List. **V codes** classify factors that influence health status or the reasons patients seek medical services when they are not ill. Examples of V codes include routine physical examinations, routine care during pregnancy, and immunizations or vaccinations.

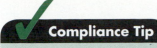

It is appropriate to use V codes:

- When a patient is not sick but receives a service for a purpose, such as an ultrasound during pregnancy.
- When a patient with a current or recurring condition receives treatments, such as physical therapy.
- When a patient has a past condition that affects current health status or has a family history of disease.

A V code can be used as either a primary code for an encounter or as an additional code. The terms that indicate the need for V codes usually have to do with a reason for an encounter other than a disease or its complications. Examples of these terms are "contact with," "history of," "follow-up," "screening," and "status."

E codes are diagnosis codes for external causes of poisonings and injuries. An E code is used *in addition to* the main code that describes the injury or poisoning itself. For example, if a person had a concussion from the impact sustained in a car accident, an E code would be used to indicate the external cause of the diagnosis. E codes are often reported on workers' compensation claims and for liability insurance, since they are used to define what happened and where it happened.

Case Study 3-3

Patient Betty Standover received an endometrial biopsy and pelvic ultrasound to monitor any changes of the endometrium that may be caused by a medication she is taking.

What type of code is used to describe the medical need for the biopsy and the ultrasound?

Answer:

_____

Case Study 3-4

Patient Frank Sherchasy fell off a ladder while on the job at Right's Painting Service. He sprained his left ankle and has a simple fracture of the right femur.

What type of code is used in addition to the main codes to describe his diagnosis?

Answer:

_____

A list of abbreviations, punctuation, symbols, typefaces, and instructional notes appears at the beginning of the ICD-9-CM. These items, called **conventions,** provide guidelines for using the ICD-9-CM system. Some key conventions are:

NOS—This abbreviation means not otherwise specified, or unspecified. This convention is used when a condition cannot be described more specifically. In general, codes with NOS should be avoided. The physician should be asked to help select a more specific code, if possible.

NEC—This abbreviation means not elsewhere classified. This convention is generally used when the ICD-9-CM does not provide a code specific enough for the patient's condition. NEC should not be used as a shortcut to avoid looking up more specific codes.

[ ] Brackets—Used around synonyms, alternative wordings, or explanations.

( ) Parentheses—Used around descriptions that do not affect the code, that is, nonessential supplementary terms.

: Colon—Used in the Tabular List after an incomplete term that needs one of the terms that follow to make it assignable to a given category.

} Brace—Encloses a series of terms, each of which is modified by the statement that appears to the right of the brace.

Includes—This note indicates that the entries following it refine the content of a preceding entry. For example, after the three-digit diagnosis code for acute sinusitis, the word *includes* is followed by the types of conditions that the code covers.

Excludes—These notes, which are italicized, indicate that an entry is not classified as part of the preceding code. The note may also give the correct location of the excluded condition.

Use additional code—This note indicates that an additional code should be used, if available.

Code first underlying disease—This instruction appears when the category is not to be used as the primary diagnosis. These codes may not be used as the first code; they must always be preceded by another code for the primary diagnosis.

FIVE STEPS TO DIAGNOSTIC CODING

Diagnostic coding follows a five-step process:

Step 1—Locate the statement of the diagnosis in the patient's medical record.

Step 2—Find the diagnosis in the ICD-9-CM's Alphabetic Index.

Step 3—Locate the code from the Alphabetic Index in the ICD-9-CM's Tabular List.

Step 4—Read all information and subclassifications to get the code that corresponds to the patient's specific disease or condition. Note fourth- or fifth-code requirements and exclusions.

Step 5—Record the diagnosis code on the insurance claim, and proofread the numbers.

Each step is explained in the following pages. Coding becomes easier with practice, but do not be tempted to take shortcuts. Every case is different, and additional terms or digits may be necessary to make a diagnosis code as specific as possible. If a step is skipped, important information may be missed. If more than one diagnosis is listed in a patient's medical record, work on only one diagnosis at a time to avoid coding errors.

Step 1. Locate the statement of the diagnosis in the patient's medical record.

First, find the place where the physician has indicated the diagnosis. This information may be located on the encounter form or elsewhere in the patient's medical record, such as in a progress note.

For example, a patient, Susan Tyne, age forty-five, comes to the office. Her medical record reads:

CC: Chest and epigastric pain; feels like a burning inside. Occasional reflux. Abdomen soft, flat without tenderness. No bowel masses or organomegaly.

Dx: Peptic ulcer.

Susan's diagnosis is peptic ulcer.

Then, if needed, decide which is the main term or condition of the diagnosis. For example, in Susan's diagnosis, the main term or condition is *ulcer*. The word *peptic* describes what type of ulcer it is.

Case Study 3-5

Patient: Hillary Baez

Dx: Complete paralysis.

What is the condition in this diagnosis?
What is the supplementary term in this diagnosis?
Answer:

_____

Case Study 3-6

Patient: Renate Martello

Dx: Heart palpitation.

What is the condition in this diagnosis?
What is the supplementary term in this diagnosis?
Answer:

_____

Case Study 3-7

Patient: Rob Blaze

Dx: Panner's disease.

What is the condition in this diagnosis?
Answer:

_____

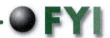

An eponym is a disease or syndrome named for an individual. An example is Graves' disease. In the ICD-9-CM, eponyms are listed both as main terms in alphabetic order and under the main terms *Disease* or *Syndrome*. A description is often included in parentheses following the eponym.

Step 2.   Find the diagnosis in the ICD-9-CM's Alphabetic Index.

Look for the condition first. Then find descriptive words that make the condition more specific. Read all cross-references to check all the possibilities for a term and its synonyms.

Suppose the diagnosis is sebaceous cyst. Look under *cyst,* the condition, rather than *sebaceous,* the descriptive word. Many entries in the Alphabetic Index are cross-referenced. For example, *sebaceous* is followed by instructions in parentheses that say "(*see also* Cyst, sebaceous)." Observe all cross-reference instructions.

Examine all subterms under the main term in the Alphabetic Index to be sure the correct term is found. Do not stop at the first one that "sounds right." When you find the correct term, make a note of the code that follows it.

For example, Figure 3-4 illustrates how to look up Susan Tyne's diagnosis of peptic ulcer. First, find the term *ulcer.* Notice that the term *peptic* is found in the list of subterms that follows the main term. After *peptic,* the term *(site unspecified)* appears. Since parentheses around a term indicates that it does not affect the code number, this is tentatively the correct code. (It must be verified by using the Tabular List.)

Make a note of the code, which is 533.9.

Step 3.   Locate the code from the Alphabetic Index in the ICD-9-CM's Tabular List.

Remember, the number to check is a code number, not a page number. The Tabular List gives codes in numerical order. Look for the number in boldfaced type. For Susan Tyne's diagnosis, look for the number 533.9 in the ICD-9-CM's Tabular List.

Ulcer, ulcerated, ulcerating, ulceration,
   ulcerative—*continued*

. . .

peptic (site unspecified) 533.9

Figure 3-4 Locating an Item in the Alphabetic Index

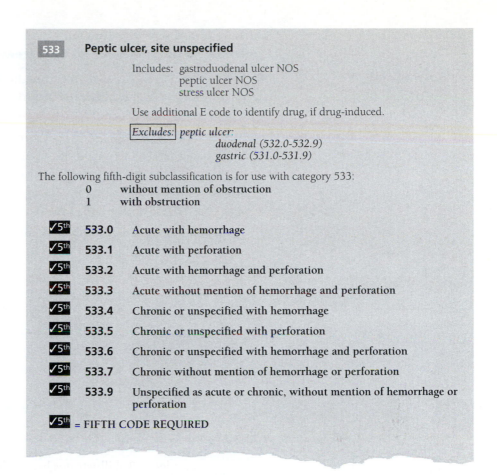

533 **Peptic ulcer, site unspecified**

Includes: gastroduodenal ulcer NOS
peptic ulcer NOS
stress ulcer NOS

Use additional E code to identify drug, if drug-induced.

Excludes: *peptic ulcer:*
duodenal (532.0-532.9)
gastric (531.0-531.9)

The following fifth-digit subclassification is for use with category 533:
0 without mention of obstruction
1 with obstruction

✓5th **533.0** Acute with hemorrhage

✓5th **533.1** Acute with perforation

✓5th **533.2** Acute with hemorrhage and perforation

✓5th **533.3** Acute without mention of hemorrhage and perforation

✓5th **533.4** Chronic or unspecified with hemorrhage

✓5th **533.5** Chronic or unspecified with perforation

✓5th **533.6** Chronic or unspecified with hemorrhage and perforation

✓5th **533.7** Chronic without mention of hemorrhage or perforation

✓5th **533.9** Unspecified as acute or chronic, without mention of hemorrhage or perforation

✓5th = FIFTH CODE REQUIRED

Figure 3-5 Locating an Item in the Tabular List

Step 4. Read all information and subclassifications to get the code that corresponds to the patient's specific disease or condition. Note fourth- or fifth-code requirements and exclusions.

Refer to Figure 3-5, which shows all the Tabular List entries that are under the three-digit code 533. Observe all instructional notations in the list.

Next to Susan Tyne's code of 533.9, the ICD-9-CM indicates "fifth code required." This note means that the correct code for the diagnosis must have five digits. In Susan Tyne's case, the diagnosis does not mention an obstruction. Therefore, the correct code is 533.90.

Note that if the ICD-9-CM indicates that a fifth digit is required, it must be included. But if it is not required, a zero or zeroes should not be added to the four-digit or three-digit code. The use of a fifth digit when it is not required makes the code invalid.

Notice also that if this diagnosis had been peptic ulcer: duodenal or gastric, it would have been excluded from the 533 code number. The italicized word *Excludes,* boxed under the main term *Peptic ulcer, site unspecified,* is an instructional note that points to alternative code numbers.

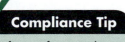

Compliance Tip

Even after performing these steps, the medical insurance specialist may not be sure the correct code has been found. In these cases, the code should be verified with the physician. Never guess a code or enter one that might not be correct.

Step 5. Record the diagnosis code on the health care claim, proofreading the numbers on the screen.

Enter the correct diagnosis code in the medical billing program (explained in detail in Chapter 6), and then proofread it. The medical insurance specialist should ask these questions:

- Are the numbers entered correctly? If numbers are transposed, the insurance carrier will receive the wrong diagnosis. Proofread the numbers on the computer screen or on the printed claim form.
- Are the codes complete? If the phone rang in the middle of coding a diagnosis, the last number of the code may have been omitted.
- Is the most specific code always used?

Case Study 3-8

Using the table shown here and the following progress notes, answer the question about this case study.

Harold Dayton's progress notes read as follows:

CC: Fatigue, chills, upset stomach, severe headache, moderate cough X 3 days, meds asa (aspirin only).

Dx: Influenza.

What is Harold Dayton's diagnosis? Use the five-step process to determine the correct ICD-9-CM diagnosis code.

Answer:

_____

Index to Diseases	Tabular List

Influenza, influenzal 487.1
   with
      bronchitis 487.1
      bronchopneumonia 487.0
      cold (any type) 487.1
      digestive manifestations 487.8
        hemoptysis 487.1
      involvement of
      gastrointestinal tract 487.8
      nervous system 487.8
      laryngitis 487. 1
      manifestations NEC 487.8
      respiratory 487.1
	487 Influenza
	487.0 With pneumonia
	487.1 With other respiratory
	    manifestations
	487.8 With other manifestations

Explore the Internet

The American Academy of Professional Coders (AAPC) is a coding association that certifies medical coders and provides information on coding issues. Using a search engine such as Google or Yahoo, visit the website of the AAPC and investigate the ways that this association keeps its members up to date about changes in procedural coding. Also review the activities of this group in your local area.

Case Study 3-9

Using the table shown here and the following progress notes, answer the questions about this case study.

Hazel Knight came to the office because of a sore, red throat. She has pus pockets in the back of her throat and has experienced fever for the past two days. A test showed streptococcal infection. Part of her examination included a blood pressure check that read 150/98. The physician diagnosed essential hypertension and streptococcal pharyngitis.

Which diagnosis is Hazel Knight's primary diagnosis?

What is the coexisting condition?

Use the five-step process to determine the correct ICD-9-CM diagnosis codes.

Answer:

_____

Primary code:

_____

Secondary code:

_____

Index to Diseases	Tabular List
essential—*see* condition	401 Essential hypertension
…	401.0 Malignant
hypertension, hypertensive (arterial) (arteriolar)(crisis) (degeneration) (disease) (essential)… .	401.1 Benign
malignant 401.0	401.9 Unspecified
benign 401.1	…
unspecified 401.9	
…	034 Streptococcal sore throat and scarlet fever
pharyngitis	
…	034.0 Streptococcal sore throat
streptococcal **034.0**	034.1 Scarlet fever

Case Study 3-10

Using the table shown here and the following progress notes, answer the questions about this case study.

Patient: Lee Yong

Patient is a fifty-eight-year-old Asian female who presents for an annual exam.

Dx: Routine health maintenance.

What is the diagnosis?

What is the correct code?

Answer:

_____

Index to Diseases	Tabular List
Health	V70 General medical examination
advice V65.4	V70.0 Routine general medical examination at health care facility
audit V70.0	
checkup V70.0	V70.1 General psychiatric examination, requested by the authority
education V65.4	
hazard (*see also* History of) V15.9	
specified cause NEC V15.89	
instruction V65.4	
services provided because … . .	

Case Study 3-11

Using the table shown here and the following progress notes, answer the question about this case study.

Patient: Ralph Kramer

Patient reported accidental injury due to the firing of a rifle by his brother during a hunting trip.

What E code should be listed following the main diagnosis code?

Answer:

_____

Index to External Causes	E Code

Accident ...
    firearm missile—*see* Shooting
...
Shooting, shot E922.9
    handgun (pistol) (revolver) E922.0 ...
    inflicted by other persons ...
    rifle (hunting) E922.2
	E922 Accident caused by firearm missile
	    E922.0 Handgun
	    E922.1 Shotgun
	    E922.2 Hunting rifle
	    E922.3 Military firearms

Professional Focus

Preview of ICD-10-CD

The tenth edition of the ICD was published by the World Health Organization in the mid-1990s. In the United States, the new *Clinical Modification* (ICD-10-CM) is being reviewed by health care professionals and is expected to be put into use. An effective date of October 1, 2011, has been proposed. The major changes include:

- The ICD-10 contains 2,033 categories of diseases, 855 more than the ICD-9. The additional codes permit more-specific reporting of diseases and newly recognized conditions.
- Codes are alphanumeric, containing a letter followed by up to five numbers.
- A sixth digit is added to capture clinical details. For example, all codes that relate to pregnancy, labor, and childbirth include a digit that indicates the patient's trimester.
- Codes are added to show which side of the body is affected when a disease or condition can be involved with the right side, the left side, or bilaterally.

Although the code numbers look different, the basic systems are very much alike. People who are familiar with the current codes will find that their training quickly applies to the new system.

Chapter Summary

1. Coding affects the payment process by giving the insurance carrier a clearly defined diagnosis that helps the carrier process the claim efficiently.

2. When a patient's medical record lists more than one diagnosis, the primary diagnosis is recorded first on the insurance claim. Additional diagnoses that occur at the same time as the primary condition and affect the patient's treatment or recovery are listed with additional diagnosis codes.

3. V codes identify encounters for reasons other than illness or injury and are used for healthy patients who are receiving routine services, for therapeutic encounters, for a problem that is not currently affecting a patient's condition, and for preoperative evaluations. E codes, which are never used as primary codes, classify the injuries resulting from various environmental events.

4. The ICD-9-CM is divided into three volumes. ICD-9-CM codes appear in lists arranged alphabetically and numerically. Medical offices use only the diagnosis codes that appear in the Tabular List (Volume 1) and the Alphabetic Index (Volume 2). ICD-9-CM procedure codes (Volume 3) are used by hospitals.

5. The five steps for analyzing diagnoses and locating the correct ICD-9-CM code are:

   (a) Locate the diagnosis in the patient's medical record.

   (b) Find the diagnosis in the ICD-9-CM's Alphabetic Index.

   (c) Locate the code from the Alphabetic Index in the ICD-9-CM's Tabular List.

   (d) Read all information and subclassifications to get the code that corresponds to the patient's specific disease or condition. Note fourth- or fifth-code requirements and exclusions.

   (e) Record the diagnosis code on the health care claim, and proofread the numbers.

Check Your Understanding

Part 1. Choose the best answer.

_____ **1.** The person who determines a patient's diagnosis is the:
  a. physician
  b. medical insurance specialist
  c. nurse

_____ **2.** The person who reports the diagnosis code on the health care claim is the:
  a. physician
  b. medical insurance specialist
  c. nurse

_____ **3.** Medical insurance specialists should proofread code numbers:
  a. to ensure accuracy
  b. to perform step 3 in the five-step coding process
  c. both a and b

_____ **4.** The person who uses the procedure codes in the ICD-9-CM (Volume 3) is the:
  a. medical insurance specialist in a medical office
  b. hospital coder
  c. both a and b

_____ **5.** The first step in the five-step process of diagnostic coding is to:
  a. record the diagnosis code on the insurance claim
  b. locate the diagnosis in the patient's encounter form or elsewhere in the medical record
  c. find the diagnosis in the ICD-9-CM's Alphabetic Index

_____ **6.** The medical insurance specialist uses the five-step diagnostic coding process:
  a. until shortcuts are discovered
  b. only during training
  c. for every diagnosis

_____ **7.** Additional diagnoses that occur at the same time as the primary condition and affect its treatment or recovery are:
  a. chief complaints
  b. coexisting conditions
  c. none of the above

_____ **8.** When assigning diagnosis codes, the medical insurance specialist uses:
  a. the Alphabetic Index
  b. the Tabular List
  c. both a and b

_____ **9.** V codes are used primarily for:
  a. emergency situations
  b. medical services having no clear diagnosis or for preventive care
  c. statistical purposes in hospital reports

_____ **10.** Diagnosis codes should be proofread to be sure they are:
  a. keyed correctly
  b. complete
  c. both a and b

Part 2. Underline the main term in the following list. Then, using the Alphabetic Index and Tabular List in the most recent ICD-9-CM available to you, code the diagnostic statements.

_____ 1. Abdominal pain

_____ 2. Acute cerebrovascular disease

_____ 3. Postoperative fibrillation

_____ 4. Night sweats

_____ 5. Singer's nodule

_____ 6. Carpal tunnel syndrome

_____ 7. Popliteal fat pad hernia

_____ 8. Harvest itch

_____ 9. Urinary incontinence without sensory awareness

_____10. Little's disease, congenital

Part 3. Using the Alphabetic Index and Tabular List in the most recent ICD-9-CM available to you, code the following diagnostic statements.

_____ 1. Breast mass

_____ 2. Muscle spasms

_____ 3. Verruca plantaris

_____ 4. Newborn vomiting

_____ 5. Herpes zoster (NOS)

_____ 6. Normal delivery

_____ 7. Menopausal syndrome

_____ 8. Diabetes, type II, uncontrolled, unspecified complication

_____ 9. Attention deficit disorder with hyperactivity

_____10. Acute pulmonary heart disease, unspecified

Part 4. Using the most recent ICD-9-CM available to you, code each of the following diagnostic statements with the correct V code or E code.

_____ 1. Routine medical health checkup of infant at health care facility

_____ 2. Fall from ladder

_____ 3. Exposure to smallpox

_____ 4. Vaccination against chickenpox

_____ 5. Accidental poisoning from motor vehicle exhaust gas

_____ **6.** HIV positive with no HIV infection symptoms or conditions

_____ **7.** Mechanical failure of equipment during kidney dialysis

_____ **8.** Accidental poisoning by gasoline

_____ **9.** Father allergic to penicillin

_____ **10.** Exposure to HIV virus but not tested for infection

Part 5. Audit the following cases to determine if the correct codes have been reported in the correct order. If a coding mistake has been made, state the correct code and your reason for assigning it.

Case 1

Chart note for Henry Blum, date of birth 11/4/57:

> Examined patient on 12/6/2010. He was complaining of a facial rash. Examination revealed sebopsoriasis and extensive seborrheic dermatitis over his upper eyebrows, nasolabial fold, and extending to the subnasal region.

The following codes were reported: 696.1, 690.1. _____

_____

Case 2

Physician's notes, 2/24/2010, patient George Kadar, DOB 10/11/1940:

> _Subjective:_ This seventy-year-old patient complains of voiding difficulties, primarily urinary incontinence. No complaints of urinary retention.
> _Objective:_ Rectal examination: enlarged prostate. Patient catheterized for residual urine of 200 cc. Urinalysis is essentially negative.
> _Assessment:_ Prostatic hypertrophy, benign.
> _Plan:_ Refer to urologist for cystoscopy.

The following code was reported: 600.0. _____

_____

Case 3

Patient: Gloria S. Diaz:

Subjective: This twenty-five-year-old female patient presents with pain in her left knee both when she moves it and when it is inactive. She denies previous trauma to this area but has had right-knee pain and arthritis in the past.

Objective: Examination revealed the left knee to be warm and slightly swollen compared to the right knee. Extension is 180 degrees; flexion is 90 degrees. Some tenderness in area.

Assessment: Left-knee pain probably due to chronic arthritis.

Plan: Daypro 600 mg 2-QD x 1 week; recheck in one week.

The following codes were reported: 719.48, 716.98. _____

_____

_____

_____

4 Procedural Coding

Learning Outcomes

After completing this chapter, you will be able to define the key terms and:

4-1 Identify the purpose and format of the Current Procedural Terminology (CPT).

4-2 Name the three key factors (components) that influence the selection of Evaluation and Management codes, and discuss E/M code assignment steps.

4-3 Compare and contrast referral and consultation services.

4-4 Recognize surgical packages and laboratory panels that are coded as single procedures.

4-5 Describe the two types of codes in the Health Care Common Procedure Coding System (HCPCS) and discuss when they should be used.

4-6 Find correct procedure codes using the CPT.

Key Terms

add-on code
bundled code
Category I code
Category II code
Category III code
Centers for Medicare and
   Medicaid Services (CMS)
code linkage
consultation

Current Procedural
   Terminology (CPT)
E/M code
established patient
global period
Health Care Common
   Procedure Coding System
   (HCPCS)
main number

modifier
new patient
panel
primary procedure
procedure code
referral
surgical package
unbundle
unlisted procedures

Why This Chapter Is Important to You

The information in this chapter will enable you to:

- Understand professional services.
- Learn to use another important reference book, the Current Procedural Terminology.
- Perform an essential step in the medical billing and payment process.

What Do You Think?

After making a diagnosis, the physician determines the proper course of treatment for the patient's health situation. As in diagnostic coding, the medical insurance specialist's role is to accurately communicate to the payer the procedures and services performed by the physician. Why is it important for the procedure codes to relate correctly to the diagnosis?

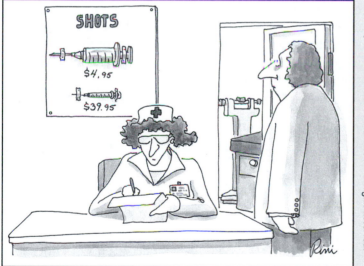

When a patient sees a physician, each procedure and service performed is reported on a health care claim using a standardized **procedure code.** Procedure codes represent medical procedures, such as surgery and diagnostic tests, and medical services, such as an examination to evaluate a patient's condition.

Medical insurance specialists verify procedure codes and use them to report physicians' services. The practice's physicians, medical coders, or—in some cases—medical insurance specialists are responsible for the selection of procedure codes. This chapter provides a basic introduction to procedural coding that will help you work effectively with health care claims and encounter forms.

On correct claims, each reported service is connected to a diagnosis that supports the procedure as necessary to investigate or treat the patient's condition. Health plans analyze this connection between the diagnostic and the procedural information, called **code linkage,** to evaluate the medical necessity of the reported charges. Correct claims also comply with many other regulations from government agencies.

Organization of the CPT

The HIPAA-required system of procedure codes is found in **Current Procedural Terminology,** published by the American Medical Association (AMA) and known as the **CPT.** An updated edition of the CPT is published every year to reflect changes in medical practice. Newly developed procedures are added, some are changed, and old ones that have become obsolete are deleted. These changes are also available in a computer file for medical offices that use a computer-based version of the CPT.

CPT **Category I codes**—which are most of the codes in CPT—are five-digit numbers. They are organized into six sections:

Section	Range of Codes
Evaluation and Management	Codes 99201–99499
Anesthesia	Codes 00100–01999
Surgery	Codes 10021–69990
Radiology	Codes 70010–79999
Pathology and Laboratory	Codes 80047–89356
Medicine	Codes 90281–99607

With the exception of the first section, the CPT is arranged in numerical order. Codes for evaluation and management are listed first, out of numerical order, because they are used most often. Each section opens with important guidelines that apply to its procedures. This material should be checked carefully before a procedure code is chosen.

Procedure codes are located by starting with the CPT's index, an alphabetical list of procedures, organs, and conditions in the back of the book (see Figure 4-1). Boldfaced main terms may be followed by descriptions and groups of indented terms. The correct code is selected by reviewing each description and indented term under the main term.

The six primary sections of the CPT are divided into subsections. These in turn are further divided into headings according to the type of test,

HIPAA Tip

New CPT codes are released around October 1 and must be used for services dated the following January 1 or later. The CPT codes as of the date of service—not the date of claim preparation—are required by HIPAA. Medical insurance specialists also update the encounter form and the medical billing software with the changed codes. Note that previous years' books should also be kept in case there is a question about already submitted insurance claims.

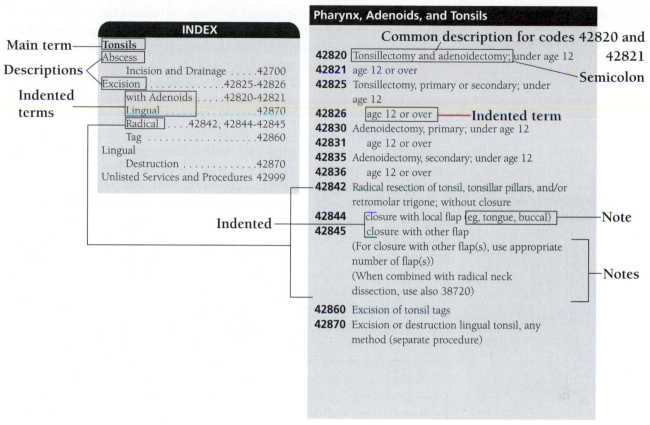

Figure 4-1 The CPT Format

service, or body system. Code number ranges included on a particular page are found in the upper-right corner. This makes locating a code faster after using the index.

In the CPT sections, four symbols are used to highlight changes or special points. A bullet, which looks like a black circle (●), indicates a new procedure code. A triangle (▲) indicates a change in the code's description. Facing triangles (▶◀) enclose other new or revised information. A plus sign (+) is used for **add-on codes,** indicating procedures that are usually carried out in addition to other procedures. For example, code 90471 covers one immunization administration, and code 90472 covers administering an additional vaccination. Add-on codes are never reported alone. They are used together with the primary code.

In CPT, the symbol ⊙ (a bullet inside a circle) next to a code means that conscious sedation is a part of the procedure that the surgeon performs. This means that, for coding to be compliant, conscious sedation is not billed in addition to the procedure. Conscious sedation is a moderate, drug-induced depression of consciousness during which patients can respond to verbal commands. This type of sedation is typically used with procedures such as bronchoscopies.

Also appearing in CPT is the symbol ⚡ (a lightning bolt). This symbol is used with vaccine codes that have been submitted to the Federal Drug Administration (FDA) and are expected to be approved for use soon. The codes cannot be used until approved, at which point this symbol is removed for the next printing of CPT. Updates are available on the American Medical Association website (www.ama-assn.org).

Format of CPT Listings

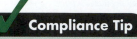
The CPT uses a particular format to show codes and their descriptions. Some descriptions are indented to show that they include a common entry from above. For example, look at the descriptions for codes 42842, 42844, and 42845 in Figure 4-1. Code 42842 is the parent code in this list. Its description begins with a capital letter. Codes 42844 and 42845 are indented, and each begins with a lowercase letter. These indented codes refer to the parent code above. The words in the description of the parent code that precede the semicolon are common to all the indented codes below it. Thus, code 42844 has the full description: "Radical resection of tonsil, tonsillar pillars, and/or retromolar trigone; closure with local flap." But if the procedure is described as "closure with other flap," the correct code would be 42845.

CPT listings may also contain notes, which are explanations for categories and individual codes. Notes often appear in parentheses after a code. Many times, notes suggest other codes that should be considered before a final code is selected. For example, the note for code 42844 in Figure 4-1 is "(e.g., tongue, buccal)," meaning that either of these terms may appear in the description of the local flap.

One or more two-digit CPT **modifiers** may be assigned to a five-digit **main number.** Modifiers are written with a hyphen before the two-digit number. The use of a modifier shows that some special circumstance applies to the service or procedure the physician performed. For example, in the Surgery section, the modifier -62 indicates that two surgeons worked together, each performing part of a surgical procedure, during an operation. Each physicians will be paid part of the amount normally reimbursed for that procedure code. Likewise, the modifier -80 indicates that the services of a surgical assistant were used, and this person's fees are a part of the claim. Appendix A of the CPT explains the proper use of each modifier. Some section guidelines also discuss the use of modifiers with the section's codes.

Unlisted Procedures, Category II Codes, and Category III Codes

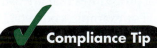
Some services or procedures occur infrequently. Others are too new to be included in the CPT. Therefore, each section provides codes to be used when a service or procedure is not listed. Codes for **unlisted procedures** are found in the guidelines at the beginning of each section, except for Anesthesiology, where the codes are found under the Other Procedures subsection. Whenever a code for an unlisted procedure is used, a special report must be attached to the health care claim. It describes the procedure, its extent, and the reason it was performed. It also gives the equipment and amount of time and effort required.

Category II codes, listed at the end of the regular (Category I) CPT codes, are used to track performance measures for a medical goal, such as reducing tobacco use. Reporting these codes on health care claims is optional, and they are not paid. They help in the development of best practices and improve documentation. These codes have an alphabetic character for the fifth digit, such as 4001F for tobacco use, smoking, assessed.

Category III codes, also listed at the end, are temporary codes for emerging technology, services, and procedures. If a Category III code exists for a service, it, rather than a unlisted code, must be used. These codes also have an alphabetic fifth digit, such as 0184T for excision of rectal tumor, TMS approach. A temporary code may become permanent and part of the regular codes if the service it identifies proves effective and is widely performed.

CODING EVALUATION AND MANAGEMENT SERVICES

To diagnose conditions and to plan treatments, physicians use a wide range of time, effort, and skill for different patients and circumstances. In the guidelines to the Evaluation and Management (**E/M codes**) section, the CPT explains how to choose the correct codes for different levels of evaluation and management services.

New or Established Patient?

Explore the Internet

New codes are released annually on the American Medical Association website and published yearly in the CPT reference. Search the AMA topics on the site, and read about new CPT Category II or III codes for the current year.

Health plans want to know whether the physician treated a **new patient** or an **established patient.** Physicians often spend more time during new patients' visits than during visits from established patients, so the E/M codes for the two types of patients are separate. For reporting purposes, a new patient is one who has not received professional services from the physician within the past three years. Medical offices commonly use the abbreviation *NP* for a new patient. An established patient is one who has seen the physician within the past three years. (Note that the current visit need not be for a problem treated previously.) Medical offices commonly use the abbreviation *EP* for an established patient. Figure 4-2 on page 76 illustrates how to decide which category fits the patient. Emergency patients are not classified as either new or established patients.

What Is the Place of Service?

The place of service (POS) is also important to know, because different E/M codes apply to services performed in a physician's office, a hospital inpatient room, a hospital emergency room, a nursing facility, an extended-care facility, and a patient's home.

Referral or Consultation?

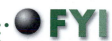

The CPT has a range of five codes each for general new-patient and established-patient encounters. The lowest-level code is often called a Level I code, on up to a Level V code. For example, code 99213 is the Level III visit code for an established patient's office encounter.

Another important item to know is whether a referral or a consultation has been provided. Sometimes one physician sends a patient to another physician for examination and treatment. For example, Martha Silvers is seen by Dr. House, her family practice physician. Ms. Silvers complains of shortness of breath (SOB) and recurring chest pain. Dr. House performs an electrocardiogram (ECG) and sends Ms. Silvers to Dr. Valentine, a cardiologist. Dr. House transfers Ms. Silvers's care for this condition to Dr. Valentine. This transfer is called a **referral.** After Dr. Valentine examines Ms. Silvers, she orders necessary tests and treatment. Since Dr. Valentine has assumed responsibility for management of Ms. Silvers's condition, the standard E/M codes for her services are used.

At other times, a physician requests advice from another physician. Suppose Dr. House asks Dr. Valentine to perform a series of tests and report the results with an opinion to him. In this case, Dr. House remains the physician in charge of the patient's care. Dr. Valentine's services are coded as a **consultation.**

Note that when a patient, not a physician, asks for a consultation with another doctor, this is called a confirmatory consultation and is coded using its own codes from the E/M section.

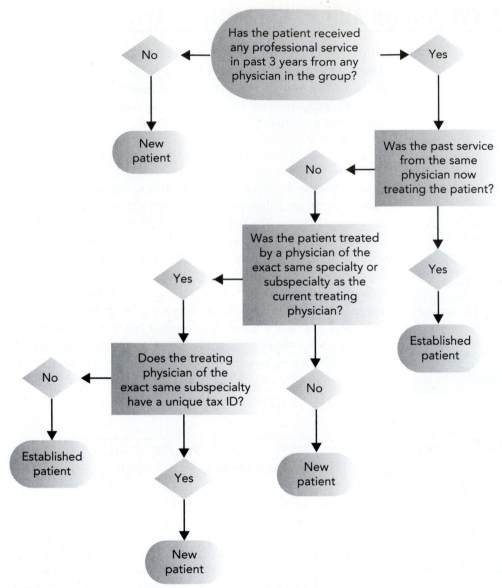

Figure 4-2 New Patient (99201-99205) Versus Established Patient (99211-99215) Flow Chart

Level of Service

The final item to decide in assigning the right E/M code is the level of service—how much work, time, and decision making were involved. These key factors documented in the patient's medical record help determine the level of service:

1. The extent of the patient history taken.
2. The extent of the examination conducted.
3. The complexity of the medical decision making.

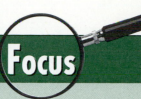

Professional Focus

Certification as a Medical Coder

A medical insurance specialist who wishes to study the field of medical coding and take an examination to earn certification as a medical coder is advised to contact one of the national accrediting associations for information. The titles of Certified Professional Coder (CPC) for physician-practice/hospital outpatient facility; Certified Professional Coder-Hospital (CPC-H); Certified Professional Coder-Payer (CPC-P) for assurance of correct review and payment of claims for reimbursement; and specialty credentials for evaluation and management, general surgery, obstetrics, and gynecology as well as an associate level for students are granted by the American Academy of Professional Coders (AAPC),

2480 South 3850 West, Suite B, Salt Lake City, UT 84120, telephone: 800-626-2633. The American Health Information Management Association (AHIMA) offers three coding certifications: the Certified Coding Associate (CCA), intended as a starting point for entering a new career as a coder; the Certified Coding Specialist (CCS); and the Certified Coding Specialist-Physician-based (CCS-P). American Health Information Management Association (AHIMA), 919 North Michigan Avenue, Suite 1400, Chicago, IL 60611-1683, telephone: 312-787-2672. Both organizations' websites contain updated information on their credentials and certification requirements.

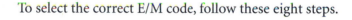

E/M Code Assignment

To select the correct E/M code, follow these eight steps.

Step 1 Determine the Category and Subcategory of Service Based on the Place of Location of Service and the Patient's Status

The list of E/M categories, such as office visits, hospital services, and preventive medicine services, is used to locate the appropriate place or type of service in the index. In the main text of the selected category, the subcategory—such as new or established patient—is then chosen.

Documentation: initial hospital visit to established patient

    Index: Hospital Services

            Inpatient Services

                Initial Care, New or Established Patient

    Code Ranges: 99221–99223

For most types of service, such as initial hospital care for an established patient, between three to five codes are listed. To select an appropriate code from this range, three key components are considered: (1) the history the physician documented, (2) the examination that was documented, and (3) the medical decisions the physician documented. (The exception to this guideline is selecting a code for counseling or coordination of care, where the amount of time the physician spends may be the only key component in some situations.)

Step 2   Determine the Extent of the History That Is Documented

History is the information the physician received by questioning the patient about the chief complaint and other signs or symptoms, about all or selected body systems, and about pertinent past history, family background, and other personal factors. If the patient is incapacitated, the history may be taken from a family member.

The history is documented in the patient medical record as follows:

History of present illness (HPI)

The history of the illness is a description of the development of the illness from the first sign or symptom that the patient experienced to the present time. It includes everything related to the illness or condition. These points about the illness or condition may be documented:

- Location *(body area of the pain/symptom)*
- Quality *(type of pain/ symptom, such as sudden or dull)*
- Severity *(degree of pain/symptom)*
- Duration *(how long the pain/symptom lasts and when it began)*
- Timing *(time of day pain/symptom occurs)*
- Context *(any situation related to the pain/symptom, such as occurs after eating)*
- Modifying factors *(any factors that alter the pain/symptom)*
- Associated signs and symptoms *(things that also happen when the pain/symptom occurs, such as the severity, location, and timing of pain, and other signs and symptoms.)*

Review of systems (ROS)

The review of systems is an inventory of body systems. These systems are:

- Constitutional symptoms *(such as fever or weight loss)*
- Eyes
- Ears, nose, mouth, and throat
- Cardiovascular (CV)
- Respiratory
- Gastrointestinal (GI)
- Genitourinary (GU)
- Musculoskeletal
- Integumentary
- Neurological
- Psychiatric
- Endocrine
- Hematologic/lymphatic
- Allergic/immunologic.

Past medical history (PMH)

The past history of the patient's experiences with illnesses, injuries, and treatments contains data about other major illnesses and injuries, operations, and hospitalizations. It also covers current medications the patient is taking, allergies, immunization status, and diet.

Family history (FH)

The family history reviews the medical events in the patient's family. It includes the health status or cause of death of parents, brothers and sisters, and children; specific diseases that are related to the patient's chief complaint or the patient's diagnosis; and the presence of any known hereditary diseases.

Social history (SH)

The facts gathered in the social history, which depend on the patient's age, include marital status, employment, and other factors.

(The histories documented after the HPI are sometimes referred to as PFSH, for past, family, and social history.)

The history that the physician decides to obtain is then categorized as one of four types on a scale from lesser to greater extent of amount of history obtained:

1. *Problem-focused:* Determining the patient's chief complaint and obtaining a brief history of the present illness
2. *Expanded problem-focused:* Determining the patient's chief complaint and obtaining a brief history of the present illness, plus a problem-pertinent system review of the particular body system that is involved
3. *Detailed:* Determining the chief complaint; obtaining an extended history of the present illness; reviewing both the problem-pertinent system and additional systems; and taking pertinent past, family, and/or social history
4. *Comprehensive:* Determining the chief complaint and taking an extended history of the present illness, a complete review of systems, and a complete past, family, and social history.

Step 3   Determine the Extent of the Examination That Is Documented

The physician may examine a particular body area or organ system or may conduct a multisystem examination. The body areas are divided into the head and face; chest, including breasts and axilla; abdomen; genitalia, groin, and buttocks; back; and each extremity.

The organ systems that may be examined are the eyes; the ears, nose, mouth, and throat; cardiovascular; respiratory; gastrointestinal; genitourinary; musculoskeletal; skin; neurologic; psychiatric; and hematologic/lymphatic/immunologic.

The examination that the physician documents is categorized as one of four types on a scale from lesser to greater extent:

1. *Problem-focused:* A limited examination of the affected body area or system
2. *Expanded problem-focused:* A limited examination of the affected body area or system and other related areas

3. *Detailed:* An extended examination of the affected body area or system and other related areas

4. *Comprehensive:* A general multisystem examination or a complete examination of a single organ system.

Step 4   Determine the Complexity of Medical Decision Making That Is Documented

The complexity of the medical decisions that the physician makes involves how many possible diagnoses or treatment options were considered; how much data information (such as test results or previous records) was considered in analyzing the patient's problem; and how serious the illness is, meaning how much risk there is for significant complications, advanced illness, or death.

The decision-making process that the physician documents is categorized as one of four types on a scale from lesser to greater complexity:

1. *Straightforward:* Minimal diagnoses options, a minimal amount of data, and minimum risk

2. *Low complexity:* Limited diagnoses options, a low amount of data, and low risk

3. *Moderate complexity:* Multiple diagnoses options, a moderate amount of data, and moderate risk

4. *High complexity:* Extensive diagnoses options, an extensive amount of data, and high risk.

Step 5   Analyze the Requirements to Report the Service Level

The descriptor for each E/M code explains the standards for its selection. For office visits and most other services to new patients, and for initial care visits, all three of the key components must be documented. This is stated in CPT as follows:

> **99203   Office or other outpatient visit** for the evaluation and management of a new patient, which require these three key components:
> - **a detailed history**
> - **a detailed examination**
> - **medical decision making of low complexity**

This means that to select code 99203, the medical record must show that a detailed history and examination were taken, and medical decision making was at least at the level of low complexity.

For most services for established patients, and for subsequent care visits, two out of three of the key components requirements must be met. For example:

> **99232   Subsequent hospital care,** per day, for the evaluation and management of a patient, which requires at least two of these three key components:
> - **an expanded problem-focused interval history**
> - **an expanded problem-focused examination**
> - **medical decision making of moderate complexity**

This means that to select code 99232, the medical record must show that two out of the three factors are documented.

Step 6   Verify the Service Level Based on the Nature of the Presenting Problem, Time, Counseling, and Care Coordination

Many descriptors mention two additional components: (1) how severe the patient's condition is, referred to as the *nature of the presenting problem,* and (2) how much time the physician typically spends directly treating the patient. These factors, while not the key components, help in selecting the correct E/M service level. For example, this wording statement appears in CPT after the 99214 code (office visit for the evaluation and management of an established patient):

> Usually, the presenting problem(s) are of moderate to high severity. Physicians typically spend 25 minutes face-to-face with the patient and/or family.

Counseling is a discussion with a patient regarding areas such as diagnostic results, instructions for follow-up treatment, and patient education. It is mentioned as a typical part of each E/M service in the descriptor, but it is not required to be documented as a key component.

Coordination of care with other providers or agencies is also mentioned. When coordination of care is provided but the patient is not present, codes from the case management and care plan oversight services subsections' codes are reported.

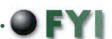

FYI

If a patient's visit is mainly about counseling and/or coordination of care regarding symptoms or illness, the length of time the physician spends is the controlling factor. If over 50 percent of the visit is spent counseling or coordinating care, time is the *main* factor. If an established patient's visit is 30 thirty minutes, for example, and 20 twenty minutes of it are spent counseling, then the E/M code is 99214.

Step 7   Verify That the Documentation Is Complete

Meeting the requirements means that the documentation must contain the record of the physician's work. When an E/M code is assigned, the patient's medical record must contain the clinical details to support it. The history, examination, and medical decision making must be sufficiently documented that the medical necessity and appropriateness of the service can be understood.

Step 8   Assign the Code

The code that has been selected is assigned. The need for any modifiers, based on the documentation of special circumstances, is also reviewed.

CODING SURGICAL PROCEDURES

Codes in the Surgery section represent groups of procedures that include all routine elements. This combination of services is called a **surgical package.** According to the Surgery section guidelines in the CPT, the procedure codes for surgical procedures include the following:

- After the decision for surgery, one related E/M encounter on the date immediately before or on the date of the procedure.
- The operation: preparing the patient for surgery, including injection of anesthesia by the surgeon (local infiltration,

metacarpal/metatarsal/digital block or topical anesthesia), and performing the operation, including normal additional procedures, such as debridement.

- Immediate postoperative care, including dictating operative notes, talking with the family and other physicians.
- Writing orders.

The procedure code for a surgical package covers a group of services that should not be listed individually. This package code is called a **bundled code.** Payers assign a fee that reimburses all the services provided under a bundled code. The period of time that is covered for follow-up care is referred to as the **global period.** For example, the global period for repairing a tendon might be set at ten days. The global period for major surgery such as an appendectomy might be set at ninety days. After the global period ends, additional services that are provided can be reported separately for additional payment.

Two types of services are not included in surgical package codes. These services are reported separately and reimbursed in addition to the surgical package fee:

- Complications or recurrences that arise after therapeutic surgical procedures.
- Care for the condition for which a diagnostic surgical procedure is performed. Routine follow-up care included in the code refers only to care related to recovery from the diagnostic procedure itself, not the condition.

When health plans pay for more than one surgical procedure performed on the same day for the same patient, they pay the full amount of the first listed surgical procedure, but they often pay less than the full amount for the other procedures. For maximum payment when multiple procedures are reported, the most complex or highest-level code—the procedure with the highest reimbursement value—should be listed first. The other procedures are listed with the modifier -51 or the modifier -59. Modifier -51 is used for multiple procedures at the same body site or system. Modifier -59 indicates distinct procedures, each fully reimbursed, rather than multiple procedures. It is usually used when the surgeon performs procedures on two different body sites or organ systems, such as the excision of a lesion on the chest as well as the incision and drainage (I & D) of an abscess on the leg.

✓ **Compliance Tip**

If each test in a panel or each procedure in a surgical package is listed separately, it will **unbundle** the panel or package. The payer's review will regroup the services under the appropriate code, which could delay payment. Note that when unbundling is done intentionally to receive more payment than is correct, the claim is likely to be considered fraudulent.

CODING LABORATORY PROCEDURES

Organ or disease-oriented **panels** listed in the Pathology and Laboratory section of the CPT include tests frequently ordered together (see Figure 4-3). A comprehensive metabolic panel, for example, includes tests for albumin, bilirubin, calcium, carbon dioxide, chloride, glucose, and other factors. Each element of the panel has its own procedure code in the Pathology and Laboratory section. However, when the tests are performed together, the code for the panel must be used, rather than listing each test separately.

ORGAN/DISEASE PANEL	
Basic Metabolic Panel	80048
General Health Panel	80050
Comprehensive Metabolic Panel	80053
Obstetric Panel	80055
Lipid Panel	80061
Acute Hepatitis Panel	80074
Hepatic Function Panel	80076

Figure 4-3 Examples of Panels in the CPT

CODING IMMUNIZATIONS

Injections and infusions of immune globulins, vaccines, toxoids, and other substances require two codes, one for giving the injection and one for the particular vaccine or toxoid that is given. For example, for an influenza shot, the administration code 90471 is used for the injection along with one of the codes for the specific vaccine, such as 90655, 90657, 90658, or 90660.

HCPCS CODES

The **Health Care Common Procedure Coding System,** commonly referred to as **HCPCS,** was developed by the **Centers for Medicare and Medicaid Services (CMS)** for use in coding services for Medicare patients (see Chapter 9). The HCPCS (pronounced hic-picks) coding system has two levels:

- Level I codes duplicate those from the CPT.
- Level II codes are issued by CMS in the *Medicare Carriers Manual.* They are called national codes and cover many supplies, such as sterile trays, drugs, and DME (durable medical equipment). Level II codes also cover services and procedures not included in the CPT. The Level II HCPCS codes have five characters, either numbers or letters or a combination of the two.

HCPCS modifiers, either two letters or a letter with a number, are also available for use. These modifiers are different from the CPT modifiers. For example, HCPCS modifiers may indicate social worker services or equipment rentals.

Examples of Level II codes are:

Explore the Internet

This year's HCPCS codes are available on the CMS website. Access this website and search for information on HCPCS by entering this term in the Search box. Locate updates to the HCPCS codes and read the general information that is posted.

Code Number	Description
A0428	Ambulance service; basic life support, non-emergency
E0112	Crutches, underarm, wood, adjustable or fixed; pair, with pads, tips, and handgrip
J0120	Injection, tetracycline, up to 250 mg

In medical offices that use the HCPCS system, regulations issued by CMS are reviewed to determine the correct code and modifier for claims.

FIVE STEPS FOR LOCATING CORRECT CPT CODES

Five steps are used for finding procedure codes in the CPT:

Step 1—Become familiar with the CPT.
Step 2—Find the services listed on the patient's encounter form.
Step 3—Look up the procedure code(s).
Step 4—Determine appropriate modifiers.
Step 5—Record the procedure code(s) on the health care claim.

Coding procedures become easier as the coder becomes more familiar with CPT codes. In fact, most medical offices use only a limited number of procedure codes. To practice using the CPT, follow the instructions below, and look up codes used in the examples to gain understanding of the format and main sections of the book.

Step 1. Become familiar with the CPT.

Read the introduction and main section guidelines and notes. For example, look at the guidelines for the Evaluation and Management section. They include definitions of key terms, such as *new and established patient, chief complaint, concurrent care,* and *counseling.* They also explain the way E/M codes should be selected.

Case Study 4-1

Study Table 1 in the guidelines for the Evaluation and Management section of the CPT.

What code range is used for emergency department services? Now turn to Appendix A. Is it correct to use modifier -24 with E/M codes? Modifier -51?
Answer:

_____

_____

_____

Step 2. Find the services listed on the patient's encounter form.

The next step is to check the patient's encounter form to see which services were performed. For E/M procedures, look for clues about the extent of history, examination, and decision making that were involved. The encounter form may also indicate the amount of time the physician spent with the patient.

For example, assume that Ms. Silvers's encounter form shows an office visit for an osteoporosis evaluation. A CAT scan is performed to test bone density, so this procedure is looked up. The evaluation and management service is also coded, based on the extent of the patient's history and examination the physician performed and the complexity of decision making.

Step 3. Look up the procedure code(s).

First, pick out a specific procedure or service, organ, or condition. Find the procedure code in the CPT's index. Remember, the number in the index is the five-digit code, not a page number. For example, to find the code for dressing change, first look alphabetically in the index for the procedure. Then, turn to the procedure code in the body of the CPT to be sure the code accurately reflects the service performed. The procedure code 15852 explains the dressing change for "other than burns" and "under anesthesia (other than local)." A dressing for a burn is listed as procedure codes 16010–16030.

Case Study 4-2

Find the correct procedure codes for the following:

Procedure: knee arthrodesis

_____

Organ: incision and drainage of kidney abscess

_____

Condition: atrial fibrillation

_____

In some cases, the patient's medical record shows an abbreviation, synonym, or eponym (the name of a person or place for which a procedure is named). For example, the record might state "treated for bone infection." In CPT's index, the entry for Infection, Bone, is followed by the instruction "See Osteomyelitis."

To code the excision of a vaginal cyst, one might first look under Excision. There is a listing for Cyst beneath Excision, followed by a list of organs, regions, or structures involved. Look for Vagina to find the code. Another way to find the code is to look under Vagina and then find the listing for Cyst Excision beneath it.

Case Study 4-3

Find the correct procedure code for the following:

Insertion, LeVeen shunt
Answer:

_____

Although it may seem tempting to record the procedure code directly from the index, resist the shortcut. Explanations and notes in the guidelines and main sections more accurately lead to finding main numbers and modifiers that reflect the services performed. That is the only way to ensure reimbursement at the highest allowed level.

Case Study 4-4

Ms. Silvers is referred to Dr. Valentine for chest pain. The patient's encounter form on her second appointment shows a cardiovascular stress test using submaximal treadmill, with continuous electrocardiographic monitoring, with physician supervision, interpretation, and report. Find the procedure code for the procedure.

Cardiovascular stress test

Answer: _____

(*Hint:* Look under the heading "Cardiology.")

To make the coding process more efficient, medical offices often list frequently used CPT codes on encounter forms. After seeing the patient, the physician checks off the appropriate procedures or services. An example is shown in Figure 4-4. On this example of a dermatology practice's encounter form, the E/M codes as well as common procedures are shown.

Step 4.   Determine appropriate modifiers.

Check section guidelines and Appendix A to find modifiers that elaborate on details of the procedure being coded. For example, a bilateral breast reconstruction requires the modifier -50. Find the code for "breast reconstruction with free flap": 19364. To show the insurance carrier that the procedure was performed on both breasts, attach the -50 modifier: 19364-50.

Case Study 4-5

Patient Amy Wan had surgery for ingrown toenails on the great toe of each foot. Find the procedure code for the service, including any applicable modifier.

Procedure code:

_____

Case Study 4-6

Patient Judi Goldfarb had a partial mastectomy of the left breast.

Procedure code:

_____

CENTRAL PRACTICE CENTER
1122 E. University Drive
Mesa, AZ 85204
602-969-4237

PATIENT NAME	APPT. DATE/TIME
Deysenrothe, Mae J.	10/06/2010 9:30am

PATIENT NO.	DX
DEYSEMA0	**1.** V70.0 Exam, Adult **2.** **3.** **4.**

DESCRIPTION	√	CPT	FEE	DESCRIPTION	√	CPT	FEE
EXAMINATION				**PROCEDURES**			
New Patient				Diagnostic Anoscopy		46600	
Problem Focused		99201		ECG Complete	√	93000	70
Expanded Problem Focused		99202		I&D, Abscess		10060	
Detailed		99203		Pap Smear		88150	
Comprehensive		99204		Removal of Cerumen		69210	
Comprehensive/Complex		99205		Removal 1 Lesion		17000	
Established Patient				Removal 2-14 Lesions		17003	
Minimum		99211		Removal 15+ Lesions		17004	
Problem Focused		99212		Rhythm ECG w/Report		93040	
Expanded Problem Focused		99213		Rhythm ECG w/Tracing		93041	
Detailed		99214		Sigmoidoscopy, diag.		45330	
Comprehensive/Complex		99215					
				LABORATORY			
PREVENTIVE VISIT				Bacteria Culture		87081	
New Patient				Fungal Culture		87101	
Age 12-17		99384		Glucose Finger Stick		82948	
Age 18-39		99385		Lipid Panel		80061	
Age 40-64	√	99386	180	Specimen Handling		99000	
Age 65+		99387		Stool/Occult Blood		82270	
Established Patient				Tine Test		85008	
Age 12-17		99394		Tuberculin PPD		86580	
Age 18-39		99395		Urinalysis	√	81000	17
Age 40-64		99396		Venipuncture		36415	
Age 65+		99397					
				INJECTION/IMMUN.			
CONSULTATION: OFFICE/ER				DT Immun		90702	
Requested By:				Hepatitis A Immun		90632	
Problem Focused		99241		Hepatitis B Immun		90746	
Expanded Problem Focused		99242		Influenza Immun	√	90660	68
Detailed		99243		Pneumovax		90732	
Comprehensive		99244					
Comprehensive/Complex		99245					
				TOTAL FEES			335.00

Figure 4-4 Encounter Form with Selected Procedure Codes

Case Study 4-7

Patient Tonisha Williams had a total abdominal hysterectomy and removal of tubes and ovaries for submucous leiomyoma of the uterus and severe polycystic disease of the ovaries.

Procedure code:

_____

Case Study 4-8

Established patient: Randy Kane
Visit to Ashworth Dermatology Clinic for recurrence of forearm rash. He is a previous patient who presented with this condition twenty days ago. I saw him for a ten-minute follow-up examination because of the flare-up. Has 4 × 6 cm rash over mid-forearm with scaly, erythematous, raised papules.

Procedure code:

_____

Case Study 4-9

Dr. LaFarge visits the home of the BeGeorgs family. She is the family physician and has taken care of the patient, Ralph, since birth. He is now thirteen years old and is recovering well from a recent broken leg. She decided to visit this established patient at home to check on possible swelling or soreness due to the cast.

Procedure code:

_____

Case Study 4-10

Juanita Escobar, age two, has an intramuscular injection for immunization with diphtheria and tetanus toxoids (DT).

Procedure codes:

_____

(*Hint:* Check the possible codes for patients' ages.)

Step 5.   Record the procedure code(s) on the health care claim.

After the procedure code is verified, it is posted to the claim. If the patient has more than one diagnosis for a single claim, the primary diagnosis is listed first (see Chapter 3). Likewise, the corresponding **primary procedure** is listed first. The primary procedure is the main service performed for the condition listed as the primary diagnosis.

The physician may perform additional procedures at the same time or in the same session as the primary procedure. If additional procedures are performed, match up each procedure with its corresponding diagnosis. If this is not done, the procedures will not be considered medically necessary, and the claim will be denied.

For example, Ms. Silvers, who saw Dr. House for chest pain and shortness of breath, also has asthma. While the patient is in the office, Dr. House renews her prescription for asthma medication along with performing the ECG. If the ECG is mistakenly shown as a procedure for asthma, the claim will be denied, because that procedure is not medically necessary for that diagnosis.

Chapter Summary

1. The purpose of the Current Procedural Terminology is to provide a standardized list of procedure codes for medical, surgical, and diagnostic services. It is divided into six sections: (a) Evaluation and Management, (b) Anesthesiology, (c) Surgery, (d) Radiology, (e) Pathology and Laboratory, and (f) Medicine (except anesthesiology).

2. The three main factors (components) that influence the level of service for coding purposes are the type and extent of (a) history, (b) examination, and (c) medical decision making. The steps for selecting correct E/M codes are to (a) determine the category and the subcategory of service, (b) determine the extent of the history, (c) determine the extent of the examination, (d) determine the complexity of medical decision making, (e) analyze the requirements to report the service level, (f) verify the service level based on the nature of the presenting problem, time, counseling, and care coordination, (g) verify that the documentation is complete, and (h) assign the code.

3. Referral services are services performed for a patient whose care has been transferred from one physician to another. Consultation services occur when an attending physician requests advice from another physician.

4. Surgical packages and laboratory panels should be coded as single procedures rather than broken into component parts.

5. The Health Care Common Procedure Coding System (HCPCS), used to code Medicare services, has codes from CPT as well as Level II codes.

6. To find correct procedure codes using the CPT:

   Step 1—Become familiar with the CPT.

   Step 2—Find the services listed on the encounter form.

   Step 3—Look up the procedure code(s) in the Index, and then cross-reference to the main section of the CPT code book.

   Step 4—Determine appropriate modifiers.

   Step 5—Record the procedure code(s) on the health care claim.

Check Your Understanding

Part 1. Fill in each blank with the correct answer. Then unscramble the bracketed letters to reveal a term that is a quick abbreviation for medical services.

1. The *Current Procedural Terminology* is better known as the ___ [__] ___.

2. This section of the CPT is found at the beginning of the book because services in it are used most often. It is called [__] __.

3. A two-digit code that describes special circumstances about a procedure is called a(n) [__] __ __ __ __ __ __ __.

4. The procedure code 23174 is found in the __ __ __ __ __ [__] __ section of the CPT.

5. A patient who has been seen by the physician within the last three years is a(n) [__] __ __ __ __ __ __ __ __ __ [__] patient.

6. A code that is used in addition to a primary procedure, shown in the CPT with a plus sign, is called a(n) __ __ __ - __ __ [__] __ __ __.

7. The __ __ [__] __ __ in the back of the CPT is an alphabetical list of procedures, organs, and conditions.

8. The six sections of the CPT are Evaluation and Management, Anesthesiology, Surgery, [__] __ __ __ __ __ __ __ __, Pathology and Laboratory, and Medicine.

9. A service performed so the physician can give advice to another physician is a(n) __ __ __ __ [__] __ __ __ __ __ [__] __.

10. A surgical __ __ [__] __ __ __ [__] is a group of related procedures and services included in the procedure code.

   A quick abbreviation for a medical service is a:

   ANSWER: __ __ __ __ __ __ __ __ __ __ __ __ __

Part 2. Using the most recent CPT code book available to you, find the following Evaluation and Management codes.

1. Follow-up visit, eight-year-old boy, nurse removes sutures from leg wound.

2. Office visit, twenty-nine-year-old female, established patient, follow-up on severe wrist sprain.

3. Initial office visit to evaluate gradual hearing loss, sixty-year-old female, history and physical examination, complete audiogram.

4. Initial office visit to evaluate forty-five-year-old male with complaint of shortness of breath and chest pain during exercise. Severe cardiovascular damage is suspected. Comprehensive history and examination performed. Physician spent about forty-five minutes with the patient.

5. Annual physical examination of established patient, male, age forty-two.

6. Emergency department visit for a new patient with rash over entire trunk after exposure to poison ivy.

7. Initial intensive care for E/M of critically ill baby, fifteen days old.

8. Home visit for E/M of established patient with congestive heart failure (CHF); caregiver phoned report of sudden difficulty breathing and profuse sweating.

9. Medical conference of physician and psychiatrist to discuss patient's care; approximately thirty minutes.

10. Patient, age twenty-eight, office visit for basic evaluation for life insurance.

Check Your Understanding (cont.)

Part 3. Using the most recent CPT code book available to you, find the following procedure codes.

1. Repair of nail bed.

2. Removal of twenty skin tags.

3. Radiologic examination, chest, two views, frontal and lateral.

4. Anesthesia for vaginal delivery.

5. Electrocardiogram, routine ECG, twelve leads, interpretation and report.

6. Glucose tolerance test (GTT), three specimens (includes glucose).

7. Modifier for unusual services beyond those usually required for the procedure.

8. Modifier for laboratory procedures performed by someone other than the treating or reporting physician.

9. Unlisted surgical procedure, nervous system.

10. Modifier for repeat radiology procedure performed by the same physician.

Part 4. Using the most recent HCPCS code book available to you, supply the correct HCPCS codes for the following.

1. Administration of hepatitis B vaccine.

2. Each composite dressing, pad size more than 48 square inches, without adhesive border.

3. Shoe lift, elevation, heel, tapered to metatarsals, per inch.

4. Screening Papanicolaou smear, cervical or vaginal, up to 3 smears, by technician under physician supervision.

5. Hot water bottle.

6. Half-length bedside rails.

7. Injection of bevacizumab, 10 mg.

8. Brachytherapy, source, palladium 103, per source.

9. Enteral nutrition infusion pump, with alarm.

10. Infusion of 1000 cc of normal saline solution.

Payment Methods: Managed Care and Indemnity Plans

Learning Outcomes

After completing this chapter, you will be able to define the key terms and:

5-1 Discuss the major types of health plans and how the various structures affect the payments that patients owe for medical services.

5-2 Describe three ways in which payments to physicians are set.

5-3 Compare the calculation of payments for participating and nonparticipating providers, and describe how balance-billing rules affect the charges that can be collected from patients.

5-4 List the types of charges for which a patient may be responsible at the time of a visit.

Key Terms

allowed charge
balance billing
capitation
capitation rate (cap rate)
consumer-driven health plan (CDHP)
discounted fee-for-service
family deductible
fee schedule
health maintenance organization (HMO)
individual deductible

network
nonparticipating (nonPAR) physician
out-of-network
out-of-pocket expenses
participating (PAR) physician
point-of-service (POS) plan
preferred provider organization (PPO)
primary care physician (PCP)

professional courtesy
referral number
relative value scale (RVS)
Resource-Based Relative Value Scale (RBRVS)
usual, customary, and reasonable (UCR)
usual fee
walkout receipt
write off (verb)

Why This Chapter Is Important to You

The information in this chapter will enable you to:

- Become familiar with contracts between physicians and health plans and with ways of calculating physicians' payments.
- Understand the charges that are often collected from patients after office encounters.

What Do You Think?

"How much will my insurance pay?" "How much will I owe?" "Why are this doctor's fees different from my previous doctor's fees?" Questions such as these are handled by medical insurance specialists every day. What steps can the specialist take to be prepared to handle these inquiries?

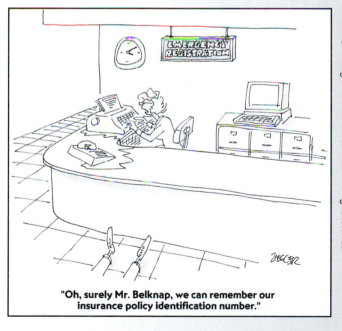

"Oh, surely Mr. Belknap, we can remember our insurance policy identification number."

TYPES OF HEALTH PLANS

Medical insurance specialists need to become familiar with the health plans that the patients seen in medical offices have. Most insured patients have medical coverage under one of the types of managed care plans, while a few have fee-for-service plans. The type of health plan affects the payments that patients must make for medical services. It also affects the way physicians are paid for providing those services.

The major types of health insurance plans are summarized in Table 5-1 and described in the following section.

Table 5-1 Comparison of Major Health Plan Types

Plan Type	Provider Options	Cost Containment	Features
Preferred Provider Organization (PPO)	Network or out-of-network providers	• Referral not required for specialists • Fees are discounted • Preauthorization for some procedures	• Higher cost for out-of-network providers • Preventive care coverage varies
Health Maintenance Organization (HMO)	Network only	• Primary care physician paid by employment contract or capitation • Specialists paid according to a contractual arrangement • No payment for out-of-network nonemergency services	• Only network provider visits covered • Covers preventive care
Point-of-Service (POS)	Network providers or out-of-network providers	• Within network, primary care physician manages care	• Lower copayments for network providers • Higher costs for out-of-network providers • Covers preventive care
Indemnity	Any provider	• Little or none • Preauthorization required for some procedures	• Higher costs • Deductibles • Coinsurance • Preventive care not usually covered
Consumer-Driven Health Plan	Usually similar to PPO	• Increases patient awareness of health care costs • Patient pays directly until high deductible is met	• High deductible • Low premium

Preferred Provider Organizations

The **preferred provider organization (PPO)** is the most popular type of managed care organization (MCO), as shown in Figure 5-1. PPOs have the largest membership because patients like the way they combine flexibility in patients' choice of physicians with reduced cost for medical services.

A PPO is a managed care organization that creates a **network** of physicians, hospitals, and other health care providers for its policyholders. The providers sign contracts with the PPO under which they agree to accept reduced fees in exchange for access to a large pool of potential patients who may choose to use their services.

Patients who belong to a PPO are encouraged, but not required, to see providers within the network. If patients receive services from **out-of-network** providers, the plan pays lower benefits. For example, a larger co-payment is usually required.

Health Maintenance Organizations

In **health maintenance organizations (HMOs),** another popular type of managed care organization, patients enroll by paying fixed premiums and very small (or no) copayments when they need services. HMOs have been popular because of their low cost, although in exchange for paying less, patients give up the flexibility of choosing their own physicians. Instead, they must use the plan's network of health care providers in order to have medical services covered under the plan's terms.

In some plans, a **primary care physician (PCP),** also known as a gate-keeper, is assigned to each patient. This physician, usually a family or internal medicine doctor, directs all aspects of the patient's care. The plan may require the PCP to authorize patients' visits to specialists. If so, the patient receives a **referral number** from the PCP that is reported to the specialist when the appointment is made.

HMOs have various contractual arrangements with providers. In some cases, physicians are employees of the HMO and work full-time seeing patients who are members of the plan. In other structures, physicians are self-employed members of the HMO's network and see both HMO policyholders and nonmember patients in their practice. In this type of structure, physicians receive a fixed payment from the HMO for each

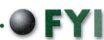

FYI

Claims with coded procedures must be filed under capitated plans even though the physician receives a salary or a set amount per patient. The CPT codes on the claim are used by the plan to adjust rates and study the quality of care that enrollees in the plan receive. The referral number is often also required on the claim.

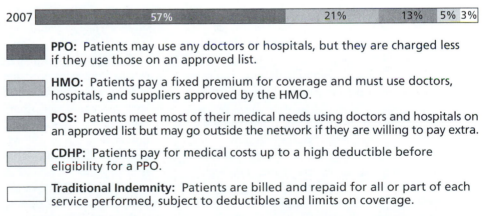

| 2007 | 57% | 21% | 13% | 5% | 3% |

PPO: Patients may use any doctors or hospitals, but they are charged less if they use those on an approved list.

HMO: Patients pay a fixed premium for coverage and must use doctors, hospitals, and suppliers approved by the HMO.

POS: Patients meet most of their medical needs using doctors and hospitals on an approved list but may go outside the network if they are willing to pay extra.

CDHP: Patients pay for medical costs up to a high deductible before eligibility for a PPO.

Traditional Indemnity: Patients are billed and repaid for all or part of each service performed, subject to deductibles and limits on coverage.

Figure 5-1 Health Plan Choices in Large Employer-Sponsored Plans
Source: Kaiser Family Foundation and Health Research and Educational Trust, 2007

member patient, rather than reimbursement for the services provided. For each patient there is a single fee, usually paid to the PCP monthly, regardless of the number of times the patient visits the physician. This way of paying is called **capitation.**

Point-of-Service Plans

Because many HMO patients do not wish to accept services from only network providers, some HMOs have become **point-of-service (POS) plans.** Patients who choose this option do not have to use only the HMO's physicians. However, if they choose to see physicians outside the HMO's network, they must pay more, such as by making larger copayments. This option makes the HMO more like a PPO in terms of choices available to the patients.

Indemnity Plans

Under traditional indemnity (fee-for-service) plans, the payments physicians receive are based on their regular charges for services, and patients owe coinsurance based on that fee. Currently, though, in many plans, the payer negotiates a discount for its members from the physician, just as in a PPO or POS plan. In fact, there is a great deal of overlap among the features of the various types of plans as payers attempt to control costs. Figure 5-2 provides an overview of the range of plans that might be offered by one payer. It shows the trade-offs for patients between the lowest price and the highest flexibility. It also lists the insurance options, such as prescription drug coverage, that patients can buy from this payer.

Professional Focus

Working as a Medical Insurance Specialist

Medical insurance specialists, also called medical billers, are employed by medical group practices. They also work in clinics, for health plans, for hospitals or nursing homes, and in other health care settings. Medical insurance specialists analyze patients' medical records and collect payments for physicians' services from health plans and from patients.

Medical insurance specialists also handle the administrative work that is part of the payment process. These activities include preparing and sending insurance claims, communicating with health plans to follow up on claims, entering charges and payments in a medical billing program, and handling bill collection. They may also gather information from patients and answer written or oral questions from both patients and payers while maintaining the confidentiality of patients' data.

Completion of a medical insurance specialist or medical assisting program at a postsecondary institution is an excellent background for an entry-level position. Professional certification, additional study, and work experience contribute to advancement to positions such as medical billing manager. Billers may also advance through specialization in a field, such as radiology billing management, or move into medical coding positions when the appropriate credentials and job skills are achieved.

	Maximum Provider Choice	◄────────────────►		Maximum Control of Cost and Quality
	Indemnity	In Network or Out of Network		In Network Only
	Managed Indemnity	**PPO/Open Access**	**Point-of-Service**	**HMO/Exclusive Provider**
Network	None; use any provider	220,000 physicians 4,300 hospitals	150,000 physicians 2,000 hospitals	150,000 physicians 2,000 hospitals
Care Managed by Primary Care Physicians (PCP)	No	No	Yes: Open access OB/GYN, behavioral, vision	Yes: Open access OB/GYN, behavioral, vision
Access to Providers	May use any provider	Use any PPO network provider; may use out-of-network providers at a higher cost	Use network providers; may use out-of-network providers at a higher cost	Must use network providers
Provider Compensation	Fee-for-service, reasonable and customary rate	**In Network:** Discounted fee-for-service **Out of Network:** Fee-for-service, reasonable and customary rate	**In Network:** Capitation and discounted fee-for-service **Out of Network:** Fee-for-service, reasonable and customary rate	Capitation and discounted fee-for-service
Options	**Prescription Drug Coverage** Behavioral Care Dental Care Vision Care Medicare HMO Life and Disability Expectant Mother			

Figure 5-2 Medical Group Plans Offered by Payer

Consumer-Driven Health Plans

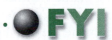

Because of the growing costs of providing health care coverage to employees, employers search for ways to control this expense. One way is to require employees to pay more of the cost themselves, such as by increasing annual premiums and copayments. Another way is to offer **consumer-driven health plans (CDHP)**. These plans were first made possible by federal laws that allow employees to avoid paying taxes on the cost of the plan on their federal income taxes, just as a federal law created individual retirement accounts (IRAs) to encourage people to save for retirement by not taxing the money saved in these accounts until it is withdrawn.

Consumer-driven health plans combine two elements. The first element is a health plan, usually a PPO, that has a high deductible (such as $1,000) and low premiums. The second element is a special "savings account" that is used to pay medical bills before the deductible has been met. The savings account, similar to an individual retirement account, lets people put aside untaxed wages that they can use to cover their out-of-pocket medical expenses. This account may be managed by the employer or by an outside institution, like a bank. Some employers contribute to employees' accounts as a benefit, while others require employees to fund them alone.

Cost control in consumer-driven health plans begins with the fact that the patient is paying for health care services directly. Both insurance companies and employers believe that paying for medical services causes patients to be careful consumers of health care. The other controls typical of a PPO, such as in-network savings, are also in effect.

SETTING FEES

Physicians have **fee schedules,** lists of fees for the procedures and services they frequently perform. These fees are called **usual fees,** meaning that the physicians charge these fees to most of their patients most of the time under typical conditions. Payers, too, set the fees that they pay providers. Most payers use one of three methods to set the fees that the health plan will pay physicians.

Usual, Customary, and Reasonable Payment Structure

Some health plans take the physicians' usual charges into account when they set their fee structures. A plan studies what many physicians have charged for similar services over a period of time. The fee that is set for each service is an average of the usual fee an individual physician charges for the service, the customary fee charged by most physicians in the community, and the reasonable fee for the service. This approach is called **usual, customary, and reasonable (UCR).**

UCR fees, for the most part, accurately reflect the charges of most physicians. However, fees may not be available for new or rare procedures. Lacking better information, a payer may set too low a fee for such procedures.

Relative Value Scale

Another method payers use to establish fees is the **relative value scale (RVS)** approach. Based on nationwide research, the relative value scale assigns numerical values to medical services. These values reflect the amount of skill and time the procedures require of physicians. For example, in an obstetrics practice, a hysterectomy has a higher RVS number than a dilation and curettage (D&C), because the hysterectomy is a more complicated surgical procedure and is considered to require more skill. To calculate the fee, the value assigned by the RVS is multiplied by a dollar conversion factor.

Resource-Based Relative Value Scale

The predominant method of setting fees is based on the Centers for Medicare and Medicaid Services (CMS) **Resource-Based Relative Value Scale (RBRVS).** This system, which is used to set the fees for services to Medicare patients, builds on the RVS method by adding factors for the provider's expenses. Instead of valuing just the skill and time, the RBRVS also has factors for how much office overhead the procedure involves and for the relative risk that the procedure presents to the patient and to the provider (essentially the malpractice insurance expense). These factors are reflected in a mathematical formula that is used to calculate the charge for every procedure and service.

Medicare's RBRVS also takes into account the differences in costs in various areas of the United States. For example, since the cost of renting an office is higher in Chicago than in rural areas of Illinois, the compensation is different in these two locations. CMS updates the RBRVS fee structure every year. To calculate a particular fee, a formula taking the factors into account is multiplied by a dollar conversion factor, which is also established annually. The RBRVS method is used by many other payers. For example, a health plan may set its fees at 120 percent of the Medicare payment.

PAYMENT METHODS

After setting the fees for scheduled benefits, health plans work out various payment arrangements with providers. For example, in some cases, physicians agree to discount their usual fees. In others, physicians receive payment for each patient rather than for services.

Most payers use one of three methods for paying providers:

1. Allowed charges.
2. Contracted fee schedule.
3. Capitation.

Payment Under an Allowed Charge Method

In the **allowed charge** (also called the allowable charge or maximum fee) approach, the health plan sets a payment for each covered service. The allowed charge is the maximum fee the health plan will pay for that particular service or procedure. A payer never pays a provider more than its allowed charge. If a provider's usual fee is higher, only the allowed charge is paid. If a provider's usual fee is lower, the payer pays that lower amount. The payer's payment is always the lower of the provider's charge and the allowable charge. For example:

The payer's allowed charge for a new patient's evaluation and management (E/M) service (CPT 99204) is $160.

Provider A Usual Charge = $180	Payment = $160
Provider B Usual Charge = $140	Payment = $140

Participating or Nonparticipating Providers

When patients have health plans that use an allowed charge payment method, physicians are paid based on whether they are participating or nonparticipating providers in that plan. A **participating physician (PAR)** has a contract with the managed care organization that requires accepting allowed charges—which are usually lower than the provider's usual fees—in return for incentives to be part of the plan, such as being paid faster. **Nonparticipating (nonPAR) physicians** have no contract with the MCO and do not agree to accept the plan's fees. Patients, of course, seek out participating physicians when they want to pay the lowest price available to them under the terms of their health plans. However, a patient may choose a nonPAR provider because of other factors, such as the physician's excellent reputation or advanced certification in a particular surgical procedure.

Balance Billing

The term **balance billing** means charging the patient for the difference between a higher usual fee and a lower allowed charge. In the example above, under balance billing, Provider A would bill the patient $20, the difference between the usual charge of $180 and the allowed charge of $160.

In most health plans that operate under allowed charge contracts, a participating provider may not balance bill the patient. Instead, the PAR provider must **write off** the difference, meaning that the amount of the difference is subtracted from the patient's bill and never collected. A nonparticipating provider often can balance bill patients. If the nonPAR provider's usual charge is higher than the allowed charge, the patient must pay the difference. However, Medicare and other government-sponsored programs have different rules for nonparticipating providers, as explained in Chapters 9–11, and these rules generally prohibit providers from balance billing patients.

Example of PAR Versus nonPAR Billing

In this example, assume that the payer's plan has an allowed charge for each procedure. The plan provides a benefit of 100 percent of the provider's usual charges up to this maximum fee. Provider A is a participating provider; Provider B does not participate and can balance bill. Provider A and Provider B both perform abdominal hysterectomies (CPT 58150). The policy's allowed charge for this procedure is $2,880.

Provider A (PAR)

Provider's usual charge	$3,100.00
Policy pays its allowed charge	$2,880.00
Provider writes off the difference between the usual charge and the allowed charge:	$220.00

Provider B (nonPAR)

Provider's usual charge	$3,000.00
Policy pays its allowed charge	$2,880.00
Provider bills patient for the difference between the usual charge and the allowed charge	$120.00 ($3,000.00 − $2,880.00)
There is no write-off.	

Contracted Fee Schedule

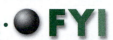

Many payers, particularly PPOs and other types of managed care plans that contract directly with providers, establish fixed fee schedules with their participating providers. These payers decide what they will pay for services in particular geographical areas. Their contracts stipulate these fixed fees for the procedures and services that the plan covers. In a particular geographical area, for example, the PPO sends practices a list of fixed fees for them to consider. If the providers join the PPO network, they enter into a contract to charge patients who are enrolled in that PPO according to that fee schedule.

When a provider is working under a contracted fee schedule, the payer's allowed charge and the provider's charge are the same. The terms of the plan determine what percentage of the charges, if any, the patients owe, and what percentage the payer covers. Participating providers can typically bill patients their usual charges for procedures and services that are not covered by the plan.

Capitation

The fixed payment for each plan member in capitation contracts, called the **capitation rate** or **cap rate,** is set by the HMO that initiates contracts with providers. The plan's contract with the PCP lists the services and procedures that are covered by the cap rate. If the services are listed, the PCP must provide them for no additional charge. For example, a typical contract with a primary care provider might include the following services:

Preventive care: well-child care, adult physical exams, gynecological exams, eye exams, and hearing exams.

Counseling and telephone calls.

Office visits.

Medical care: medical care services such as therapeutic injections and immunizations, allergy immunotherapy, electrocardiograms, and pulmonary function tests.

Local treatment of first-degree burns, application of dressings, suture removal, excision of small skin lesions, removal of foreign bodies or cerumen from external ear.

These services are covered in the per-member charge for each plan member who selects the PCP. Noncovered services can be billed to patients using the provider's usual rate. Plans often require the provider to notify the patient in advance that a service is not covered and to state the fee for which the patient will be responsible.

PATIENTS' CHARGES

Insured individuals have a variety of financial responsibilities under their health plans. Usually, a periodic premium payment is required. There are five other types of payments that patients may be obligated to pay: deductibles, copayments, coinsurance, noncovered (excluded) and over-limit services, and balance billing. The amounts that a patient pays are referred to as the insured's **out-of-pocket expenses.**

Deductibles

Most payers require policyholders to pay their deductibles before the insurance benefits begin. For example, a plan may require a patient to pay the first $200 of physician charges each year. Payments for noncovered (excluded) services—those that the policy does not cover—do not count toward a deductible. Some plans require an **individual deductible,** which must be met for each individual—whether the policyholder or a covered dependent—who has an encounter. In other cases, there is a **family deductible** that can be met by the combined payments to providers for any covered member(s) of the insured's family.

Copayments

Many health care plans require patient copayments (copays). Copayments are always due and collected at the time of service. Copayments may be different for various types of services. Usually, a copay is stated as a dollar amount, such as $15 for an office visit or $10 for a prescription drug. After checking with the health plan, many offices have a policy of telling patients who are scheduling visits what copays they will owe at the time of service so that they are prepared to pay.

Coinsurance

Many payers require coinsurance. Noncapitated health care plans such as PPOs usually require patients to pay a greater percentage of the charges of out-of-network providers than of plan providers. For example, a patient may owe 20 percent of the charge when using a network member but 40 percent of the charge of a physician who is out of the network.

Noncovered (Excluded) and Over-Limit Services

All payers require patients to pay for noncovered (excluded) services. Providers generally can charge their usual fees for these services. Likewise, in managed care plans that set limits on the annual (or other period) usage of covered services, patients are responsible for usage beyond the allowed number. For example, if one preventive physical examination is permitted annually, additional preventive examinations

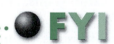

Patients who are enrolled in consumer-driven health plans (CDHPs) have the highest deductibles of any plan type. Because these plans are growing in popularity, medical insurance specialists must be aware of and prepare for collecting these payments at the time of service.

Sample Agreement for Patient Payment of Excluded Services

Service to be performed: _____

Estimated charge: _____

Date of planned service: _____

Reason for exclusion: _____

I, _____, a patient of _____, understand the service described above is excluded from my health insurance. I am responsible for payment in full of the charges for this service.

Figure 5-3 Sample Agreement for Patient Payment of Noncovered (Excluded) Services

are paid for by the patient. Figure 5-3 shows an example of an agreement used by medical offices to notify patients of the expected fees for excluded services.

Balance Billing

Patients may be responsible for the amount of the usual charge that exceeds the payer's allowed charge.

WHEN PATIENTS' CHARGES MUST BE PAID

There are different procedures for collecting payments, depending on participation contracts. Some charges are collected up front at the time of service, while others are billed later.

Charges from PAR Providers

When a patient has an encounter with a participating provider, the provider files the health care claim, receives reimbursement directly from the payer, and agrees to accept the payer's allowed charge. After the payer's payment is posted, patients are sent bills for charges that payers deny, do not pay, or pay only partially.

The following types of patient charges are collected at the time of service rather than billed later:

- Copayments.
- Usual fees for services that are excluded under the patient's plan.
- Usual fees for services to patients performed by nonparticipating providers (except for government-sponsored programs) and HMO out-of-network providers.

If the patient makes a payment at the time of service, the medical billing program is used to print a **walkout receipt,** which summarizes the services and charges for that day as well as any payment the patient made (see Figure 5-4 on page 104).

Charges from NonPAR Providers

When a patient has an encounter with a nonparticipating provider, the procedure is usually different. To avoid the difficulty of collecting patient payments at a later date, a practice may either (1) require the patient to assign benefits, so that the physician receives the payment, or (2) require payment in full at the time of service.

If the provider has not accepted assignment and is not going to file a claim for a patient, the patient may use the walkout receipt to report the charges and payments to the insurance company. In this case, the insurance company repays the patient (or insured) after the deductible is met, according to the terms of the plan. In other cases, the medical office collects payment from the patient and then sends a claim to the insurance company for the patient. The insurance company sends a check to the patient with an explanation of benefits, with a copy to the provider. In still other cases, patients arrange to be billed for payments due. In this case, the billing program issues an invoice when the practice's bills are generated (see Chapter 7).

Central Practice Center
1122 E. University Drive
Mesa, AZ 85204
(602)969-4237

Page: 1

10/1/2010

Patient:	Walter Williams
	17 Mill Rd
	Chandler, AZ 85246-4567
Chart #:	WILLIWA0
Case #:	8

Instructions:
Complete the patient information portion of your insurance claim form. Attach this bill, signed and dated, and all other bills pertaining to the claim. If you have a deductible policy, hold your claim forms until you have met your deductible. Mail directly to your insurance carrier.

Date	Description	Procedure	Modify	Dx 1	Dx 2	Dx 3	Dx 4	Units	Charge
10/1/2010	EP Problem Focused	99212		401.1	780.7			1	46.00
10/1/2010	EOG Complete	93000		401.1	780.7			1	70.00
10/1/2010	Aetna Copayment	AETCPAY						1	-15.00

Provider Information

Provider Name:	Christopher Connolly M.D.
License:	37C4629
Commercial PIN:	
SSN or EIN:	161234567

Total Charges:	$ 116.00
Total Payments:	-$ 15.00
Total Adjustments:	$ 0.00
Total Due This Visit:	**$ 101.00**
Total Account Balance:	$ 101.00

Assign and Release: I hereby authorize payment of medical benefits to this physician for the services described above. I also authorize the release of any information necessary to process this claim.

Patient Signature: _____   Date: _____

Figure 5-4 Sample Walkout Receipt

Consumer-Driven Health Plan Deductibles

As a rule, deductibles are hard for medical offices to collect. Patients see more than one provider, so it can be difficult for the office to know whether the patient has met the deductible. Many offices wait for the payer's RA/EOB to tell them what the patient owes.

However, in CDHPs, deductibles are very high and make up a big part of the medical office's cash flow. For this reason, many offices collect these payments at the time of service. Many offices inform patients with these plans of this fact well before the visit so they are prepared to pay.

Medical Office Financial Policy

Patients should always be reminded of their financial obligations under their plans, including their obligations on denied claims. The practice's financial policy regarding payment for services is usually either displayed on the wall of the reception area or included in a new patient information packet. The policy should explain what is required of the patient and when payment is due.

Estimating Patients' Charges

Many times, patients want to know what their bills will be. To estimate charges, the medical insurance specialist contacts the patient's health plan and verifies:

- The patient's deductible amount and whether it has been paid in full, the covered benefits, and coinsurance or other patient financial obligations.
- The payer's allowed charges or the contracted fees for the services that the provider anticipates providing.

If the patient's request comes after the encounter, the medical insurance specialist can use the encounter form to tell the payer what CPT codes are going to be reported on the patient's claim to learn the likely payer reimbursement.

Professional Courtesy

Professional courtesy describes a number of billing practices. A physician may waive all or part of the fee for services provided to the physician's office staff, other physicians, and/or their families. The term has come to also mean the waiver of coinsurance obligations or other out-of-pocket expenses for physicians or their families (i.e., "insurance only" billing). Since Medicare and most private payers do not permit a physician to bill for the treatment of immediate family or household members, many physician practices consult with their attorneys to clarify their professional courtesy arrangements.

Discounts to Uninsured and Low-Income Patients

In billing for services, many physician practices take into account their patients' ability to pay. Under HIPAA, it is permissible for physicians to offer discounts to their uninsured and low-income patients. As in the case of professional courtesy, the practice's criteria for determining who receives a discount should be documented in the compliance plan.

Chapter Summary

1. The leading type of health plan, the preferred provider organization (PPO), creates a network of providers for its policyholders. Patients pay premiums and copayments and may have to satisfy deductibles. PPOs pay lower benefits, such as requiring larger copayments, when patients receive services from providers who do not belong to the network. Patients in a health maintenance organization (HMO) pay low fees, usually a premium and a copayment, but must use the services of HMO providers to be covered. Patients in point-of-service (POS) plans have options to see providers outside of the network for higher fees. Fee-for-service (indemnity) plan holders pay annual premiums, deductibles, and coinsurance for visits. A consumer-driven health plan (CDHP) combines a high-deductible plan and a PPO; patients are responsible for a large initial deductible, which may be drawn from an employer-managed account.

2. Payments to physicians are based on the usual, customary, and reasonable (UCR) method; the relative value scale (RVS) method; or the Resource-Based Relative Value Scale (RBRVS) method.

3. Payers pay participating providers according to the allowed charge, contracted fee schedule, or cap rate. Nonparticipating physicians are usually paid according to their usual fees. If balance billing is allowed, the physician may collect the difference between a higher usual fee and the lower fee the health plan pays. Usually, only nonparticipating physicians can balance bill private-plan patients; government programs often prohibit this activity.

4. Patients may be responsible for copayments, excluded services, over-limit usage, and coinsurance. Patients often must also meet deductibles before receiving benefits. Under some conditions, patients may also be obligated to pay the difference between a provider's higher usual fee and a payer's lower allowed charge.

Part 1. Choose the best answer.

_____ **1.** The only type of managed care organization that employs physicians directly is:
    a. a health maintenance organization (HMO)
    b. a preferred provider organization (PPO)
    c. a consumer-driven health plan (CDHP)

_____ **2.** In an HMO, the primary care physician is:
    a. the first physician who recommends surgery for a patient who later gets a second opinion
    b. the first physician to diagnose a patient's illness
    c. the physician who supervises all aspects of a patient's health care

_____ **3.** A physician who is a participant in a program must write off:
    a. deductibles
    b. denied or excluded charges
    c. charges in excess of the allowed amount

_____ **4.** The method that Medicare uses to establish allowed charges is:
    a. UCR
    b. RBRVS
    c. capitation

_____ **5.** The fee for a service that is charged by a provider for most patients is called the:
    a. cap rate
    b. usual fee
    c. write off

_____ **6.** Balance billing means to bill the patient for the difference between the:
    a. cap rate and the allowed amount
    b. UCR fee and the usual fee
    c. allowed amount and the usual fee

_____ **7.** The amount that an insured person must pay annually before receiving benefits from the health plan is called the:
    a. deductible
    b. cap rate
    c. allowed charge

_____ **8.** If a participating physician's usual fee is $400 and the allowed amount is $350, what amount is written off?
    a. zero
    b. $50
    c. $75

_____ **9.** The RBRVS fee-calculation method for a procedure takes into account:
    a. the time and skill of the physician
    b. regional cost differences
    c. both a and b

_____ **10.** A point-of-service option in an HMO plan allows patients:
    a. to see doctors not in the plan for an additional cost
    b. to visit doctors anywhere in the United States
    c. to select their own specialists at no additional cost

Part 2. A patient shows the following insurance identification card to the medical insurance specialist:

Connecticut HealthPlan

I.D.#:	1002.9713
Employee:	DANIEL ANTHONY
Group #:	A0000323
Eff. date:	03/01/2004
Status:	Dependent Coverage? F
In-network:	$10 Co-Pay
Out-of-network:	$250 Ded; 80%/20%

Front of card

IMPORTANT INFORMATION
Notice to Members and Providers of Care
To avoid a reduction in your hospital benefits, you are responsible for obtaining certification for hospitalization and emergency admissions. The review is required regardless of the reason for hospital admission. For specified procedures, Second Surgical Opinions may be mandatory.
For certification, call Utilization Management Services at 800-837-8808:
• At least 7 days in advance of Scheduled Surgery of Hospital Admissions.
• Within 48 hours after Emergency Admissions or on the first business day following weekend or holiday Emergency Admissions.

CONNECTICUT HEALTHPLAN C/O
WEISS   Robert S. Weiss
& Company
Silver Hill Business Center
500 S. Broad Street
P.O. Box 1034
Meriden, CT 06450
(800) 466-7900

THIS CARD IS FOR IDENTIFICATION ONLY AND DOES NOT ESTABLISH ELIGIBILITY FOR COVERAGE BY CONNECTICUT HEALTH PLAN. Please refer to your insurance booklet for further details.

Back of card

A. What copayment is due when the patient sees a network physician?

B. What payment rules apply when the patient sees an out-of-network physician?

C. What rules apply when the patient needs to be admitted to the hospital?

Part 3. Based on the following information, answer the questions in each case.

A. A patient's insurance policy states:

Annual deductible: $300.00

Coinsurance: 70–30

This year, the patient has made payments totaling $533.00 to all providers. Today, the patient has an office visit (fee: $80.00). The patient presents a credit card for payment of today's bill. What is the amount that the patient should pay?

B. A patient is a member of a health plan with a 15 percent discount from the provider's usual fees and a $10.00 copay. The days' charges are $480.00. What are the amounts that the plan and the patient each pay?

C. A patient is a member of a health plan that has a 20 percent discount from the provider and a 15 percent copay. If the day's charges are $210.00, what are the amounts that the plan and the patient each pay?

Health Care Claim Preparation

Learning Outcomes

After completing this chapter, you will be able to define the key terms and:

6-1 Describe the process of using medical billing programs to prepare health care claims.

6-2 Discuss the content of the patient information section of the CMS-1500 claim.

6-3 Discuss the content of the physician or supplier information section of the CMS-1500 claim.

6-4 Briefly describe the information contained in the five major sections of the HIPAA claim.

6-5 Compare billing provider, pay-to provider, rendering provider, and referring provider.

6-6 Discuss the importance and use of claim control numbers and line-item control numbers on HIPAA claims.

Key Terms

837P claim
administrative code set
billing provider
carrier block
claim attachment
claim control number
claim filing indicator code
claim frequency code (claim submission reason code)
CMS-1500 claim

condition code
database
data element
destination payer
HIPAA claim
individual relationship code
legacy number
line item control number
National Uniform Claim Committee (NUCC)

outside laboratory
pay-to provider
place of service (POS) code
qualifier
referring provider
rendering provider
service line information
subscriber
taxonomy code
transactions

Why This Chapter Is Important to You

The information in this chapter will enable you to:

- Understand the information that is needed to prepare complete, accurate health care claims.
- Gain practice with case studies similar to situations you will encounter in a medical office.
- Learn the methods used to transmit correct health care claims.

What Do You Think?

To complete health care claims, medical insurance specialists work constantly with numbers—billing software, Web sites, diagnosis codes, procedure codes, fees and charges, identification numbers, preauthorization numbers, and more. Why is it important to know how to use available resources in the medical office to research or verify information? What role do accurate data entry and proofreading have in this process?

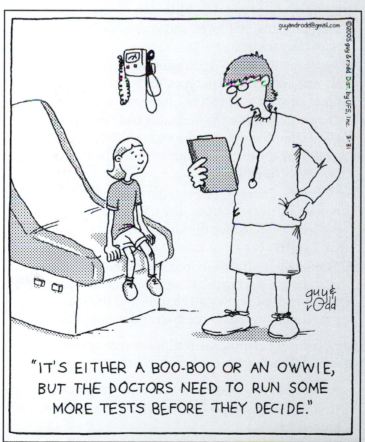

"IT'S EITHER A BOO-BOO OR AN OWWIE, BUT THE DOCTORS NEED TO RUN SOME MORE TESTS BEFORE THEY DECIDE."

PREPARING CLAIMS USING MEDICAL BILLING PROGRAMS

Health care claims are a critical type of communication between providers and payers on behalf of patients. Understanding how medical offices prepare and transmit claims is important for success as a medical insurance specialist. Claim processing is a major task, but today's technology makes it possible to create, send, and track a large volume of claims efficiently and effectively.

Billing Program Databases

Medical billing programs increase efficiency because repeatedly used data are stored in **databases**—collections of related facts—and quickly accessed. For example, the office's frequently used diagnosis and procedure codes, as well as fee schedules, are entered once and then stored. A medical insurance specialist who is posting (that is, entering) the information from the encounter form does not have to enter a complete code and its description. That information has already been stored, so the correct code can be chosen from a list on the screen.

The major databases in billing programs are:

- *Provider*—The provider database has information about the licensed medical professional staff members who work in the medical office, such as names, office addresses, and National Provider IDs.
- *Patient/Guarantor*—The data from each patient information form are stored in the patient/guarantor database. These data include the patient's unique account number and personal information: name, address, phone number, birth date, Social Security number, gender, marital status, employer, and guarantor (the insured person if other than the patient).
- *Insurance Carriers*—The insurance carrier database contains the names, addresses, plan types, and other data about the major health plans used by the practice's patients.
- *Diagnosis Codes*—The diagnosis code database contains the ICD-9-CM codes that indicate the reasons services are provided. The codes stored are those most frequently used by the office. Additional codes can easily be entered.
- *Procedure Codes*—The procedure code database contains the data needed to create charges. The CPT codes most often used by the office are selected for this database. Like the ICD codes, additional CPT codes are easy to enter if needed.
- *Transactions*—**Transactions** are all the financial aspects of visits— charges and payments. The transaction database stores information about each patient's visit charges and the related diagnoses and procedures, as well as received and outstanding payments.

When preparing claims, medical insurance specialists work with billing programs, following these steps:

- Record patients' insurance and demographic information.
- Record diagnoses, procedures, charges, and payments for patients' encounters.
- Create and transmit claims to payers.

Recording Patients' Information

The first step in preparing claims is recording patients' information from new or updated patient information forms and patients' insurance cards. A new record must be created for a new patient, and facts about established patients may need to be updated.

Recording Diagnoses, Procedures, Charges, and Payments for Patients' Encounters

After the patient's visit with the medical professional staff, the diagnosis codes and the procedure codes are recorded in the billing program. The provider the patient saw is selected from the billing program's list of the practice's physicians and other staff members. The appropriate transactions for the visit are also entered. The source of the codes, charges, and payment information is the encounter form. The patient's appropriate insurance coverage for this visit is also selected. Usually, it is the patient's main (primary, if the patient has more than one plan) health plan, but if the case is for a workers' compensation claim, that insurance is selected.

Creating and Transmitting Claims to Payers

When all required data have been entered and checked, the medical insurance specialist instructs the billing program to create a claim for the appropriate payer. Following its programmed instructions, the program draws the needed facts from the stored information and organizes these data elements into a claim file. Claims generated by billing programs can be transmitted as electronic claims to payers, or the claims can be printed and mailed to the payers. Most health care claims are submitted electronically, not on paper. (This final task is covered in Chapter 7.)

Notes on Data Entry

Although medical billing programs increase efficiency and reduce errors, they are not more accurate than the individual who is entering the data. If people make mistakes while entering data, the information the computer produces will be incorrect. Computers are very precise and also very unforgiving. While the human brain knows that *flu* is short for *influenza,* the computer regards them as two distinct conditions. If a computer user accidentally enters a name as *Orourke* instead of *O'Rourke,* a person might know what is meant; the computer does not. It would probably respond with a message such as "No such patient exists in the database."

Many human errors occur during data entry, such as pressing the wrong key on the keyboard. Other errors are a result of a lack of computer literacy—not knowing how to use a program to accomplish tasks. For this reason, having proper training in data-entry techniques, so that errors are caught, and knowing how to use computer programs are both essential for medical insurance specialists. Follow these tips for accurate data entry when entering data in medical billing programs:

- Do not use prefixes for people's names, such as Mr., Ms., or Dr.
- Unless required by a particular insurance carrier, do not use special characters such as hyphens, commas, or apostrophes.
- Use only valid data in all fields.

- Enter the required number of characters for each data element, such as four numbers for the year, but do not worry about the format. Most billing programs or claim transmission programs automatically reformat data such as dates correctly.

HEALTH CARE CLAIMS

The HIPAA-mandated electronic transaction for claims (HIPAA X12 837 Health Care Claim or Equivalent Encounter Information) is often called the **HIPAA claim** or the **837P claim.** The electronic HIPAA claim is based on the **CMS-1500 claim,** formerly the HCFA-1500, which is a paper claim form. The information on the paper claim and on the electronic transaction, with a few exceptions, is the same.

This book covers the way to fill out the paper claim before showing how to fill out the HIPAA claim, because this is a good way to understand the data that claims generally require. Of course, the CMS-1500 is not usually filled out by transferring information directly from other office forms, like the patient information and encounter forms. Instead, claims are created using a medical billing program, which makes it easy to update, correct, and manage the claim process.

Claim Background

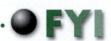

Medical insurance specialists become familiar with the information most often required on claims so that they can efficiently research missing information and respond to payers' questions. Memorization is not required, but good thinking and organizational skills are.

The CMS-1500 was for many years the universal health claim, meaning that it was accepted by most payers. The familiar red-and-black printed form was typed or computer-generated and mailed to payers. The method of sending claims changed with the increased use of information technology (IT) in physician practices. HIPAA, with its emphasis on electronic transactions, has essentially made the use of IT mandatory. HIPAA requires electronic transmission of claims except from very small practices and those that never send any kind of electronic health care transactions (see Chapter 2). Only these providers can still mail or fax paper claims. Electronic transmission of the HIPAA claim is mandated for all other physician practices.

HIPAA has changed the way things work on the payer side, too. Payers may not require providers to make changes or additions to the content of the HIPAA claim. Further, they cannot refuse to accept the standard transaction or delay payment of any proper HIPAA transaction, claims included.

Claim Content

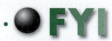

The NUCC can be expected to continue to update the CMS-1500 form. Be sure to check with payers about the correct form to use for their claims.

The **National Uniform Claim Committee (NUCC),** led by the American Medical Association, determines the content of both HIPAA and CMS-1500 claims. The current version of the CMS-1500 form was updated by the NUCC to allow reporting the National Provider Identifier (NPI). The new version has spaces for using both the NPI and other types of identifying numbers, called **legacy numbers.** An example of a legacy number is the UPIN, which was formerly assigned by Medicare to providers.

COMPLETING THE CMS-1500 CLAIM

The current CMS-1500 claim contains thirty-three form locators (FLs), or information boxes, as shown in Figure 6-1 (on page 116). Form locators 1 through 13 refer to the patient and the patient's insurance coverage. This information is entered based on the patient information form and the patient insurance card. Form locators 14 through 33 contain information about the provider and the patient's condition, including diagnoses, procedures, and charges. This information is entered from the encounter form and clinical documentation.

Carrier Block

The **carrier block** is located in the upper right of the CMS-1500. It allows for a four-line address for the payer. If the payer's address requires just three lines, leave a blank line in the third position:

> ABC Insurance Company
> 567 Willow Lane
> Franklin IL 60605

Note that commas, periods, or other punctuation are not used in the address. However, when entering a 9-digit Zip code, the hyphen is included (for example, 60609-4563).

Patient Information

The items in this part of the CMS-1500 claim form identify the patient and the insured, the health plan, and assignment of benefits/release information.

Form Locator 1: Type of Insurance

1. MEDICARE	MEDICAID	TRICARE CHAMPUS	CHAMPVA	GROUP HEALTH PLAN	FECA BLK LUNG	OTHER
(Medicare #)	(Medicaid #)	(Sponsor's SSN)	(Member ID#)	(SSN or ID)	(SSN)	(ID)

Form locator 1 is used to indicate the patient's type of insurance coverage. Five specific government programs are listed (Medicare, Medicaid, TRICARE/CHAMPUS, CHAMPVA, FECA Black Lung), as well as Group Health Plan and Other. If the patient has group contract insurance, Group Health Plan is selected. The Other box indicates health insurance including individual health plans, HMOs, commercial insurance, automobile accident, liability, and workers' compensation.

Form Locator 1a: Insured's ID Number

1a. INSURED'S I.D. NUMBER	(FOR PROGRAM IN ITEM 1)

The insured's ID number is the identification number of the person who holds the policy or the dependent patient if this person has been issued a unique identifier by the payer. Form locator 1a records the insurance identification number that appears on the insurance card of the person who holds the policy (who may or may not be the patient).

1500

HEALTH INSURANCE CLAIM FORM

APPROVED BY NATIONAL UNIFORM CLAIM COMMITTEE 08/05

☐☐ PICA   PICA ☐☐

| 1. MEDICARE ☐ (Medicare #) | MEDICAID ☐ (Medicaid #) | TRICARE CHAMPUS ☐ (Sponsor's SSN) | CHAMPVA ☐ (Member ID#) | GROUP HEALTH PLAN ☐ (SSN or ID) | FECA BLK LUNG ☐ (SSN) | OTHER ☐ (ID) | 1a. INSURED'S I.D. NUMBER   (For Program in Item 1) |

2. PATIENT'S NAME (Last Name, First Name, Middle Initial)

3. PATIENT'S BIRTH DATE   MM | DD | YY   SEX   M ☐   F ☐

4. INSURED'S NAME (Last Name, First Name, Middle Initial)

5. PATIENT'S ADDRESS (No., Street)

6. PATIENT RELATIONSHIP TO INSURED   Self ☐   Spouse ☐   Child ☐   Other ☐

7. INSURED'S ADDRESS (No., Street)

CITY   STATE

8. PATIENT STATUS   Single ☐   Married ☐   Other ☐
Employed ☐   Full-Time Student ☐   Part-Time Student ☐

CITY   STATE

ZIP CODE   TELEPHONE (Include Area Code) (   )

ZIP CODE   TELEPHONE (INCLUDE AREA CODE) (   )

9. OTHER INSURED'S NAME (Last Name, First Name, Middle Initial)

10. IS PATIENT'S CONDITION RELATED TO:

11. INSURED'S POLICY GROUP OR FECA NUMBER

a. OTHER INSURED'S POLICY OR GROUP NUMBER

a. EMPLOYMENT? (CURRENT OR PREVIOUS)   ☐ YES   ☐ NO

a. INSURED'S DATE OF BIRTH   MM | DD | YY   SEX   M ☐   F ☐

b. OTHER INSURED'S DATE OF BIRTH   MM | DD | YY   SEX   M ☐   F ☐

b. AUTO ACCIDENT?   ☐ YES   ☐ NO   PLACE (State) ___

b. EMPLOYER'S NAME OR SCHOOL NAME

c. EMPLOYER'S NAME OR SCHOOL NAME

c. OTHER ACCIDENT?   ☐ YES   ☐ NO

c. INSURANCE PLAN NAME OR PROGRAM NAME

d. INSURANCE PLAN NAME OR PROGRAM NAME

10d. RESERVED FOR LOCAL USE

d. IS THERE ANOTHER HEALTH BENEFIT PLAN?   ☐ YES   ☐ NO   **If yes**, return to and complete item 9 a-d.

READ BACK OF FORM BEFORE COMPLETING & SIGNING THIS FORM.
12. PATIENT'S OR AUTHORIZED PERSON'S SIGNATURE I authorize the release of any medical or other information necessary to process this claim. I also request payment of government benefits either to myself or to the party who accepts assignment below.

SIGNED _____   DATE _____

13. INSURED'S OR AUTHORIZED PERSON'S SIGNATURE I authorize payment of medical benefits to the undersigned physician or supplier for services described below.

SIGNED _____

14. DATE OF CURRENT: MM | DD | YY   ◄ ILLNESS (First symptom) OR INJURY (Accident) OR PREGNANCY(LMP)

15. IF PATIENT HAS HAD SAME OR SIMILAR ILLNESS. GIVE FIRST DATE   MM | DD | YY

16. DATES PATIENT UNABLE TO WORK IN CURRENT OCCUPATION   FROM MM | DD | YY   TO MM | DD | YY

17. NAME OF REFERRING PHYSICIAN OR OTHER SOURCE

17a.
17b. NPI

18. HOSPITALIZATION DATES RELATED TO CURRENT SERVICES   FROM MM | DD | YY   TO MM | DD | YY

19. RESERVED FOR LOCAL USE

20. OUTSIDE LAB?   ☐ YES   ☐ NO $ CHARGES

21. DIAGNOSIS OR NATURE OF ILLNESS OR INJURY. (Relate Items 1,2,3 or 4 to Item 24e by Line)
1. ___ . ___   3. ___ . ___
2. ___ . ___   4. ___ . ___

22. MEDICAID RESUBMISSION CODE   ORIGINAL REF. NO.

23. PRIOR AUTHORIZATION NUMBER

24. A. DATE(S) OF SERVICE From MM DD YY To MM DD YY	B. PLACE OF SERVICE	C. EMG	D. PROCEDURES, SERVICES, OR SUPPLIES (Explain Unusual Circumstances) CPT/HCPCS MODIFIER	E. DIAGNOSIS POINTER	F. $ CHARGES	G. DAYS OR UNITS	H. EPSDT Family Plan	I. ID. QUAL.	J. RENDERING PROVIDER ID.#
1									NPI
2									NPI
3									NPI
4									NPI
5									NPI
6									NPI

25. FEDERAL TAX I.D. NUMBER   SSN ☐ EIN ☐

26. PATIENT'S ACCOUNT NO.

27. ACCEPT ASSIGNMENT? (For govt. claims, see back)   ☐ YES   ☐ NO

28. TOTAL CHARGE $

29. AMOUNT PAID $

30. BALANCE DUE $

31. SIGNATURE OF PHYSICIAN OR SUPPLIER INCLUDING DEGREES OR CREDENTIALS (I certify that the statements on the reverse apply to this bill and are made a part thereof.)

SIGNED _____   DATE _____

32. SERVICE FACILITY LOCATION INFORMATION

a. NPI   b.

33. BILLING PROVIDER INFO & PHONE # (   )

a. NPI   b.

NUCC Instruction Manual available at: www.nucc.org

Figure 6-1 CMS-1500 Claim

BECAUSE THIS FORM IS USED BY VARIOUS GOVERNMENT AND PRIVATE HEALTH PROGRAMS, SEE SEPARATE INSTRUCTIONS ISSUED BY APPLICABLE PROGRAMS.

NOTICE: Any person who knowingly files a statement of claim containing any misrepresentation or any false, incomplete or misleading information may be guilty of a criminal act punishable under law and may be subject to civil penalties.

REFERS TO GOVERNMENT PROGRAMS ONLY

MEDICARE AND CHAMPUS PAYMENTS: A patient's signature requests that payment be made and authorizes release of any information necessary to process the claim and certifies that the information provided in Blocks 1 through 12 is true, accurate and complete. In the case of a Medicare claim, the patient's signature authorizes any entity to release to Medicare medical and nonmedical information, including employment status, and whether the person has employer group health insurance, liability, no-fault, worker's compensation or other insurance which is responsible to pay for the services for which the Medicare claim is made. See 42 CFR 411.24(a). If item 9 is completed, the patient's signature authorizes release of the information to the health plan or agency shown. In Medicare assigned or CHAMPUS participation cases, the physician agrees to accept the charge determination of the Medicare carrier or CHAMPUS fiscal intermediary as the full charge, and the patient is responsible only for the deductible, coinsurance and noncovered services. Coinsurance and the deductible are based upon the charge determination of the Medicare carrier or CHAMPUS fiscal intermediary if this is less than the charge submitted. CHAMPUS is not a health insurance program but makes payment for health benefits provided through certain affiliations with the Uniformed Services. Information on the patient's sponsor should be provided in those items captioned in "Insured"; i.e., items 1a, 4, 6, 7, 9, and 11.

BLACK LUNG AND FECA CLAIMS

The provider agrees to accept the amount paid by the Government as payment in full. See Black Lung and FECA instructions regarding required procedure and diagnosis coding systems.

SIGNATURE OF PHYSICIAN OR SUPPLIER (MEDICARE, CHAMPUS, FECA AND BLACK LUNG)

I certify that the services shown on this form were medically indicated and necessary for the health of the patient and were personally furnished by me or were furnished incident to my professional service by my employee under my immediate personal supervision, except as otherwise expressly permitted by Medicare or CHAMPUS regulations.

For services to be considered as "incident" to a physician's professional service, 1) they must be rendered under the physician's immediate personal supervision by his/her employee, 2) they must be an integral, although incidental part of a covered physician's service, 3) they must be of kinds commonly furnished in physician's offices, and 4) the services of nonphysicians must be included on the physician's bills.

For CHAMPUS claims, I further certify that I (or any employee) who rendered services am not an active duty member of the Uniformed Services or a civilian employee of the United States Government or a contract employee of the United States Government, either civilian or military (refer to 5 USC 5536). For Black-Lung claims, I further certify that the services performed were for a Black Lung-related disorder.

No Part B Medicare benefits may be paid unless this form is received as required by existing law and regulations (42 CFR 424.32).

NOTICE: Any one who misrepresents or falsifies essential information to receive payment from Federal funds requested by this form may upon conviction be subject to fine and imprisonment under applicable Federal laws.

NOTICE TO PATIENT ABOUT THE COLLECTION AND USE OF MEDICARE, CHAMPUS, FECA, AND BLACK LUNG INFORMATION
(PRIVACY ACT STATEMENT)

We are authorized by CMS, CHAMPUS and OWCP to ask you for information needed in the administration of the Medicare, CHAMPUS, FECA, and Black Lung programs. Authority to collect information is in section 205(a), 1862, 1872 and 1874 of the Social Security Act as amended, 42 CFR 411.24(a) and 424.5(a) (6), and 44 USC 3101;41 CFR 101 et seq and 10 USC 1079 and 1086; 5 USC 8101 et seq; and 30 USC 901 et seq; 38 USC 613; E.O. 9397.

The information we obtain to complete claims under these programs is used to identify you and to determine your eligibility. It is also used to decide if the services and supplies you received are covered by these programs and to insure that proper payment is made.

The information may also be given to other providers of services, carriers, intermediaries, medical review boards, health plans, and other organizations or Federal agencies, for the effective administration of Federal provisions that require other third parties payers to pay primary to Federal program, and as otherwise necessary to administer these programs. For example, it may be necessary to disclose information about the benefits you have used to a hospital or doctor. Additional disclosures are made through routine uses for information contained in systems of records.

FOR MEDICARE CLAIMS: See the notice modifying system No. 09-70-0501, titled, 'Carrier Medicare Claims Record,' published in the Federal Register, Vol. 55 No. 177, page 37549, Wed. Sept. 12, 1990, or as updated and republished.

FOR OWCP CLAIMS: Department of Labor, Privacy Act of 1974, "Republication of Notice of Systems of Records," Federal Register Vol. 55 No. 40, Wed Feb. 28, 1990, See ESA-5, ESA-6, ESA-12, ESA-13, ESA-30, or as updated and republished.

FOR CHAMPUS CLAIMS: PRINCIPLE PURPOSE(S): To evaluate eligibility for medical care provided by civilian sources and to issue payment upon establishment of eligibility and determination that the services/supplies received are authorized by law.

ROUTINE USE(S): Information from claims and related documents may be given to the Dept. of Veterans Affairs, the Dept. of Health and Human Services and/or the Dept. of Transportation consistent with their statutory administrative responsibilities under CHAMPUS/CHAMPVA; to the Dept. of Justice for representation of the Secretary of Defense in civil actions; to the Internal Revenue Service, private collection agencies, and consumer reporting agencies in connection with recoupment claims; and to Congressional Offices in response to inquiries made at the request of the person to whom a record pertains. Appropriate disclosures may be made to other federal, state, local, foreign government agencies, private business entities, and individual providers of care, on matters relating to entitlement, claims adjudication, fraud, program abuse, utilization review, quality assurance, peer review, program integrity, third-party liability, coordination of benefits, and civil and criminal litigation related to the operation of CHAMPUS.

DISCLOSURES: Voluntary; however, failure to provide information will result in delay in payment or may result in denial of claim. With the one exception discussed below, there are no penalties under these programs for refusing to supply information. However, failure to furnish information regarding the medical services rendered or the amount charged would prevent payment of claims under these programs. Failure to furnish any other information, such as name or claim number, would delay payment of the claim. Failure to provide medical information under FECA could be deemed an obstruction.

It is mandatory that you tell us if you know that another party is responsible for paying for your treatment. Section 1128B of the Social Security Act and 31 USC 3801-3812 provide penalties for withholding this information.

You should be aware that P.L. 100-503, the "Computer Matching and Privacy Protection Act of 1988", permits the government to verify information by way of computer matches.

MEDICAID PAYMENTS (PROVIDER CERTIFICATION)

I hereby agree to keep such records as are necessary to disclose fully the extent of services provided to individuals under the State's Title XIX plan and to furnish information regarding any payments claimed for providing such services as the State Agency or Dept. of Health and Human Services may request.

I further agree to accept, as payment in full, the amount paid by the Medicaid program for those claims submitted for payment under that program, with the exception of authorized deductible, coinsurance, co-payment or similar cost-sharing charge.

SIGNATURE OF PHYSICIAN (OR SUPPLIER): I certify that the services listed above were medically indicated and necessary to the health of this patient and were personally furnished by me or my employee under my personal direction.

NOTICE: This is to certify that the foregoing information is true, accurate and complete. I understand that payment and satisfaction of this claim will be from Federal and State funds, and that any false claims, statements, or documents, or concealment of a material fact, may be prosecuted under applicable Federal or State laws.

According to the Paperwork Reduction Act of 1995, no persons are required to respond to a collection of information unless it displays a valid OMB control number. The valid OMB control number for this information collection is 0938-0008. The time required to complete this information collection is estimated to average 10 minutes per response, including the time to review instructions, search existing data resources, gather the data needed, and complete and review the information collection. If you have any comments concerning the accuracy of the time estimate(s) or suggestions for improving this form, please write to: CMS, Attn: PRA Reports Clearance Officer, 7500 Security Boulevard, Baltimore, Maryland 21244-1850.

Figure 6-1 CMS-1500 Claim *(continued)*

Form Locator 2: Patient's Name

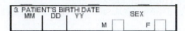

The patient's name is the name of the person who received the treatment or supplies, listed exactly as it appears on the insurance card. Do not change the spelling, even if the card is incorrect. The order in which the name should appear is last name, first name, and middle initial. Use commas to separate the last name, first name, and middle initial.

Form Locator 3: Patient's Birth Date/Sex

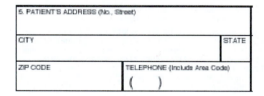

The patient's birth date and sex (gender) help identify the patient; this information distinguishes persons with similar names. Enter the patient's date of birth in eight-digit format (MM/DD/CCYY). Note that all four digits for the year are entered, even though the printed form indicates only two characters (YY). Use zeros before single digits. Enter an X in the correct box to indicate the sex of the patient. Leave this box blank if the patient's gender is unknown.

Form Locator 4: Insured's Name

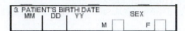

In FL 4, enter the full name of the person who holds the insurance policy (the insured). If the patient is a dependent, the insured may be a spouse, parent, or other person. If the insured is the patient, enter SAME. Use commas to separate the last name, first name, and middle initial.

Form Locator 5: Patient's Address

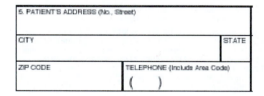

Form locator 5 contains the patient's address and telephone number. The address includes the number and street, city, state, and ZIP code. The first line is for the street address; the second line, the city and state; the third line, the ZIP code and phone number. Use a two-digit state abbreviation and a nine-digit ZIP code if it is available. Do not use a space or hyphen as a separator within the telephone number.

Note that the patient's address refers to the patient's permanent residence. A temporary address or school address should not be used.

Form Locator 6: Patient's Relationship to Insured

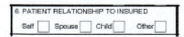

In FL 6, enter the patient's relationship to the insured who is listed in FL 4. Choosing *self* indicates that the insured is the patient. *Spouse* indicates that the patient is the husband or wife or qualified partner as defined by the insured's plan. *Child* means that the patient is the minor dependent as defined by the insured's plan. *Other* means that the patient is someone other than the insured, the spouse, or the child, which may include employee, ward, or dependent as defined by the insured's plan.

Form Locator 7: Insured's Address

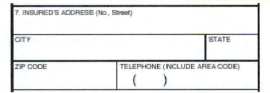

The insured's address refers to the insured's permanent residence, which may be different from the patient's address (FL 5). Enter the address and telephone number of the person who is listed in FL 4. If the insured's address is the same as the patient's, enter SAME. This form locator does not need to be completed if the patient is the insured person.

Form Locator 8: Patient Status

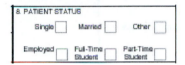

Enter an X in the box for the patient's marital status and for the patient's employment or student status. Choosing *employed* indicates that the patient has a job. *Full-time student* means that the patient is registered as a full-time student as defined by the postsecondary school or university. *Part-time student* means that the patient is registered as a part-time student as defined by the postsecondary school or university.

Form Locator 9: Other Insured's Name

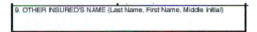

An entry in the other insured's name box indicates that there is a holder of another policy that may cover the patient. When additional group health coverage exists, enter the insured's name (the last name, first name, and middle initial of the enrollee in another health plan if it is different from that shown in FL 2). Otherwise, use SAME.

    Example: If a husband is covered by his employer's group policy and also by his wife's group health plan, enter the wife's name in FL 9.

Form Locator 9a: Other Insured's Policy or Group Number

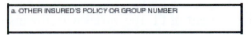

Enter the policy or group number of the other insurance plan. Do not use a hyphen or space as a separator with the policy or group number.

Form Locator 9b: Other Insured's Date of Birth

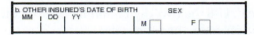

Enter the eight-digit date of birth (MM/DD/CCYY) and the sex of the other insured indicated in FL 9. Leave the box for the gender blank if not known.

Form Locator 9c: Employer's Name or School Name

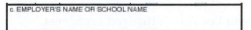

Enter the name of the other insured's employer or school. This box identifies the name of the employer or school attended by the other insured indicated in FL 9.

Form Locator 9d: Insurance Plan Name or Program Name

d. INSURANCE PLAN NAME OR PROGRAM NAME

Enter the other insured's insurance plan or program name. This box identifies the name of the plan or program of the other insured indicated in FL 9.

Form Locator 10a–10c: Is Patient Condition Related to:

10. IS PATIENT'S CONDITION RELATED TO:

a. EMPLOYMENT? (CURRENT OR PREVIOUS)
☐ YES ☐ NO
b. AUTO ACCIDENT? PLACE (State)
☐ YES ☐ NO ☐
c. OTHER ACCIDENT?
☐ YES ☐ NO

This information indicates whether the patient's illness or injury is related to employment, auto accident, or other accident. Choosing *employment* (current or previous) indicates that the condition is related to the patient's job or workplace. *Auto accident* means that the condition is the result of an automobile accident. *Other accident* means that the condition is the result of any other type of accident.

When appropriate, enter an X in the correct box to indicate whether one or more of the services described in FL 24 are for a condition or injury that occurred on the job or as a result of an automobile or other accident. The state postal code must be shown if YES is checked in FL 10b for Auto Accident. Any item checked YES indicates that there may be other applicable insurance coverage that would be primary, such as automobile liability insurance. Primary insurance information must then be shown in FL 11.

Form Locator 10d: Reserved for Local Use

10d. RESERVED FOR LOCAL USE

The content of FL 10d varies with the insurance plan. For example, some plans require the word *Attachment* in this form locator if there is a **claim attachment,** an additional form or medical record item needed to process the claim. Check instructions from the applicable public or private payer regarding the use of this field.

When required by payers to provide a *condition code,* enter it in this field. Use the two-digit *qualifier* BG to indicate that the following is a condition code, then the code.

In agreement with the NUBC (the organization that controls the hospital claim form, which will be covered in Chapter 15), **condition codes** for abortion and sterilization are approved for use for professional claims and can be reported in field 10d. Condition codes are two-digit numeric or alphanumeric codes used to report a special condition or unique circumstance about a claim. The qualifier code BG goes before these codes to show that a condition code follows.

The following condition codes are valid for the CMS-1500 and 837P claims:

AA   Abortion Performed due to Rape

AB   Abortion Performed due to Incest

AC   Abortion Performed due to Serious Fetal Genetic Defect, Deformity, or Abnormality

AD   Abortion Performed due to a Life Endangering Physical Condition Caused by, Arising from, or Exacerbated by the Pregnancy Itself

AE   Abortion Performed due to Physical Health of Mother that is not Life Endangering

AF   Abortion Performed due to Emotional/Psychological Health of the Mother

AG   Abortion Performed due to Social or Economic Reasons

AH   Elective Abortion

AI   Sterilization

Example of a complete entry:

BGAA

Form Locator 11: Insured's Policy Group or FECA Number

11. INSURED'S POLICY GROUP OR FECA NUMBER

Enter the insured's policy or group number as it appears on the insured's health care identification card. If FL 4 is completed, this entry should also be completed.

The insured's policy group or FECA number is the alphanumeric identifier for the health, auto, or other insurance plan coverage. The FECA (Federal Employees' Compensation Act) number is the nine-digit alphanumeric identifier assigned to a patient who is an employee of the federal government claiming work-related condition(s) under the Federal Employees Compensation Act.

Form Locator 11a: Insured's Date of Birth/Sex

a. INSURED'S DATE OF BIRTH	SEX
MM DD YY	M ☐ F ☐

The insured's date of birth and sex (gender) refers to the birth date and gender of the insured as indicated in FL 1a. These data are needed when the insured and the patient are different individuals. Enter the insured's eight-digit birth date (MM/DD/CCYY) and sex.

Form Locator 11b: Employer's Name or School Name

b. EMPLOYER'S NAME OR SCHOOL NAME

Enter the name of the insured's employer or the school attended by the insured who is indicated in FL 1a.

Form Locator 11c: Insurance Plan Name or Program Name

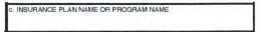

Enter the insurance plan or program name of the insured who is indicated in FL 1a. Note that some payers require an identification number of the primary insurer rather than the name in this field.

Form Locator 11d: Is There Another Health Benefit Plan?

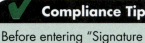

Select Yes if the patient is covered by additional insurance. If the answer is Yes, form locators 9a through 9d must also be completed. If the patient does not have additional insurance, select No. If not known, leave 11d blank.

Form Locator 12: Patient's or Authorized Person's Signature

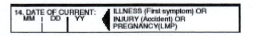

Enter "Signature on File" or "SOF" if the patient/insured's signature is on file for the release of any medical or other information necessary to process the claim. Otherwise, this form locator is for the legal signature. When legal signature is entered, also enter the date an authorization was signed in six-digit format (MM/DD/YY) or eight-digit format (MM/DD/CCYY).

Form Locator 13: Insured or Authorized Person's Signature

This entry authorizes payment of medical benefits directly to the provider of the services listed on the claim. Enter "Signature on File," "SOF," or legal signature and the date signed, as appropriate. If there is no signature on file, leave blank or enter "No Signature on File."

Physician or Supplier Information

The items in this part of the CMS-1500 claim form identify the health care provider, describe the services performed, and give the payer additional information to process the claim.

Form Locator 14: Date of Current Illness or Injury or Pregnancy

Enter the six-digit or eight-digit date for the first date of the present illness, injury, or pregnancy. For pregnancy, use the date of the last menstrual

1500

HEALTH INSURANCE CLAIM FORM

APPROVED BY NATIONAL UNIFORM CLAIM COMMITTEE 08/05

PICA | PICA | CARRIER

1. MEDICARE [X] (Medicare #) MEDICAID [ ] (Medicaid #) TRICARE CHAMPUS [ ] (Sponsor's SSN) CHAMPVA [ ] (Member ID#) GROUP HEALTH PLAN [ ] (SSN or ID) FECA BLK LUNG [ ] (SSN) OTHER [ ] (ID)

1a. INSURED'S I.D. NUMBER (For Program in Item 1): 079650202A

2. PATIENT'S NAME (Last Name, First Name, Middle Initial): JONES, DAVID, H

3. PATIENT'S BIRTH DATE MM DD YY: 05 29 1936 SEX M [X] F [ ]

4. INSURED'S NAME (Last Name, First Name, Middle Initial): SAME

5. PATIENT'S ADDRESS (No., Street): 765 SOUTH BLVD

6. PATIENT RELATIONSHIP TO INSURED: Self [X] Spouse [ ] Child [ ] Other [ ]

7. INSURED'S ADDRESS (No., Street): SAME

CITY: NEW YORK STATE: NY

8. PATIENT STATUS: Single [X] Married [ ] Other [ ]; Employed [ ] Full-Time Student [ ] Part-Time Student [ ]

CITY STATE

ZIP CODE: 20010 TELEPHONE (Include Area Code): (212) 5551444

ZIP CODE TELEPHONE (INCLUDE AREA CODE) ( )

9. OTHER INSURED'S NAME (Last Name, First Name, Middle Initial)

10. IS PATIENT'S CONDITION RELATED TO:

11. INSURED'S POLICY GROUP OR FECA NUMBER

a. OTHER INSURED'S POLICY OR GROUP NUMBER

a. EMPLOYMENT? (CURRENT OR PREVIOUS) [ ] YES [X] NO

a. INSURED'S DATE OF BIRTH MM DD YY SEX M [ ] F [ ]

b. OTHER INSURED'S DATE OF BIRTH MM DD YY SEX M [ ] F [ ]

b. AUTO ACCIDENT? [ ] YES [X] NO PLACE (State)

b. EMPLOYER'S NAME OR SCHOOL NAME

c. EMPLOYER'S NAME OR SCHOOL NAME

c. OTHER ACCIDENT? [ ] YES [X] NO

c. INSURANCE PLAN NAME OR PROGRAM NAME

d. INSURANCE PLAN NAME OR PROGRAM NAME

10d. RESERVED FOR LOCAL USE

d. IS THERE ANOTHER HEALTH BENEFIT PLAN? [ ] YES [X] NO *If yes,* return to and complete item 9 a-d.

READ BACK OF FORM BEFORE COMPLETING & SIGNING THIS FORM.

12. PATIENT'S OR AUTHORIZED PERSON'S SIGNATURE I authorize the release of any medical or other information necessary to process this claim. I also request payment of government benefits either to myself or to the party who accepts assignment below.

SIGNED SOF DATE

13. INSURED'S OR AUTHORIZED PERSON'S SIGNATURE I authorize payment of medical benefits to the undersigned physician or supplier for services described below.

SIGNED SOF

PATIENT AND INSURED INFORMATION

Figure 6-2 Completed CMS-1500 Claim, Form Locators 1–13 (Medicare Patient)

period (LMP) as the first date. This date refers to the first date of onset of illness, the actual date of injury, or the LMP for pregnancy.

Form Locator 15: If Patient Has Had Same or Similar Illness

15. IF PATIENT HAS HAD SAME OR SIMILAR ILLNESS. GIVE FIRST DATE MM DD YY

Enter the first date the patient had the same or a similar illness. The form locator is asking whether the patient previously had a related condition. A previous pregnancy is not a similar illness. Leave blank if unknown.

Form Locator 16: Dates Patient Unable to Work in Current Occupation

16. DATES PATIENT UNABLE TO WORK IN CURRENT OCCUPATION FROM MM DD YY TO MM DD YY

If the patient is employed and is unable to work in his or her current occupation, a six-digit or eight-digit date must be shown as the "from–to" dates that the patient is unable to work. "Dates patient unable to work in current occupation" refers to the time span the patient is or was unable to work. An entry in this field may indicate employment-related insurance coverage.

Form Locator 17: Name of Referring Physician or Other Source

17. NAME OF REFERRING PROVIDER OR OTHER SOURCE

Table 6-1 Qualifiers for Non-NPI (Other ID) Numbers

Code	Definition
0B	State License Number
1B	Blue Shield Provider Number
1C	Medicare Provider Number
1D	Medicaid Provider Number
1G	Provider UPIN Number
1H	CHAMPUS Identification Number
EI	Employer's Identification Number
G2	Provider Commercial Number
LU	Location Number
N5	Provider Plan Network Identification Number
SY	Social Security Number (The Social Security number may not be used for Medicare.)
X5	State Industrial Accident Provider Number
ZZ	Provider Taxonomy

The name of the **referring provider,** ordering provider, or other source must be shown if the service or item was ordered or referred by a provider. The entry should have the name (first name, middle initial, last name) and credentials of the professional who referred or ordered the service or supply on the claim.

Form Locator 17a and 17b: ID Number of Referring Physician (split field)

17a.	
17b. NPI#	

The non-NPI ID number (for 17a) of the referring provider, ordering provider, or other source is the payer-assigned unique identifier of the physician or other health care provider. The non-NPI of the referring provider, ordering provider, or other source is put in FL 17a above the dotted line. The **qualifier** (a code indicating what the number represents) should also be reported above the dotted line and on the left side of the box before the Other ID# is entered. The NUCC defines the qualifiers shown in Table 6-1 on page 124. The NPI is entered in 17b.

Form Locator 18: Hospitalization Dates Related to Current Services

18. HOSPITALIZATION DATES RELATED TO CURRENT SERVICES					
	MM	DD	YY	MM	DD	YY
FROM				TO		

The hospitalization dates related to current services refer to an inpatient stay and indicate the admission and discharge dates associated with the services on the claim.

If the services are needed because of a related hospitalization, enter the admission and discharge dates of that hospitalization in FL 18. For patients still hospitalized, the admission date is listed in the From box, and the To box is left blank.

Form Locator 19: Reserved for Local Use

```
19. RESERVED FOR LOCAL USE
```

Refer to instructions from the payer regarding the use of this field. Some payers ask for certain identifiers in the field. If identifiers are reported in this field, the appropriate qualifiers describing the identifier should be used (see Table 6-1 on page 124).

An example of local is the Medicare use of FL 19 to hold modifiers beyond the four that fit. If there are more than four modifiers to be included with FL 24D, three of them plus modifier -99 go in 24D, and the additional modifiers go in FL 19.

Form Locator 20: Outside Lab? $Charges

```
20. OUTSIDE LAB?          $ CHARGES
      [ ] YES   [ ] NO
```

"Outside lab? $ charges" indicates that services have been rendered by an independent provider as indicated in FL 32 and shows the related costs.

Complete this item when billing for laboratory services. Enter an X in Yes if the reported service was performed by an **outside laboratory.** If Yes is checked, enter the purchase price under "charges." A yes response indicates that the laboratory service was performed by an entity other than the entity billing for the service. A check mark in No indicates that no purchased lab services are included on the claim. When Yes is annotated, FL 32 must be completed. When billing for multiple purchased lab services, each service should be submitted on a separate claim.

Form Locator 21: Diagnosis or Nature of Illness or Injury (relate items 1, 2, 3, or 4 to item 24e by line)

```
21. DIAGNOSIS OR NATURE OF ILLNESS OR INJURY. (RELATE ITEMS 1,2,3 OR 4 TO ITEM 24E BY LINE)

1. L___.__                               3. L___.__

2. L___.__                               4. L___.__
```

ICD-9-CM codes that describe the patient's condition are entered in priority order. The first code listed is the primary diagnosis. Additional codes for secondary diagnoses are used only when the diagnoses are directly related to the services being provided. When entering the number, include a space (accommodated by the period) between the two sets of numbers. If entering a code with more than 3 beginning digits (e.g., E codes), enter the fourth digit *above* the period.

Relate lines 1, 2, 3, and 4 to the lines of service in FL 24e by line number. The codes used should specify the highest level of detail possible, including the use of a fifth digit when appropriate.

Form Locator 22: Medicaid Resubmission and/or Original Reference Number

```
22. MEDICAID RESUBMISSION
    CODE            ORIGINAL REF. NO.
```

Medicaid resubmission means the code and original reference number assigned by the destination payer or receiver to indicate a previously submitted claim or encounter. List the original reference number for resubmitted claims. Please refer to the most current instructions from the applicable public or private payer regarding the use of this field (e.g., code). When resubmitting a claim, enter the appropriate bill frequency code left justified in the left-hand side of the field.

7- Replacement of prior claim

8- Void/cancel of prior claim

This Item Number is not intended for use for original claim submissions.

Form Locator 23: Prior Authorization Number

23. PRIOR AUTHORIZATION NUMBER

The prior authorization number refers to the payer-assigned number authorizing the service(s). Enter any of the following: prior authorization number or referral number, as assigned by the payer for the current service, or the Clinical Laboratory Improvement Amendments (CLIA) number or the mammography pre-certification number. Do not enter hyphens or spaces within the number.

Section 24

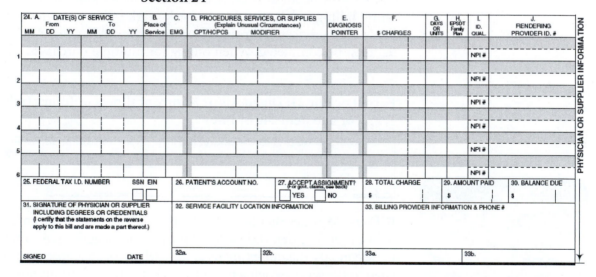

The term **service line information** describes section 24 of the claim, the part that reports the procedures—that is, the services—performed for the patient. Each item of service line information has a procedure code and a charge, with additional information as detailed below.

The six service lines in section 24, which contains FLs 24A through 24J, are divided horizontally to fit both the NPI and a non-NPI identifier when required, as well as to permit the submission of supplemental information to support the billed service. For example, when billing HCPCS codes for products such as drugs, the payer may require an indicator (N4) and the National Drug Code. The non-NPI identifier or supplemental information is to be placed in the upper shaded section of 24C through 24J.

Form Locator 24A: Dates of Service

24. A.	DATE(S) OF SERVICE					
	From			To		
MM	DD	YY		MM	DD	YY
1						
2						
3						
4						
5						
6						

Date(s) of service indicate the actual month, day, and year the service was provided. "Grouping services" refers to a charge for a series of identical services without listing each date of service.

Enter the from and to date(s) of service: If there is only one date of service, enter that date under From. Leave To blank or reenter the From date. If grouping services, the place of service, procedure code, charges, and individual provider for each line must be identical for that service line. Grouping is allowed only for services on consecutive days. The number of days must correspond to the number of units in FL 24G.

Form Locator 24B: Place of Service

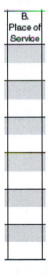

In 24B, enter the appropriate two-digit code from the place of service code list for each item used or service performed. A **place of service (POS)** code describes the location where the service was provided. It is also called the facility type code. Table 6-2 on page 128 shows typical codes for medical office claims.

Table 6-2 Selected Place of Service Codes

Code	Definition
11	Office
12	Home
22	Outpatient hospital
23	Emergency room—hospital
24	Ambulatory surgical center
31	Skilled nursing facility
81	Independent laboratory

Form Locator 24C: EMG

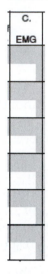

The form locator is EMG, for emergency indicator, as defined by federal or state regulations or programs, payer contracts, or HIPAA claim rules. Generally, an emergency situation is one in which the patient requires immediate medical intervention as a result of severe, life-threatening, or potentially disabling conditions. Check with the payer to determine whether the emergency indicator is necessary. If it is required, enter Y (yes) or N (no) in the unshaded bottom portion of the field.

Form Locator 24D: Procedures, Services, or Supplies

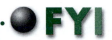
Enter the CPT or HCPCS code(s) and modifier(s) (if applicable) from the appropriate code set in effect on the date of service. State-defined procedure and supply codes are needed for workers' compensation claims.

Form Locator 24E: Diagnosis Pointer

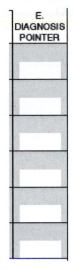

The diagnosis pointer refers to the line number from FL 21 that provides the link between diagnosis and treatment. In FL 24E, enter the diagnosis code reference number (pointer) as shown in FL 21 to relate the date of service and the procedures performed to the primary diagnosis. When multiple diagnoses are related to one service, the reference number for the primary diagnosis should be listed first; other applicable diagnosis reference numbers should follow. The reference number(s) should be a 1, or a 2, or a 3, or a 4; or multiple numbers as explained. Do not enter ICD-9-CM diagnosis codes in 24E.

Form Locator 24F: $ Charges

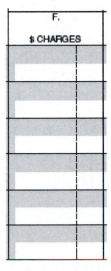

Form locator 24F lists the total billed charges for each service line in FL 24D. A charge for each service line must be reported. If the claim reports an encounter with no charge, such as a capitated visit, a value of zero (0) may be used.

The numbers should be entered without dollar signs and decimals. If the services are for multiple days or units, the number of days or units must be multiplied by the charge to determine the entry in FL 24F. This is done automatically when a billing program is used to create the claim.

Form Locator 24G: Days or Units

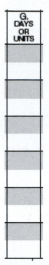

The item *days or units* refers to the number of days corresponding to the dates entered in 24A or units as defined in CPT or HCPCS. Enter the number of days or units. This field is most commonly used for multiple visits, units of supplies, anesthesia units or minutes, or oxygen volume. If only one service is performed, the numeral 1 must be entered. Enter numbers right justified in the field. No leading zeros are required. If reporting a fraction of a unit, use the decimal point.

Form Locator 24H: EPSDT Family Plan

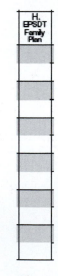

The Medicaid EPSDT/family plan identifies certain services that may be covered under some state plans (see Chapter 10).

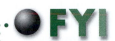

FYI

Even though the NPI has been fully implemented, it is assumed that there will always be providers who do not have NPIs and who may have non-NPI identifiers that need to be reported on their claim forms.

Form Locators 24I (ID Qualifier) and 24J (Rendering Provider ID#)

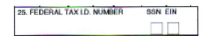

Form locator 24I works together with FL 24J. These boxes are used to enter an ID number for the **rendering provider**—the individual who is providing the service. This identifier is required only if the rendering provider is not the billing provider shown in FL 33.

If the number is an NPI, it goes in FL 24J in the nonshaded area next to the 24I NPI label. If the number is a non-NPI, the qualifier identifying the type of number goes in FL 24I next to the number in 24J. Refer to Table 6-1 for the common qualifiers.

Form Locator 25: Federal Tax ID Number

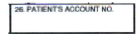

Enter the physician's Social Security number or Employer Identification Number (EIN) in FL 25. Mark the appropriate box (SSI or EIN). Do not use hyphens in numbers.

Form Locator 26: Patient's Account No.

Enter the patient account number used by the billing program to help identify the patient and post payments when working with RAs/EOBs.

Form Locator 27: Accept Assignment?

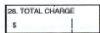

Enter a capital X in the correct box. "Yes" means that the provider agrees to accept assignment under the terms of Medicare.

Form Locator 28: Total Charge

Form locator 28 lists the total of all charges in form locator 24F, lines 1 through 6. Do not use dollar signs or commas. If the claim is to be submitted on paper and there are more services to be billed, put *continued* here and put the total charge on the last claim form page.

Form Locator 29: Amount Paid

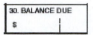

Enter the amount that the patient has paid toward this claim. If no payment was made, enter "none" or 0.00.

Form Locator 30: Balance Due

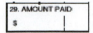

Check with the payer regarding the use of this field. Generally, for fee-for-service plans, subtract the amount in FL 29 from the amount in FL 28, and enter the balance in FL 30. Do not use dollar signs or commas.

Form Locator 31: Signature of Physician or Supplier Including Degrees or Credentials

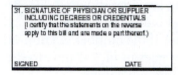

Enter the provider's or supplier's signature, the date of the signature, and the provider's credentials (such as MD).

Form Locator 32: Service Facility Location Information

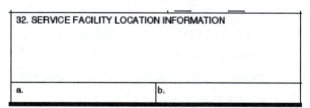

If the information in Form Locator 33 is different from Form Locator 32, enter the name, address, city, state, and Zip code of the location where the services were rendered. In 32a, enter the NPI of the service facility location. In 32b, enter the two-digit qualifier for a non-NPI number.

Form Locator 33: Billing Provider Information

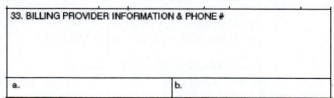

The **billing provider** is the organization or person transmitting the claim to the payer. This term is used to distinguish between a billing provider and the **pay-to provider,** the organization or person that should receive payment. (Note that if the pay-to provider is also the rendering provider, no rendering provider is reported.)

This distinction is necessary because physician practices often hire other firms, such as billing services and clearinghouses, to send their claims. When this is done, the outside organization is the billing provider, and the practice is the pay-to provider that receives the payment from the insurance carrier. If a practice sends claims directly to the payer, it is both the billing provider and the pay-to provider, so there is no additional pay-to provider to report.

Enter the provider's or supplier's billing name, address, ZIP code, phone number, NPI, non-NPI number, and appropriate qualifier. Note that no punctuation is used in the address, other than a hyphen for a 9-digit Zip code. Also, no space or hyphen is used as a separator within the phone number or between the qualifier and non-NPI identifier. The NPI should be placed in FL 33a. Enter the identifying non-NPI number of the billing provider in box 33b. The appropriate qualifier describing that the number is a non-NPI identifier is reported to the left of the non-NPI number in FL 33b. If the billing provider is a group, then the rendering provider NPI goes in FL24J. If the billing provider is a solo practitioner, then Form Locator 24J is left blank. The referring provider NPI goes in FL 17b.

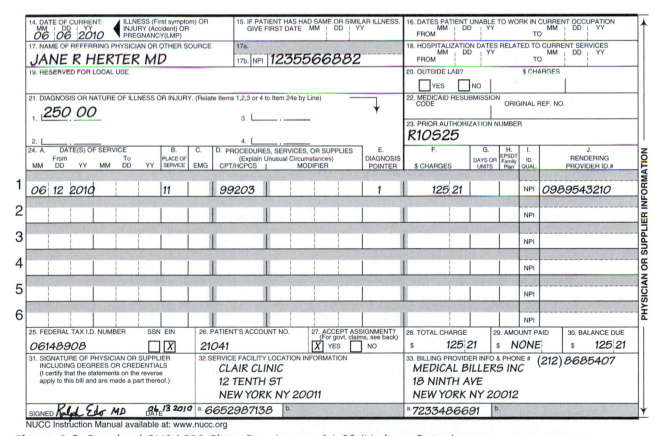

Figure 6-3 Completed CMS-1500 Claim, Form Locators 14–33 (Medicare Patient)

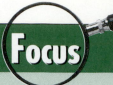

Professional Focus

Billing Services

A billing service is a company that provides data entry and claim processing services to providers for a fee. Many small practices do not have the time, knowledge, or staff available to create and process claims in-house. Some large practices may decide, too, that they would rather not develop the expertise necessary for health care claim preparation and transmission. A billing service offers a viable alternative. The medical office gives the billing service the information it needs to create claims, including patient information forms, insurance cards, and encounter forms. The billing service staff member inputs the data, creates claims, and submits claims either directly to payers or to a clearinghouse, which performs an edit and then submits the claims in HIPAA format.

A Note on Taxonomy Codes

HIPAA Tip

The taxonomy codes are one of the nonmedical or nonclinical **administrative code sets.** These code sets, which are maintained by the NUCC, are business-related, in contrast to medical code sets such as the ICD and CPT. Although not required by HIPAA to appear on a claim, as is an ICD code, if one of these codes is used it must be on the NUCC list.

Other ID number may be completed with a **taxonomy code** as well as a legacy number. (If two numbers are reported, they should be separated by three blank spaces.) A taxonomy code is a ten-digit number that stands for a physician's medical specialty. The type of specialty may affect the physician's pay, usually because of the payer's contract with the physician. For example, nuclear medicine is usually a higher-paid specialty than is internal medicine. An internist who is also certified in nuclear medicine would report the nuclear medicine taxonomy code when billing for that service and use the internal medicine taxonomy code when reporting internal medicine claims. Most billing programs store a taxonomy-code database.

Summary of Claim Information

Table 6-3 (on pages 134–136) summarizes the information that is required for the correct completion of the CMS-1500 claim.

Table 6-3 Summary of CMS-1500 Claim Completion

Form Locator	Content
1	**Medicare, Medicaid, CHAMPUS, CHAMPVA, FECA Black Lung, Group Health Plan,** or **Other:** Enter the type of insurance.
1a	**Insured's ID Number:** The insurance identification number that appears on the insurance card of the policyholder.
2	**Patient's Name:** As it appears on the insurance card.
3	**Patient's Birth Date/Sex:** Date of birth in eight-digit format; appropriate selection for male or female.
4	**Insured's Name:** The full name of the person who holds the insurance policy (the insured). If the patient is a dependent, the insured may be a spouse, parent, or other person. If the insured is the patient, enter "Same."
5	**Patient's Address:** Address includes the number and street, city, state, ZIP code, and telephone number.
6	**Patient's Relationship to Insured:** Self, spouse, child, or other. *Self* means that the patient is the policyholder.

(Table 6-3 Continued)

7	**Insured's Address:** Address and telephone number of the person listed in FL 4. If the insured's address is the same as the patient's, enter "Same."
8	**Patient Status:** Marital status and employment status—employed, full-time student, or part-time student.
9	**Other Insured's Name:** If there is additional insurance coverage, the insured's name.
9a	**Other Insured's Policy or Group Number:** The policy or group number of the other insurance plan.
9b	**Other Insured's Date of Birth:** Date of birth and sex of the other insured.
9c	**Employer's Name or School Name:** Other insured's employer or school.
9d	**Insurance Plan Name or Program Name:** Other insured's insurance plan or program name.
10a–10c	**Is Patient Condition Related to:** To indicate whether the patient's condition is the result of a work injury, an automobile accident, or another type of accident.
10d	**Reserved for Local Use:** Varies with the insurance plan.
11	**Insured's Policy Group or FECA Number:** As it appears on the insurance identification card.
11a	**Insured's Date of Birth/Sex:** The insured's date of birth and sex if the patient is not the insured.
11b	**Employer's Name or School Name:** Insured's employer or school.
11c	**Insurance Plan Name or Program Name:** Of the insured.
11d	**Is There Another Health Benefit Plan?** Yes if the patient is covered by additional insurance. If yes, FL 9a–9d must also be completed.
12	**Patient's or Authorized Person's Signature:** If the patient's or authorized representative's signature authorizing release of information is on file, the words "Signature on file" or "SOF" are entered. The patient/insured may instead sign and date the form.
13	**Insured or Authorized Person's Signature:** The words "Signature on File" or "SOF" are entered, or the form is signed/dated, to indicate that the patient or patient's representative authorizes payments from the insurance carrier to be made directly to the provider.
14	**Date of Current Illness or Injury or Pregnancy:** The date that symptoms first began for the current illness, injury, or pregnancy. For pregnancy, enter the date of the patient's last menstrual period (LMP).
15	**If Patient Has Had Same or Similar Illness:** Date when the patient first consulted the provider for treatment of the same or a similar condition.
16	**Dates Patient Unable to Work in Current Occupation:** Dates the patient has been unable to work.
17	**Name of Referring Physician or Other Source:** Name of the physician or other source who referred the patient to the billing provider.
17a	**ID Number of Referring Physician:** Identifying number(s) for the referring physician.
18	**Hospitalization Dates Related to Current Services:** If the services provided are needed because of a related hospitalization, the admission and discharge dates are entered. For patients still hospitalized, the admission date is listed in the From box, and the To box is left blank.
19	**Reserved for Local Use**
20	**Outside Lab? $Charges:** Completed if billing for outside lab services.
21	**Diagnosis or Nature of Illness or Injury:** ICD-9-CM codes in priority order.
22	**Medicaid Resubmission:** Medicaid-specific.
23	**Prior Authorization Number:** If required by payer, report the assigned number.
24A	**Dates of Service:** Date(s) service was provided.
24B	**Place of Service:** A place of service (POS) code describes the location at which the service was provided.
24C	**EMG:** Payer-specific code.
24D	**Procedures, Services, or Supplies:** CPT or HCPCS codes and applicable modifiers for services provided.
24E	**Diagnosis Pointer:** Using the numbers (1, 2, 3, 4) listed to the left of the diagnosis codes in FL 21, enter the diagnosis for the each service listed in FL 24D.
24F	**$ Charges:** For each service listed in FL 24D, enter charges without dollar signs and decimals.
24G	**Days or Units:** The number or days or units.
24H	**EPSDT Family Plan:** Medicaid-specific.
24I and J	**ID Qualifier and ID Numbers** (such as NPI)—completed if different than entered in box 33.
25	**Federal Tax ID Number:** Physician's or supplier's Social Security number or Employer Identification Number (EIN).
26	**Patient's Account No.:** Patient account number used by the practice's accounting system.
27	**Accept Assignment?** For Medicare claims, if the physician accepts Medicare assignment, select Yes. If not, select No.
28	**Total Charge:** Total of all charges in FL 24F.
29	**Amount Paid:** Amount of the payments received for the services listed on this claim.

(Table 6-3 Continued)

Form
Locator   Content

30   **Balance Due:** May be payer-specific; generally balance resulting from subtracting the amount in FL 29 from the amount in FL 28 or left blank.

31   **Signature of Physician or Supplier Including Degrees or Credentials:** Provider's or supplier's signature, the date of the signature, and the provider's credentials (such as MD).

32   **Service Facility Location Information:** Complete if different from the billing provider information in FL 33.

33   **Billing Provider Information:** Billing office name, address, telephone number, and ID numbers.

COMPLETING THE HIPAA CLAIM

M ost of the information reported on the CMS-1500 is also used to complete the HIPAA claim. Billing programs are set up to automatically supply the various items of information for electronic claims. There are some different terms used in instructions for the HIPAA claim, though, and some additional data must be relayed to the payer. This section covers those terms and data items as it presents the basic organization of the HIPAA claim.

Claim Organization

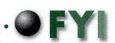

Certain information from the CMS-1500 is *not* needed on the HIPAA claim. Following is a partial list:
- Patient's/insured's telephone number(s)
- Patient's employment or student status
- Insured's marital status and gender

The HIPAA claim contains many **data elements.** Examples of data elements are a patient's first name, middle name or initial, and last name. Although these data elements are essentially the same as those used to complete a CMS-1500, they are organized in a different way. This organization is efficient for electronic transmission, rather than for use on a paper form.

The elements are structured in the five major sections, or levels, of the claim:

1. Provider.
2. Subscriber (guarantor, insured, policyholder) and patient (the subscriber or another person).
3. Payer.
4. Claim details.
5. Services.

Table 6-4 on pages 136–138 shows all the data elements that can be reported. Review this table as you read the rest of theis section.

Table 6-4 HIPAA Claim Data Elements

PROVIDER, SUBSCRIBER, PATIENT, PAYER

Billing Provider	Country Code
Last or Organization Name	Secondary Identifiers, such as State License Number
First Name	Contact Name
Middle Name	Communication Numbers
Name Suffix	Telephone Number
Primary Identifier: NPI	Fax
Address 1	E-mail
Address 2	Telephone Extension
City Name	Taxonomy Code
State/Province Code	Currency Code
ZIP Code	

(Table 6-4 Continued)

Pay-to Provider

Last or Organization Name
    First Name
    Middle Name
    Name Suffix
Primary Identifier: NPI
Address 1
Address 2
City Name
State/Province Code
ZIP Code
Country Code
Secondary Identifiers, such as State License Number
Taxonomy Code

Subscriber

Insured Group or Policy Number
Group or Plan Name
Insurance Type Code
Claim Filing Indicator Code
Last Name
First Name
Middle Name
Name Suffix
Primary Identifier
    Member Identification Number
    National Individual Identifier
    IHS/CHS Tribe Residency Code
Secondary Identifiers
    HIS Health Record Number
    Insurance Policy Number
    SSN
Patient's Relationship to Subscriber
Other Subscriber Information
Birth Date
Gender Code
Address Line 1
Address Line 2
City Name
State/Province Code
Zip Code
Country Code

Patient

Last Name
First Name
Middle Name
Name Suffix
Primary Identifier
    Member ID Number
    National Individual Identifier
Address 1
Address 2
    City Name
    State/Province Code
Zip Code
Country Code
Birth Date
Gender Code
Secondary Identifiers

    IHS Health Record Number
    Insurance Policy Number
    SSN
Death Date
Weight
Pregnancy Indicator

Responsible Party

Last or Organization Name
First Name
Middle Name
Suffix Name
Address 1
Address 2
City Name
State/Province Code
Zip Code
Country Code

Payer

Payer Responsibility Sequence Number Code
Organization Name
Primary Identifier
    Payer ID
    National Plan ID
Address 1
Address 2
City Name
State/Province Code
Zip Code
Secondary Identifiers
    Claim Office Number
    NAIC Code
    TIN
Assignment of Benefits
Release of Information Code
Patient Signature Source Code
Referral Number
Prior Authorization Number

Claim Level

Claim Control Number (Patient Account Number)
Total Submitted Charges
Place of Service Code
Claim Frequency Code
Provider Signature on File
Medicare Assignment Code
Participation Agreement
Delay Reason Code
Onset of Current Symptoms or Illness Date
Similar Illness/Symptom Onset Date
Last Menstrual Period Date
Admission Date
Discharge Date
Patient Amount Paid
Claim Original Reference Number
Investigational Device Exemption Number
Medical Record Number
Note Reference Code
Claim Note

(Table 6-4 Continued)

PROVIDER, SUBSCRIBER, PATIENT, PAYER

Diagnosis Code 1–8
Accident Claims
   Accident Cause
      Auto Accident
      Another Party Responsible
      Employment Related
      Other Accident
   Auto Accident State/Province Code
   Auto Accident Country Code
   Accident Date
   Accident Hour

Rendering Provider

Last or Organization Name
First Name
Middle Name
Name Suffix
Primary Identifier: NPI
Taxonomy Code
Secondary Identifiers

Referring/PCP Providers

Last or Organization Name
First Name
Middle Name
Name Suffix
Primary Identifier: NPI
Taxonomy Code
Secondary Identifiers
Proc

Service Facility Location

Type Code
Last or Organization Name
Primary Identifier: NPI
Address 1
Address 2
City Name
State/Province Code
Zip Code
Country Code
Secondary Identifiers

SERVICE LINE INFORMATION

Procedure Type Code
Procedure Code
Modifiers 1–4
Line Item Charge Amount
Units of Service/Anesthesia Minutes
Place of Service Code
Diagnosis Code Pointers 1–4
Emergency Indicator
Copay Status Code
Service Date Begun
Service Date End
Shipped Date

Onset Date
Similar Illness or Symptom Date
Referral/Prior Authorization Number
Line Item Control Number
Ambulatory Patient Group
Sales Tax Amount
Postage Claimed Amount
Line Note Text
Rendering/Referring/PCP Provider at the Service
   Line Level
Service Facility Location at the Service Line
Level

Provider Information

> **HIPAA Tip**
>
> The correct medical code sets are those valid at the time the health care is provided. The correct administrative code sets are those valid at the time the transaction—such as the claim—is started.

Like the CMS-1500, the HIPAA claim requires data on these types of providers, as applicable:

- Billing provider.
- Pay-to provider.
- Rendering provider.
- Referring provider.

For each provider, an NPI and possibly non-NPI numbers with the qualifiers as shown in Table 6-1 are reported. The billing provider contact name and telephone number are required data elements.

Subscriber Information

The HIPAA claim uses the term **subscriber** for the insurance policyholder or guarantor; this term is the same as *insured* on the CMS-1500 claim. The subscriber may be the patient or someone other than the patient. If the subscriber and patient are not the same person, data elements about the patient are also required. The name and address of any responsible party—an entity or person other than the subscriber or patient who has financial responsibility for the bill—are reported if applicable.

Claim Filing Indicator Code

A **claim filing indictor** code is an administrative code used to identify the type of health plan, such as a PPO. One of the claim filing indicator codes shown in Table 6-5 is reported. These codes are valid until a National Payer ID system becomes law. (Under HIPAA, a standard health plan identifier system must eventually be created, like the National Provider ID system has been. Each plan's number will be its National Payer ID. It is also called the National Health Plan ID.)

Table 6-5 Claim Filing Indicator Codes

Code	Definition
01	Self-pay
02	Central certification
03	Other nonfederal programs
04	Preferred provider organization (PPO)
05	Point of service (POS)
06	Exclusive provider organization (EPO)
07	Indemnity insurance
08	Health maintenance organization (HMO) Medicare risk plan
AM	Automobile medical
BL	Blue Cross and Blue Shield
CH	CHAMPUS (TRICARE)
CI	Commercial insurance company
DS	Disability
HM	Health maintenance organization
LI	Liability
LM	Liability medical
MB	Medicare Part B
MC	Medicaid
OF	Other federal program
TV	Title V
VA	Department of Veteran's Affairs plan
WC	Workers' compensation health claim
ZZ	Unknown

Relationship of Patient to Subscriber

The HIPAA claim allows for a more detailed description of the relationship of the patient to the subscriber than does the CMS-1500. When the patient and the subscriber are not the same person, an **individual relationship** code is required to specify the patient's relationship to the subscriber. The current list of choices is shown in Table 6-6.

Table 6-6 Relationship Codes

Code	Definition
01	Spouse
04	Grandfather or grandmother

(Table 6-6 Continued)

05	Grandson or granddaughter
07	Nephew or niece
09	Adopted child
10	Foster child
15	Ward
17	Stepson or stepdaughter
19	Child
20	Employee
21	Unknown
22	Handicapped dependent
23	Sponsored dependent
24	Dependent of a minor dependent
29	Significant other
32	Mother
33	Father
34	Other adult
36	Emancipated minor
39	Organ donor
40	Cadaver donor
41	Injured plaintiff
43	Child where insured has no financial responsibility
53	Life partner
G8	Other relationship

Other Data Elements

If another individual (called "other subscriber") might be involved in paying the claim, that person's birth date, gender, and address must be reported. Also, patient-specific information may be reported if applicable, such as:

- *Patient Death Date*—The date of death is required when the patient is known to be deceased and the provider knows the date on which the patient died.
- *Weight.*
- *Pregnancy Indicator Code*—If the patient is pregnant, a *Y* for yes is required when mandated by law.

HIPAA Tips

- Patient information forms and electronic medical records should be designed to record the relationship of the patient to the insured according to HIPAA categories, so that the data can be included on the HIPAA claim.
- The patient's address is a required data element, so if it is not known, "Unknown" should be entered.

Payer Information

This section of the HIPAA claim contains information about the payer to whom the claim is going to be sent, called the **destination payer.** A payer responsibility sequence number code identifies whether the insurance carrier is the primary (P), secondary (S), or tertiary (T) payer. This code is used when more than one insurance plan is responsible for payment, a situation that is covered in Chapter 7. The T code is used for the payer of last resort, such as Medicaid (see Chapter 10 for an explanation of "payer of last resort").

Claim Information

The claim information section of the HIPAA claim reports information related to just that particular claim. For example, an accident description is included if the patient's visit is the result of an accident. Data elements about the rendering provider—if not the same as the billing provider or the pay-to provider—are supplied. If another provider referred the patient for care, the claim reports data elements about the referring physician or primary care physician (PCP).

Claim Control Number

A **claim control number,** unique for each claim, is assigned by the medical office sending the claim. The maximum number of characters is twenty. The claim control number will appear on payments that come from payers (see Chapter 7), so it is very important for tracking purposes.

Although sometimes called the patient account number, the claim control number should not be the same as the practice's account number for the patient. It may, however, incorporate the account number. For example, if the account number is A1234, a three-digit number might be added for each claim, beginning with A1234001.

Claim Frequency Code

The **claim frequency code,** also called the **claim submission reason code,** for physician practice claims indicates whether this claim is one of the following.

Code   Definition

1   *Original Claim*—The initial claim sent for the patient, date of service, and procedure.
7   *Replacement of Prior Claim*—Used if an original claim is being replaced with a new claim.
8   *Void/Cancel of Prior Claim*—Used to completely eliminate a submitted claim.

First claims are always 1. Payers do not usually allow for corrections to be sent after a claim has been submitted; instead, an entire new claim is transmitted. When a claim is replaced, the original claim number (Claim Original Reference Number) is reported.

Diagnosis Codes and Pointers

The HIPAA claim permits up to eight ICD-9-CM codes to be reported. The order of entry is not regulated. Each diagnosis code must be directly related to the patient's treatment.

Up to four of these codes can be linked to each procedure code that is reported. A total of four diagnosis codes can be linked to each service line procedure. At least one diagnosis code must be linked to the procedure code. Codes two, three, and four may also be linked, in declining level of their importance to the patient's treatment.

Service Line Information

HIPAA Tip

A claim payer should receive only what is needed to process a claim. If an attachment has PHI related to another patient, those data must be marked over or deleted. Information about other dates of service or conditions not pertinent to the claim should also be crossed through or deleted.

The HIPAA claim has the same elements as the CMS-1500 at the service line level. Different information for a particular service line, such as a prior authorization number that applies only to that service, can be supplied at the service line level.

Claims for various payers require additional data elements. These include Medicare claims (Chapter 9), EPSDT/Medicaid claims (Chapter 10), and workers' compensation (Chapter 12).

Line Item Control Number

A **line item control number** is a unique number assigned by the sender to each service line. Like the claim control number, it is used to track payments from the insurance carrier, but for a particular service rather than for the entire claim.

Claim Attachments

A HIPAA transaction standard for electronic health care claim attachments is under review. When it is adopted, payers will be required to accept all attachments that are submitted by providers according to the standard. Claim attachments may include lab results, specialty consultation notes, and discharge notes.

Explore the Internet

There are three important websites for HIPAA claims:
- National Uniform Claim Committee—for the CMS-1500 claim format
- CMS – for updated place of service codes
- Washington Publishing Company for all administrative code sets, including taxonomy codes (under HIPAA-related code lists)

Visit each site and find the location of updated information.

Chapter Summary

1. Medical billing programs are used in most medical offices to prepare health care claims. The program's databases are set up with data about the physicians, common diagnosis and procedure codes, fee schedules, and payers. To create a claim, the medical insurance specialist (a) records the patient's information, based on a new or updated patient information form and insurance card; (b) records services, charges, and payments based on the patient's encounter form; and (c) instructs the program to create and transmit the claim.

2. The upper portion of the CMS-1500 claim form (form locators 1 through 13) lists demographic information about the patient and specific information about the patient's insurance coverage.

3. The lower portion of the CMS-1500 claim form (form locators 14 through 33) contains information about the provider or supplier and the patient's condition, including the diagnoses, procedures, and charges.

4. The HIPAA claim has five major sections: (a) provider, (b) subscriber/patient, (c) payer, (d) claim information, and (e) services. Most of the information from the billing program that is gathered for CMS-1500 claims is included on the HIPAA claim. Additional data elements include claim filing indicator code, individual relationship code, claim control number, claim submission reason code, and line item control number.

5. The billing provider is the entity that is transmitting the claim to the payer, usually a billing service or a clearinghouse. The pay-to provider receives the payment from the insurance carrier. A rendering provider is a physician who provides the patient's treatment but is not the pay-to provider entity. A referring provider has sent the patient for treatment.

6. The unique claim control numbers and line-item control numbers that are assigned by the sender are important because they appear on payments and other transactions that are returned by payers.

Part 1. Match each term below with its correct definition.

A. billing provider

B. claim control number

C. destination payer

D. line item control number

E. pay-to provider

F. POS code

G. referring provider

H. rendering provider

I. subscriber

J. taxonomy code

_____ **1.** Unique number assigned by the sender to a claim.

_____ **2.** Unique number assigned by the sender to each service line on a claim.

_____ **3.** Physician who has sent the patient to the billing or pay-to provider.

_____ **4.** Stands for the type of provider specialty.

_____ **5.** Entity providing patient care for this claim if other than the billing or pay-to provider.

_____ **6.** Entity that is to receive payment for the claim.

_____ **7.** Stands for the type of facility in which services reported on the claim were provided.

_____ **8.** Insurance carrier that is to receive the claim.

_____ **9.** Entity that is sending the claim to the payer.

_____**10.** The insurance policyholder or guarantor for the claim.

Part 2. Choose the best answer.

_____ **1.** If a physician uses a billing service to prepare and transmit its health care claims, which entity is the pay-to provider?
   a. billing service
   b. physician
   c. referring provider

_____ **2.** Medical billing programs store information such as patients' names in:
   a. transactions
   b. audit/edit reports
   c. databases

_____ **3.** Medical offices restrict access to patients' protected health information by limiting it to those who:
   a. are staff members
   b. need the information
   c. process HIPAA claims

_____ **4.** The name of the paper claim form is:
   a. HIPAA 837
   b. CMS-1492
   c. CMS-1500

_____ **5.** Which organization is in charge of the content of claims?
  a. CMS
  b. NUCC
  c. HIPAA

_____ **6.** On a HIPAA claim, the line item control number is in the:
  a. claim information section
  b. provider information section
  c. services section

_____ **7.** If the subscriber and the patient are not the same person, what type of code describes this?
  a. relationship code
  b. place of service code
  c. National Payer ID

_____ **8.** Which type of code describes the medical specialty of a provider?
  a. pay-to code
  b. taxonomy code
  c. relationship code

_____ **9.** What is the minimum number of diagnosis codes that must appear for each service line?
  a. one
  b. two
  c. four

_____ **10.** The correct medical code sets are those valid at the time the health care is provided. The correct _____ are those valid at the time the transaction—such as the claim—is started.
  a. diagnosis code set
  b. administrative code sets
  c. neither a nor b

Part 3. Read the cases below and answer the questions.

A. Joan McNavish, a sixty-one-year-old retiree, is covered by her husband's insurance policy. Her husband Ray is still working and receives health benefits through his employer, Rockford Valley Concrete, which has a PPO plan. In this case, who is the subscriber and who is the patient?

_____

B. Sherry Denise Cleaver is a patient in the medical office where you work. This information appears on her patient information and encounter forms:

Name: Sherry Denise Cleaver
Established Patient
Birth Date: July 1, 2009
Marital Status: Single
Responsible Person: James T. Cleaver
Relationship to Patient: Father
Insured's Plan: BMA PPO

Diagnosis of otitis media, left, on May 13, 2010; the charge is $22 for a CPT 99211. The medical office collected a copayment of $10 and waits for payment directly from the insurance companies on assigned claims.

Supply the following data elements:
Subscriber: _____
Patient: _____
Relationship of Patient to Subscriber: _____
Claim Filing Indicator Code: _____
Total Charge: _____
Amount Collected: _____
Place of Service Code:_____
Diagnosis Code: _____
Date of Service: _____
Procedure Code/Charge: _____

C. The following information appears on a series of encounter forms for patient Daniel M. Williams. You are preparing a claim for the three encounters.

Patient: Daniel M. Williams (EP)
Insurance: Aetna POS
Insured: Marla Y. Jones (grandmother)

Date: 6-14-10
T-101 P-90 R-18 BP 132/76 WT 175
CC: Swollen neck glands, fever, headache, general malaise since this morning.
Dx: Epidemic parotitis.
Rx: Rest, fluids, Tylenol for headache prn. Return in 5 days for recheck.
Services and Charges: Office visit, problem-focused history and exam, straightforward decision making: $65.

Date: 6-19-10
T-101 P-88 R-18 BP 130/60
CC: Fever, pain, and swelling of right testicle.
Dx: Orchitis, complication of epidemic parotitis.
Rx: Ampicillin 500 mg. #16; IM Ampicillin 500 mg. Return 2 days for recheck.
Services and Charges: Office visit, problem-focused history and exam, straightforward decision making: $65.
Intramuscular (IM) administration of antibiotic (Ampicillin) 500 mg, $20.

Date: 6-21-10
T-98.8 P-80 R-16 BP 132/74
Rx: Recheck, improvement, continue meds, recheck in 2 weeks.
Dx: Orchitis.
Services and Charges: Office visit, problem-focused history and exam, straightforward decision making: $65.

Supply the following data elements:
Subscriber: _____
Patient: _____
Relationship: _____
Claim Filing Indicator Code: _____
Total Charge: _____
Place of Service Code: _____
Diagnosis Codes: _____

Service Line Information:
Date of Service: _____
Procedure Code/Charge: _____
Diagnosis:

Date of Service: _____
Procedure Code/Charge: _____
Diagnosis: _____

Date of Service: _____
Procedure Code/Charge: _____
Diagnosis: _____

Date of Service: _____
Procedure Code/Charge: _____
Diagnosis: _____

D. The following information is in the file of patient Martha M. Butler. You are preparing a claim for the encounters.

Name: Martha M. Butler (EP)
Insurance Medicare Part B

Date: 4-19-2010
T-98.8 P-68 R-15 BP 178/98 WT 155
CC: This a.m. while going to get mail pt. fell on sidewalk; a neighbor brought her in c/o pain and disability in left hip area, SOB, chest pain.
Exam: Pt. in distress, X-ray L hip two views—negative, ECG T-wave inversion.
Lab: Cardiac enzymes, electrolytes.
Dx: Sprained L hip, essential hypertension, R/O angina pectoris.
Rx: Injection 2.0 cc Norflex IM, moist heat, Norflex tablets #12, Inderal capsules 80 mg #30.
Return in 3 days for lab results and recheck.

Date: 4-22-2010
T-98.6 P-68 R-15 BP 150/88
Lab Results: Within normal limits.
Exam: Hip improving, ECG negative.
Dx: Essential hypertension, angina pectoris.
Rx: Continue prescribed meds. Nitrostat tablets, one tab dissolved under tongue at first sign of angina attack.

List of Fees for Service:
Date: 4-19-2010
Dx: Sprained L hip, essential hypertension.
Services and Charges:
Office visit, detailed history and detailed exam, decision making of moderate complexity: $80.
X-ray L hip, complete, two views, $90.
Therapeutic Intramuscular Injection 2.0 cc Norflex IM, $12.
ECG routine, 12 leads, interpretation and report, $55.

Date: 4-22-2010
Dx: Essential hypertension, angina pectoris.
Services and Charges: Office visit, problem-focused history and exam, straightforward decision making: $65.

Supply the following data elements:
Subscriber/Patient: _____
Claim Filing Indicator Code: _____
Total Charge: _____
Place of Service Code: _____
Diagnosis Codes: _____

Service Line Information_____
Date of Service: _____
Procedure Code/Charge: _____
Diagnosis: _____

Date of Service: _____
Procedure Code/Charge: _____
Diagnosis: _____

Date of Service: _____
Procedure Code/Charge: _____
Diagnosis: _____

Date of Service: _____
Procedure Code/Charge: _____
Diagnosis: _____

Date of Service: _____
Procedure Code/Charge: _____
Diagnosis: _____

Claim Transmission, RA/EOB Follow-Up, and Collections

Learning Outcomes

After completing this chapter, you will be able to define the key terms and:

7-1 Identify the three major methods of electronic claim transmission.

7-2 Describe the claim determination process used by health plans.

7-3 Follow five steps to process RAs/EOBs from health plans.

7-4 Discuss common reasons for and appeals of reduced and denied payments.

7-5 Discuss the coordination of benefits process used to determine the patient's primary and additional insurance coverage.

7-6 Describe the patient billing and collections processes.

7-7 Be prepared to handle patients' inquiries about insurance and billing problems.

Key Terms

accounts receivable (AR)	determination	patient ledger
adjudication	downcoding	patient statement
adjustments	edit	primary insurance
appeal	electronic data	real-time claims adjudication
audit/edit claim response	interchange (EDI)	(RTCA)
birthday rule	electronic funds transfer (EFT)	secondary insurance
clean claim	insurance aging report	uncollectible account
coordination of benefits (COB)	patient aging report	

Why This Chapter Is Important to You

The information in this chapter will enable you to:

- Solve common payment problems.
- Understand how health plans can help with questions about claims.
- Increase your confidence by learning to answer patients' common questions about claims and bills.
- Check payers' RAs/EOBs for accurate and complete payment.
- Understand insurance benefit statements and explain them to patients.

What Do You Think?

One of the critical goals of a medical insurance specialist is to have claims approved and paid promptly by insurance carriers. Another goal is to help ensure prompt payments from patients. What steps can the specialist take to avoid claim rejection and to speed correct reimbursement from carriers and patients?

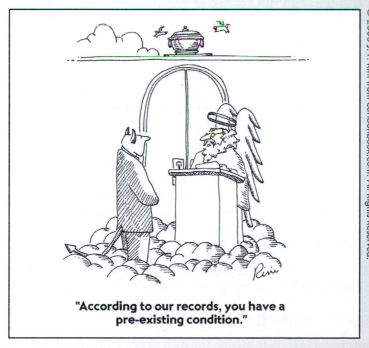

"According to our records, you have a pre-existing condition."

After claims have been prepared and reviewed, the final step is to transmit them to the payer using the billing program.

Electronic Data Interchange

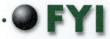

Transmitting HIPAA claims involves **electronic data interchange**, or **EDI.** EDI is the computer-to-computer exchange of routine business information using publicly available standards. HIPAA requires a particular EDI format, called the X12, for transmission. It also requires keeping patients' protected health information (PHI) secure and private when claims are sent.

Methods of Sending Claims

The billing program claim screen is used to monitor the transmission process. There are three major methods of transmitting claims electronically: clearinghouses, direct transmission, and direct data entry (DDE).

Clearinghouses

Most providers pay clearinghouses (described in Chapter 2) to receive their claims and put them in the correct EDI format for HIPAA transmission. Clearinghouses must receive all required data elements because they are prohibited by HIPAA from creating or modifying data content. This means that they cannot themselves fix errors on a claim but instead must transmit the claim back to the sender for correction.

To ensure clean claims, programs called claim scrubbers are used to make sure that all claims are complete and accurate.

Clearinghouses perform edits on claims before sending them to payers. An **edit** is a computer check for missing data, such as the birth date of a patient, or mistakes, like outdated codes. An **audit/edit claim response** is returned electronically by the clearinghouse to the provider. It lists the problems that would cause the claim to be rejected by the payer and asks the sender to correct the errors. When this has been done and correct claim information is sent, the clearinghouse transmits the **clean claim** to the appropriate payer. (Claims with missing information or that fail other edit screens, such as use of a gender-specific procedure code for a patient of the wrong sex, are called dirty claims.)

Direct Transmission

Some providers and payers exchange transactions directly. This method might be worth the expense of setting up for a practice's major payers, like Medicare.

Direct Data Entry (DDE)

Another option is DDE, in which the office uses an Internet-based service connected to the payer into which the claim's data elements are keyed. Like direct transmission, this method involves a high level of technical knowledge and investment at the medical office.

HEALTH PLAN CLAIM PROCESSING BY PAYERS

Clean claims increase the probability of being paid in full and on time. Claims that payers pay late, decide not to pay, or pay at a reduced level have a negative effect on **accounts receivable,** (AR) the practice's flow of income from payers and patients. To follow up on claims, medical insurance specialists need to understand the process that payers follow to examine claims and determine payments, which is called **adjudication.** The flow of information in this process is shown in Figure 7-1.

Claim Processing by Payers

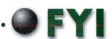

Paper claims are mailed to payers, who usually use a technology called optical character recognition, or OCR, to scan claims (not to be confused with the abbreviation OCR for the Office for Civil Rights in Chapter 2).

When a payer has accepted a health care claim as complete and on time, the claims department answers two major questions:

1. Are benefits due according to the patient's policy?
2. Were the services provided medically necessary?

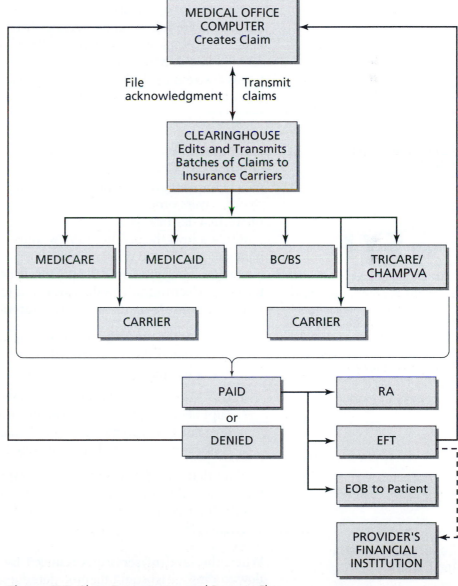

Figure 7-1 Claim Determination and Payment Flow

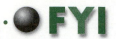
The first items checked are the subscriber's and patient's policy identification numbers. Then the payer ensures that policy payments, such as premiums, are up to date and that the policy is in effect for the date of service. Correct spelling of names and use of names as they appear in the payer's master file are essential. A nickname or typographical error can make it very difficult to identify a person covered by a policy or contract.

The claim is reviewed by a claims examiner and sometimes by a medical professional. Procedure codes are compared with the policy's schedule of benefits to see whether the reported services are covered. The examiner may decide to hold the claim and ask the treating physician for additional clinical information. In this case, the examiner may request documentation to check:

- Where the service took place.
- Whether the treatments were appropriate and a logical outcome of the facts and conditions shown in the medical record.
- That services provided were accurately reported.

After the case is examined, a payment **determination** is made—a decision whether to (1) pay the claim, (2) deny the claim, or (3) reduce the payment for the claim. If the claims examiner decides that the claim falls within normal guidelines and is complete, the claim is paid. If it is complete but not reimbursable, the claim is denied. If the examiner determines that any of the services the patient received were at too high a level for the related diagnosis, the examiner may assign a lower-level code to the service and pay a lower amount than was billed.

Real-time Claims Adjudication

Some major payers offer medical offices the capability of **real-time claims adjudication (RTCA).** RTCA is likely the billing model that will be most widely implemented in the future. Instead of claim processing that takes weeks, payers process these transactions in seconds and follow with payments in a day or two.

RTCA allows the practice to view, at the time of service, what the health plan will pay for the visit and what the patient will owe. The process is to (1) create the claim while the patient is being checked out, (2) transmit the claim electronically to the payer, and (3) receive an immediate ("real-time") response from the payer. This response:

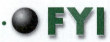
- Informs the practice if there are any errors in the claim, so these can be fixed and the claim immediately resent for adjudication.
- States whether the patient has met the plan's deductible.
- Provides the patient's financial responsibility.
- Supplies an explanation of benefits for this patient, so that any questions the patient has about denial of coverage or payment history can be immediately answered.

Note that the RTCA does not generate a "real-time" payment—that follows usually within 24 hours. This brief waiting period is also a great improvement over the time it normally takes payers to send payments.

Reduced Payments for Claims

When the level of service is reduced by the claims examiner—called **downcoding**—it is because the procedure does not link correctly to the diagnosis.

Perhaps the procedure's place of service is an emergency department, but the patient's problem is not considered an emergency. Claims may also be downcoded because the documentation fails to support the level of service claimed. For example, if the physician has coded a high-level evaluation and management service for a patient who presents with an apparently straightforward problem, the claims examiner is likely to request the encounter documentation. The medical record should contain information about the type of medical history and examination done as well as the complexity of the medical decision making that was performed. If the documentation does not support the service, the examiner downcodes the E/M code to a level considered appropriate.

Denied Claims

Claims may be denied because the services are not covered by the patient's contract with the insurance carrier. Common examples are when the patient's diagnosis is related to a noncovered preexisting condition or when an illness or disorder is specified in the policy as not covered or excluded. The insurance carrier will not pay for services for preexisting conditions or exclusions, but the physician may bill the patient for them.

When payment is denied, both the physician and the patient are notified by the insurance carrier. The medical insurance specialist should follow up with a letter to the patient explaining what action is being taken. In cases of preexisting conditions and canceled coverage, the patient is responsible for the bill. Any specific written correspondence received from the insurance company should be filed with the patient's records. If the patient has questions, the information from the insurance company may help resolve them.

Overdue Claims

> **HIPAA Tip**
>
> Medical offices use a HIPAA transaction called the claim status inquiry to electronically follow up with payers. The payer responds with the status of the claim.

Just as medical offices are required to file claims within a certain period of time, health plans have contractual agreements to pay claims within a period of time from receipt. Claims must be monitored until payments are received. Most offices follow up on claim status seven to fourteen days after claims are transmitted.

To avoid late payments, medical insurance specialists regularly review the **insurance aging report.** This report shows the ages of unpaid claims—that is, how much time has passed since the claims were filed (see Figure 7-2 on page 154).

In addition to regular claim follow-up, other reasons for contacting the insurance carrier are:

- The carrier notifies the medical office that a claim is being investigated. This might be due to preexisting conditions, workers' compensation, or other reasons. After a period of thirty days from the carrier's notice, however, follow-up should be done.
- An unclear denial of payment or an incorrect payment is received.
- Payment is received with no indication of the amount of the allowed charge or how much the patient is responsible for.
- The carrier asks for more information to process the claim. For example, a claim may contain an unlisted CPT code. In response, the payer asks for a special report (a narrative description) on the procedure or precise details of the service provided.

```
                              Central Practice Center
                             Primary Insurance Aging
                                November 30, 2010

Date of                    - Past -     - Past -     - Past -     - Past -     - Past -       Total
Service   Procedure        0 to 30      31 to 60     61 to 90     91 to 120    121 +        Balance

Aetna Choice (AET00)                                                                    (602)777-1000

WILLIWA0  Walter Williams                   SS: 401-26-9939
Birthdate: 9/4/1936            Policy: ABC103562239              Group: BDC1001

Claim: 59       Initial Billing Date: 10/4/2010      Last Billing Date: 10/4/2010

10/1/2010   99212          $0.00        $46.00       $0.00        $0.00        $0.00        $46.00
10/1/2010   93000          $0.00        $70.00       $0.00        $0.00        $0.00        $70.00
                           $0.00       $116.00       $0.00        $0.00        $0.00       $116.00

        Insurance Totals:  $0.00       $116.00       $0.00        $0.00        $0.00       $116.00


Anthem BCBS PPO (ANT01)                                                                  (602)888-1000

WINDOTI0  Timmy H. Window                    SS: 321-32-3440
Birthdate: 3/2/1997            Policy: XGS00096 14933            Group: 041886000

Claim: 66       Initial Billing Date: 10/15/2010     Last Billing Date: 10/15/2010

10/15/2010  99212          $0.00        $46.00       $0.00        $0.00        $0.00        $46.00
10/15/2010  69210          $0.00        $63.00       $0.00        $0.00        $0.00        $63.00
                           $0.00       $109.00       $0.00        $0.00        $0.00       $109.00

        Insurance Totals:  $0.00       $109.00       $0.00        $0.00        $0.00       $109.00


Cigna HMO Plus (CIG00)                                                                   (602)666-3001

PEREZCA0  Carmen Perez                       SS: 140-24-6113
Birthdate: 5/15/1934           Policy: 140603312X               Group:

Claim: 58       Initial Billing Date: 10/4/2010      Last Billing Date: 10/4/2010

10/1/2010   99213          $0.00        $62.00       $0.00        $0.00        $0.00        $62.00
                           $0.00        $62.00       $0.00        $0.00        $0.00        $62.00

        Insurance Totals:  $0.00        $62.00       $0.00        $0.00        $0.00        $62.00
```

Figure 7-2 Example of Insurance Aging Report

Professional Focus

Career Opportunities with Health Plans

Customer Service Representative

Customer service representatives handle written, e-mail, and telephone inquiries from physicians and policyholders about referrals, billing requirements, claim submission, preauthorization for procedures or hospital admissions, coverage issues, eligibility for benefits, copayment requirements, and balance billing. They are trained on the plans that are offered by the payer, and they must be familiar with the organization of their company so that they can correctly direct inquiries.

Claims Examiner

Claims examiners (also called claims analysts) work with the payer's computer system to process claims. They are trained to apply the payer's rules for determining medically necessary procedures and for bundling or global period coverage. They contact providers for information needed to complete claims, review and check claims attachments, and determine whether to pay, deny, or partially pay a claim.

PROCESSING THE RA/EOB

The RA/EOB sent by the payer to the medical office summarizes the determinations for a number of claims. See Figure 7-3 on page 156 for an example of an RA/EOB received by a medical office. (The document the patient receives covers just the patient's determination, as shown in Figure 1-4 on page 12.) For each claim on the RA/EOB, the claim control number, patient, dates of service, types of service, and charges are shown, along with an explanation of the way the amount of the benefit payment was determined. RAs/EOBs cover claims for a number of patients, and payments may not be made for every service line on a particular claim.

When a RA/EOB is received, usually electronically, the medical insurance specialist reviews it for accuracy and completeness. The amount of the payment depends on the practice's contract with the payer. Seldom do the practice's fee and the payer's fee match exactly. Most payers have their own fee schedules for contractual arrangements on fees.

The medical billing program is used to locate each claim listed on the RA/EOB, following these steps:

1. Match the claim control number, patient's name, and date of service with the payer's payments.
2. Check the patient data, plan, and listed procedures against the claim. Note any mismatched or missing information so that the claim can be corrected.
3. Compare the payment for each procedure with the expected amount. If a physician participates in the plan, the difference between what the physician charged on the claim and the allowed charge may be described as disallowed, nonallowed, not eligible for payment, or something similar. The disallowed amount may be listed as a separate item. If not, it can be calculated by subtracting the allowed charge from the amount the physician charged.
4. Read the carrier's explanations for unpaid, reduced, or denied claims. If the carrier's action is not warranted, the claim may be resubmitted or appealed, as described later in this chapter.
5. Determine the amounts of any write-offs that must be entered as adjustments in the patient's account. Also note the balance due from the patient or refund due to the patient (if the patient paid in advance or overpaid on the account).

Payment deposit is handled according to office practices. It may be a check or a notice of an electronic deposit called an **electronic funds transfer (EFT).** This type of payment is deposited directly in the practice's bank account.

If the patient has not assigned benefits to the provider, a benefits statement and the payment are sent directly to the patient. Even if no payment is due, a benefits explanation is usually sent. For example, if the physician's charges were applied to the patient's deductible, the physician does not receive a check. However, the health plan still sends a benefits statement.

Anthem Blue Cross Blue Shield
900 West Market Street
Phoenix, AZ 84209

Date: 6/22/2010

	Patient's name	Dates of service from - thru	POS	Proc	Qty	Charge amount	Allowed amount	Patient coins.	Amt paid provider	Patient balance
	Claim number 0347914									
4-101	Daiute, Angelo X	06/17/10 - 06/17/10	11	36415	1	$11.00	$8.00	$1.60	$6.40	$1.60
4-102	Daiute, Angelo X	06/17/10 - 06/17/10	11	80050	1	$98.00	$90.00	$9.00	$81.00	$9.00
4-103	Daiute, Angelo X	06/17/10 - 06/17/10	11	81000	1	$12.00	$10.00	$1.00	$9.00	$1.00
4-104	Daiute, Angelo X	06/17/10 - 06/17/10	11	93000	1	$51.00	$50.00	$5.00	$45.00	$5.00
4-105	Daiute, Angelo X	06/17/10 - 06/17/10	11	99386	1	$123.00	$76.00	$15.20	$60.80	$15.20
	Claim number 0347915									
5-101	Daiute, Brian G	06/17/10 - 06/17/10	11	99383	1	$98.00	$90.00	$9.00	$81.00	$9.00
5-102	Daiute, Brian G	06/17/10 - 06/17/10	11	90711	1	$74.00	$70.00	$14.00	$56.00	$14.00
	Claim number 0347916									
6-101	Daiute, Mary F	06/17/10 - 06/17/10	11	36415	1	$11.00	$8.00	$1.60	$6.40	$1.60
6-102	Daiute, Mary F	06/17/10 - 06/17/10	11	80050	1	$98.00	$90.00	$9.00	$81.00	$9.00
6-103	Daiute, Mary F	06/17/10 - 06/17/10	11	81000	1	$12.00	$10.00	0.00	$10.00	0.00
6-104	Daiute, Mary F	06/17/10 - 06/17/10	11	93000	1	$51.00	$50.00	$5.00	$45.00	$5.00
6-105	Daiute, Mary F	06/17/10 - 06/17/10	11	99386	1	$123.00	$76.00	$15.20	$60.80	$15.20
6-106	Daiute, Mary F	06/17/10 - 06/17/10	11	88150	1	$212.00	$212.00	0.00	0.00	$212.00**
	Claim number 0347917									
7-101	Daiute, Rosemary B	06/17/10 - 06/17/10	11	99384	1	$122.00	$64.00	$12.80	$51.20	$12.80
7-102	Daiute, Rosemary B	06/17/10 - 06/17/10	11	90707	1	$82.00	$82.00	$8.20	$73.80	$8.20
7-103	Daiute, Rosemary B	06/17/10 - 06/17/10	11	90702	1	$30.00	$26.00	$2.60	$23.40	$2.60

**Total for patient exceeds annual maximum for DME.

* * * * * * * * Check #109876 is attached in the amount of $690.80 * * * * * * * *

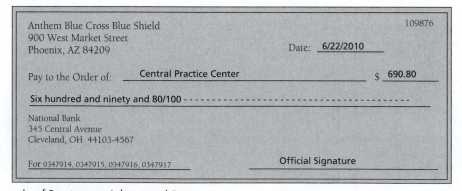

Figure 7-3 Example of Remittance Advice and Payment

APPEALS

When an incorrect payment is received, the carrier should be contacted. The carrier may have made a mistake and not entered the code that was submitted, which requires an adjustment to the payment. Sometimes the physician considers the carrier's reimbursement for services to be inadequate or incorrect. In either case, a claim rejection can be appealed. A claim **appeal** is a written request for a review of payment. It is a formal way of asking the insurance carrier to reconsider its claim determination.

An appeal is usually filed in the following situations:

- The physician did not file for preauthorization in a timely manner due to unusual circumstances.
- The physician thinks that the payment received for a procedure is inadequate.
- The physician disagrees with the carrier's decision about a patient's preexisting condition.
- Unusual circumstances affected the medical treatment.

A letter requesting an appeal of an inadequate payment might be worded as follows: "I am requesting special reconsideration of the disallowance for patient Mary Amamot, Case #1728564. A copy of the RA is enclosed for your review. I am also enclosing a list of fees that our research determined other plans allow for this CPT code. Your maximum allowed fees are below what comparable plans pay. We are certain our fees are cost-efficient and are based on the current relative value. Please inform us of your decision by calling or writing. We will contact you if we have not received an answer within thirty days."

If, after an appeal, the health plan denies what the physician considers fair compensation for services, the physician may want a peer review, in which an objective, unbiased group of physicians determines what payment is adequate for services provided. Another level of appeal is directed to the state's insurance commissioner. Each state has such an insurance regulatory agency, which is a liaison between the patient and the health plan and between the physician and the health plan. Physician, health plan, or patient may appeal to the insurance commissioner if any feels unfairly treated.

PATIENT BILLING AND COLLECTIONS

When the patient completes an office visit, the medical insurance specialist enters the transactions in the medical billing program. As patients' charges and payments are posted, the billing program also updates the **patient ledger,** or patient account record, a collection of all the financial activity in each patient's account.

If the physician has not accepted assignment and is not going to file a claim for an insured patient, the patient is usually required to pay at the end of the visit. When the physician accepts assignment and is going to file a claim, the patient usually does not pay fees other than a required copayment or deductible at the time of service. The amount of the copayment is entered and subtracted from the balance due. Then the health care claim for the service is created and transmitted to the payer.

Later, when insurance payments are received for patients, those payments are also posted to the patient's account and reduce the balance that the patient owes.

Other Insurance Plans: Coordination of Benefits

Some patients have more than one insurance policy. A patient may have coverage under more than one group plan, such as a person who has both employer-sponsored insurance and a policy from union membership. The primary plan is billed first. Then, when the RA/EOB is received, the second plan can be billed.

Determining the Primary Plan

The medical insurance specialist must determine which plan is primary. A person may have **primary insurance** coverage from an employer, but also be covered as a dependent under a spouse's insurance, making the spouse's plan the person's **secondary insurance.**

A common issue involves determining which of two parents' plans is primary for a child. If both parents cover dependents on their plans, the child's primary insurance is usually determined by the **birthday rule.** This rule states that the parent whose day of birth is earlier in the calendar year is primary. For example, Rachel Foster's mother and father both work and have employer-sponsored insurance policies. Her father, George Foster, was born on October 7, 1971, and her mother, Myrna, was born on May 15, 1972. Since the mother's date of birth is earlier in the calendar year (although the father is older), her plan is Rachel's primary insurance. The father's plan is secondary for Rachel.

Coordination of Benefits

Table 7-1 summarizes the facts that are used to determine which plan is primary. Determining the primary policy is important because under state and/or federal law, insurance policies contain a provision called **coordination of benefits (COB).** The coordination of benefits provision ensures that when a patient is covered under more than one policy, maximum appropriate benefits are paid, but without duplication.

If the patient has signed an assignment of benefits statement, it is the provider's responsibility to supply the information about the secondary insurance coverage to the primary payer. This information is included in the claim to the primary payer. When the primary payer's RA/EOB is received, the medical insurance specialist prepares another claim for the secondary payer, which reports the amount the first insurance policy paid and the patient's balance. The primary RA/EOB is attached to a HIPAA claim (or in some case, a CMS-1500 paper claim) and sent to the additional health plan. On the paper claim, for example, this amount appears in FL 29: Amount Paid, in place of a patient payment.

Form Locator 29: Amount Paid

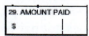

After both carriers have made payments, any unpaid bills are submitted to the patient.

Table 7-1 Determining Primary Coverage

☐ If the patient has only one policy, it is primary.

☐ If the patient has coverage under two plans, the plan that has been in effect for the patient for the longest period of time is primary. However, if an active employee has a plan with the present employer and is still covered by a former employer's plan as a retiree or a laid-off employee, the current employer's plan is primary.

☐ If the patient is also covered as a dependent under another insurance policy, the patient's plan is primary.

☐ If an employed patient has coverage under the employer's plan and additional coverage under a government-sponsored plan, such as Medicare, the employer's plan is primary.

☐ If a retired patient is covered by a spouse's employer's plan and the spouse is still employed, the spouse's plan is primary, even if the retired person has Medicare.

☐ If the patient is a dependent child covered by both parents' plans and the parents are not separated or divorced (or if the parents have joint custody of the child), the primary plan is determined by the birthday rule

☐ If two or more plans cover dependent children of separated or divorced parents who do not have joint custody of their children, the children's primary plan is determined in this order:
—The plan of the custodial parent.
—The plan of the spouse of the custodial parent (if the parent has remarried).
—The plan of the parent without custody.

Patient Statements

> **✔ Compliance Tip**
>
> Transactions should not be deleted in the patient billing program because doing so could be interpreted by an auditor as a fraudulent act. Instead, corrections, changes, and write-offs are made with **adjustments** to existing transactions. The adjusting entries give both the medical office and the patient a history of events in case there is a billing inquiry or an audit.

Patients owe amounts corresponding to their health plan coverage. A patient may owe a coinsurance payment. Patients also owe for services not covered by the policy. For these, the amount due from the patient is the amount that the physician charged—the usual fee. Since the services are not under contract, no allowed charges are in effect. The patient owes the entire physician's fee, which the physician may collect from the patient.

After all payer payments have been received on claims, the medical insurance specialist uses the medical billing program to update **patient statements,** or bills. The patient statements are mailed to patients who have balances due on their accounts after insurance payments have been received. Practices usually prepare and mail patient statements on a regular basis. For example, twice a week bills are sent to certain groups of patients, such as alphabetical groupings. This way of billing, called cycle billing, might be set up as follows: Monday, last names beginning with A through D, Wednesday E through H, the following Monday, I though L, and so on.

Follow the example of patient Karen Giroux, with a visit on October 7, 2010, and an RA posted on October 8, 2010. Figure 7-4 (on page 160) shows the transaction screen of the medical billing program after the visit has been posted. Figure 7-5 shows the ledger, illustrating the entry of the transactions for the office visit and the payment (on page 160). The patient statement shown in Figure 7-6 (on page 161) is sent to the patient and shows the balance that is owed. When patient payments are received, they are recorded in the billing program.

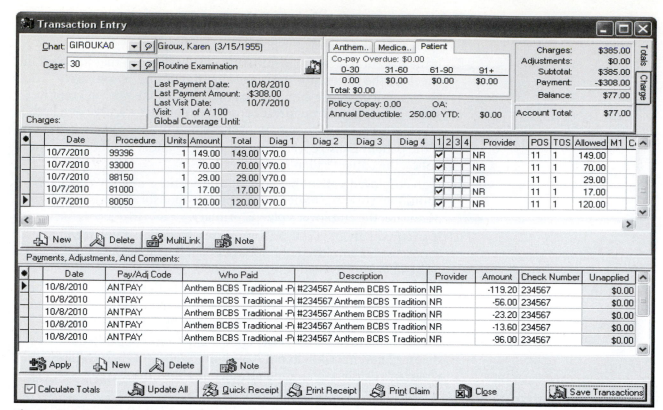

Figure 7-4 Transaction Screen

Central Practice Center
Patient Account Ledger
As of 10/31/2010

Entry	Date	POS	Description	Procedure	Document	Provider	Amount
GIROUKA0	Karen Giroux				(555)683-5364		
	Last Payment: -308.00		On: 10/8/2010				
75	10/7/2010	11		99396	1010070000	NR	149.00
76	10/7/2010	11		93000	1010070000	NR	70.00
77	10/7/2010	11		88150	1010070000	NR	29.00
78	10/7/2010	11		81000	1010070000	NR	17.00
79	10/7/2010	11		80050	1010070000	NR	120.00
80	10/8/2010		#234567 Anthem BCBS Traditic ANTPAY		1010070000	NR	-119.20
81	10/8/2010		#234567 Anthem BCBS Traditic ANTPAY		1010070000	NR	-56.00
82	10/8/2010		#234567 Anthem BCBS Traditic ANTPAY		1010070000	NR	-23.20
83	10/8/2010		#234567 Anthem BCBS Traditic ANTPAY		1010070000	NR	-13.60
84	10/8/2010		#234567 Anthem BCBS Traditic ANTPAY		1010070000	NR	-96.00
	Patient Totals						**77.00**
	Ledger Totals						**77.00**

Figure 7-5 Patient Ledger

The Collection Process

The collection process really begins with effective communications with patients about their responsibility to pay for services. When patients understand the charges and agree to pay them in advance, collecting the payments is not usually a problem. Most patients pay their bills on time. However, every practice has some patients who do not pay their bills when they receive their

Central Practice Center
1122 E. University Drive
Mesa, AZ 85204
602-969-4237

Statement Date	Chart Number	Page
10/29/2010	GIROUKA0	1

Make Checks Payable To:

Central Practice Center
1122 E. University Drive
Mesa, AZ 85204
602-969-4237

Karen Giroux
14A West Front St
Brooklyn, OH 44144-1234

Date of Last Payment: 10/8/2010	Amount: -96.00	Previous Balance:	0.00

Patient: Karen Giroux   Chart Number: GIROUKA0   Case: Routine Examination

Dates	Procedure	Charge	Paid by Primary	Paid by Secondary	Paid By Guarantor	Adjustments	Remainder
10/07/10	99396	149.00	-119.20	0.00		0.00	29.80
10/07/10	93000	70.00	-56.00	0.00		0.00	14.00
10/07/10	88150	29.00	-23.20	0.00		0.00	5.80
10/07/10	81000	17.00	-13.60	0.00		0.00	3.40
10/07/10	80050	120.00	-96.00	0.00		0.00	24.00

Amount Due
77.00

Figure 7-6 Patient Statement

monthly statements. Patients' reasons for not paying range from forgetfulness or inability to pay to dissatisfaction with the services or charges.

Medical insurance specialists are often responsible for collections from patients. The **patient aging report** printed by the patient billing program is the starting point, since it shows which patients' payments are due or overdue (termed *past due*). Figure 7-7 (on page 162) shows an example of a patient aging report. The aging begins on the date of the bill. For each account, an aging report shows the name of the patient, the last payment, and the amount of charges in each of these categories:

- *Current*—0 to 30 days.
- *Past*—31 to 60 days.

FYI

If patients have large bills that they must pay over time, a financial arrangement for a series of payments may be made. Such arrangements may be governed by specific laws in each state. If the practice's financial policy permits finance charges on late accounts, it is acceptable to apply them. The amount of the finance charge must comply with appropriate federal and state laws.

Central Practice Center
Patient Aging Applied Payment
by Date From
As of December 01, 2010

Chart # Name	Birthdate	Current 0 - 30	Past 31 - 60	Past 61 - 90	Past 91 +	Total Balance
ESTEPWIO Estephan, Wilma	3/14/1940	0.00	5.60	0.00	0.00	5.60
Last Pmt: -22.40 On: 10/8/2010	(602)683-5272					
GIROUKAO Giroux, Karen	3/15/1945	0.00	77.00	0.00	0.00	77.00
Last Pmt: -96.00 On: 10/9/2010	(602)683-5364					
PEREZCAO Perez, Carmen	5/15/1934	0.00	0.00	42.00	0.00	42.00
Last Pmt: -20.00 On: 10/1/2010	(602)692-3314					
PORCEJEO Porcelli, Jennifer	7/5/1970	0.00	61.00	0.00	0.00	61.00
Last Pmt: -15.00 On: 10/13/2010	(602)709-0388					
WILLIWAO Williams, Walter	9/4/1936	0.00	0.00	101.00	0.00	101.00
Last Pmt: -15.00 On: 10/1/2010	(602)936-0216					
WINDOTIO Window, Timmy H	3/2/1997	0.00	89.00	0.00	0.00	89.00
Last Pmt: -20.00 On: 10/15/2010	(602)239-3004					
Report Aging Total		$0.00	$232.60	$143.00	$0.00	$375.60
Percent of Aging Total		0.0%	61.9%	38.1%	0.0%	100.0%

Figure 7-7 Example of Patient Aging Report

- *Past*—61 to 90 days.
- *Past*—Over 91 days.

Each office sets its own procedures for the collection process. Large bills have priority over smaller ones. Usually, an automatic reminder notice and a second statement are mailed when a bill has not been paid within thirty days after it was issued. Some medical offices phone a patient with a thirty-day overdue account. If the bill is not then paid, collection letters are generated at intervals, each more stringent in tone and more direct in approach. Examples of collection letters are shown in Figure 7-8. Some medical offices use small claims court or outside collection agencies to pursue significant unpaid bills.

Writing Off Uncollectible Accounts

If no payment has been made after the collection process, the medical insurance specialist follows the office policy on bills it does not expect to collect. Usually, if all collection attempts have been exhausted and the cost of pursuing payment is greater than the amount to be collected, the process is ended. In this case, the amount is called an **uncollectible account** or bad debt and is written off from the expected revenues.

Communicating with Patients

Patients with complaints and problems with their health plans often need a go-between to contact the carrier and get questions answered. A medical insurance specialist with expertise and objectivity can build good will for the physician's office by using problem-solving and communication skills to fulfill this role. The first step in answering patients' inquiries about claims is to find out exactly what the problem is. Ask the patient whether he or she has:

- Contacted the health plan.
- Talked to the service representative.
- Reviewed the policy.

Date:
Patient:
Acct. #:
Balance Due: $

Dear

Your insurance company has paid its portion of your bill. You are now responsible for the remaining balance. Full payment is due, or you must contact this office within 10 days to make suitable payment arrangements. As an added payment option, you may pay by credit card, using the payment form below.

Sincerely,

<Employee signature>
Employee Name and Title

(a)

Date:
Patient:
Acct. #:
Balance Due: $

Dear

This is a reminder that your account is overdue. If there are any problems we should know about, please telephone or stop in at the office. A statement is attached showing your past account activity.

Your prompt payment is requested.

Sincerely,

<Employee signature>
Employee Name and Title

(b)

Figure 7-8 Examples of Collection Letters (a) First Letter (b) Second Letter (c) Third Letter

Date:
Patient:
Acct. #:
Balance Due: $

Dear

Your account is seriously past due and has been placed with our in-house collection department. Immediate payment is needed to keep an unfavorable credit rating from being reported on this account. If you are unable to pay in full, please call to make acceptable arrangements for payment. Failure to respond to this notice within 10 days will precipitate further collection actions.

Sincerely,

<Employee signature>
Employee Name and Title

(c)

Figure 7-8 Examples of Collection Letters (a) First Letter (b) Second Letter (c) Third Letter (*continued*)

Explore the Internet

The National Committee for Quality Assurance (NCQA), an independent nonprofit organization, rates health plans. Working with the health care industry, NCQA developed standardized performance measures that provide employers and consumers with information about each plan's effectiveness in preventing and treating disease, patients' access to care, and members' satisfaction with care. Visit the NCQA website and research the rating of your health plan or of a family member's health plan.

Often, the answer is no. The patient may not understand the insurance policy or may be confused about the rules of an HMO. On other occasions, the payer has made an error, and the patient is correct.

Understandably, patients get upset when they receive unexpected large bills or incorrect payments or when payments are delayed. The medical insurance specialist is the patients' advocate with the health plan. Sometimes the problem is just a misunderstanding because the patient does not know the right questions to ask, does not understand the answers, or is unaware that benefits have changed. In other situations, the patient may accuse the office staff of billing incorrectly. In these cases, try to listen carefully for the facts without letting feelings interfere.

If the patient has already called the health plan but is still upset or confused, the medical insurance specialist should call again and listen carefully to the explanation. The patient may have been too stressed to understand it. Explaining the solution again to the patient may help clear up misunderstandings.

Following are some techniques to use when explaining insurance issues to patients:

- Volunteer to explain. Speak slowly and calmly.
- Use simple language. Try to avoid insurance jargon.
- Explain more than once when necessary.
- Ask the patient "Do you understand?" or say "Perhaps I can explain that better."
- Remember, patients are under stress. Use respect and care.

Chapter Summary

1. Three methods for claim transmittal are (a) direct transmission, in which the claim is sent by EDI directly to the payer's computer system, (b) via a clearinghouse, which transmits the data file to the payer in correct format, and (c) direct data entry, in which the provider keys data elements directly into the payer's computer system rather than transmitting them via EDI. Most medical offices use clearinghouses to send their claims in HIPAA EDI format. Clearinghouses, which must follow proper practices for privacy and security of PHI, help providers and payers communicate using HIPAA transactions. They take nonstandard EDI communications and convert them to HIPAA-standard communications.

2. A claim is examined to determine whether benefits are due to a patient according to the policy and whether the services the patient received were medically necessary. At times, additional clinical information is required to process a claim. If the payer offers real-time claims adjudication, the patient's obligation may be determined at the close of the visit.

3. The five steps for processing RAs/EOBs are to (a) match the claim control number, patient's name, and date of service with the payer's payments; (b) check the patient data, plan, and listed procedures against the claim; (c) compare the payment for each procedure with the expected amount; (d) read the carrier's explanations for unpaid, reduced, or denied claims and decide whether resubmission or appeal is warranted; and (e) determine the amounts of any write-offs that must be entered as adjustments in the patient's account and note the balance due from the patient.

4. Health plans may reduce or deny claims because the patient is not currently enrolled or up-to-date with required premiums, the services are not covered by the patient's policy or are deemed not medically necessary, or the linkage between diagnoses and procedures does not satisfy the payer. The physician or the patient may decide to appeal the payer's determination. An appeal is the process of reviewing benefit reimbursement questions. If an appeal does not resolve a reimbursement issue, a peer review by an unbiased group of physicians may be requested. Appeals may also be resolved by asking the state insurance commissioner to make a ruling.

5. Primary insurance coverage is determined when more than one policy is in effect. This determination is based on coordination of benefits rules. The primary plan is billed first, then the secondary plan. Claims to secondary plans inform the payer what the primary plan has paid.

6. After an office visit, the new charges are entered into the patient's account in the billing program. If the physician is not filing a claim for the patient, the patient is charged for the services, often paying at the end of the visit. If the physician is filing a claim, the patient pays a copayment if required at the time of service and then is billed for the balance due after the insurance carrier's payment is recorded. After patient bills are sent, the collections process is used to collect overdue payments.

7. Often, patients do not understand insurance billing issues. The medical insurance specialist should offer to help patients resolve them. When explaining an insurance issue to a patient, speech should be slow and calm, and simple language should be used. It may be necessary to explain information more than once.

Check Your Understanding

Part 1. Choose the best answer.

_____ **1.** It has been thirty days since a claim was filed, and no response has arrived from the carrier. The best thing to do is:
   a. wait another ten days
   b. inform the physician
   c. contact the health plan

_____ **2.** A mistake on a claim already paid is discovered. The medical insurance specialist should:
   a. write off the unpaid amount
   b. rebill according to the payer's instructions
   c. send the patient a bill

_____ **3.** A claim was denied. Which of the following was not the reason?
   a. preexisting condition
   b. coverage cancellation
   c. vacationing carrier representative

_____ **4.** A letter from the carrier states that not enough information was submitted to process a claim. The medical insurance specialist should:
   a. make sure all the necessary information is provided
   b. send the letter to the patient
   c. make a note in the patient's record to rebill in thirty days

_____ **5.** The RA/EOB summarizes payments for:
   a. a single patient
   b. a single claim
   c. multiple patients and claims

_____ **6.** Collections are done on bills that are classified as:
   a. current
   b. written off
   c. past due

_____ **7.** Which report is used by billers to follow up on late claims from health plans?
   a. patient aging
   b. insurance aging
   c. patient ledger

_____ **8.** The abbreviation _EFT_ means
   a. electric forwarding transmission
   b. eventual follow-up of transfer
   c. electronic funds transfer

_____ **9.** Uncollectible accounts are:
   a. reported to health plans
   b. written off
   c. reported to CMS

_____ **10.** When more than one insurance plan covers a patient, determining which is primary is based on:
   a. coordination of benefits
   b. the HIPAA Privacy Rule
   c. determination

Part 2. Determine the primary plan.

A. George Rangley enrolled in the ACR plan in 2008 and in the New York Health plan in 2006.

George's primary plan:_____

B. Mary is the child of Gloria and Craig Bivilaque, who are divorced. Mary is a dependent under both Craig's and Gloria's plans. Gloria has custody of Mary.

Mary's primary plan: _____

C. Karen Kaplan's date of birth is 10/11/1970; her husband Carl was born on 12/8/1971. Their child Ralph was born on 4/15/2000. Ralph is a dependent under both Karen's and Carl's plans.

Ralph's primary plan: _____

D. Belle Estaphan has medical insurance from Internet Services, from which she retired last year. She is on Medicare but is also covered under her husband Bernard's plan from Orion International, where he works.

Belle's primary plan: _____

E. Jim Larenges is covered under his spouse's plan and also has medical insurance through his employer.

Jim's primary plan: _____

Part 3. Calculate the balances due from the four patients listed in Figure 7-3 on page 156.

A. Angelo Daiute
B. Brian Daiute
C. Mary F. Daiute
D. Rosemary B. Daiute

Part 4. Determine the amount due from the patient of a PAR physician based on the following information from the RA/EOB, explaining your reasoning.

Charges	$25.00
Disallowed:	$ 3.42
Allowed Charge:	$21.58
Deductible:	0
Coinsurance:	$10.00
Amount Due from Carrier:	$11.58
Additional Amount Due from Patient:	$ _____

CHAPTER 8

Blue Cross and Blue Shield

Learning Outcomes

After completing this chapter, you will be able to define the key terms and:

8-1 Discuss the history and structure of the Blue Cross and Blue Shield Association.

8-2 Describe four key features of Blue Cross and Blue Shield member plans.

8-3 Compare the responsibilities of physicians who do and do not participate in Blue Cross and Blue Shield member plans.

8-4 Explain the BlueCard Program.

8-5 Describe important data to obtain from a subscriber's Blue Cross and Blue Shield card.

8-6 State two reasons to complete claim forms within established time limits.

Key Terms

BlueCard Program
BlueCard Worldwide
Blue Cross
Blue Cross and Blue Shield
   Association (BCBS)

Blue Shield
certificate
Federal Employee Health
   Benefits (FEHB) plan
Flexible Blue

home plan
host plan
member plan
nationwide plan
out-of-area program

Why This Chapter Is Important to You

The information in this chapter will enable you to:

- Learn about an important insurance carrier that you will frequently work with as a medical insurance specialist.
- Learn rules for processing claims for the Blue Cross and Blue Shield BlueCard Program and BlueCard Worldwide program.
- Become familiar with terms that apply to Blue Cross and Blue Shield coverage.

What Do You Think?

Blue Cross and Blue Shield is a national association with affiliated plans in each state. If a new patient presents a Blue Cross and Blue Shield card, how does the medical insurance specialist verify insurance coverage?

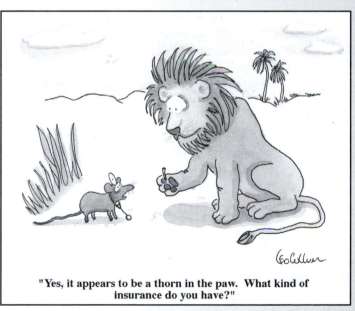

"Yes, it appears to be a thorn in the paw. What kind of insurance do you have?"

INTRODUCTION TO BLUE CROSS AND BLUE SHIELD

The **Blue Cross and Blue Shield Association (BCBS)** is a group of individual, independently licensed local companies. The association itself is not an insurance provider. Instead, it licenses the Blue Cross and Blue Shield brands and membership standards to the individual health plans. Blue Cross and Blue Shield companies that provide this coverage are known as **member plans.**

The Blue Cross and Blue Shield Association was developed from two kinds of health care programs: **Blue Cross,** which covered hospital services, and **Blue Shield,** which covered physician services. Today, Blue Cross has expanded its coverage from inpatient care to include benefits for outpatient and home care services as well as other kinds of institutional care. Blue Shield plans, in addition to physician services, offer specialty plans for dental, vision, mental health, prescription, and hearing services and other outpatient benefits. These plans may be added to an existing BCBS plan, or they may be purchased as stand-alone plans.

The first Blue Cross plan was founded in 1929 at Baylor University in Dallas, Texas. Teachers there agreed to pay $6 a year in exchange for twenty-one days of care at the university hospital, should the need arise. The first Blue Shield plan, founded in 1939 to provide physician services, was known as the California Physicians' Service. Its membership was restricted to individuals who earned less than $3,000 per year. The first members paid a monthly premium of $1.70.

Soon after these plans began, additional employee groups and health care providers joined, and similar programs were started in other communities. Today, there are more than forty independent plans with a total enrollment of over 100 million people. About 66 percent of the members are in preferred provider organizations (PPOs), 13 percent in indemnity plans, another 16 percent in health maintenance organizations (HMOs), and 5 percent in point-of-service plans. Blue Cross and Blue Shield companies also offer a consumer-driven health plan (CDHP) called **Flexible Blue.** This plan combines a comprehensive PPO plan with either a health savings account, a health reimbursement arrangement, or a flexible spending account. Also part of the CDHP are online decision-support resources.

The Blue Cross and Blue Shield Association represents member plans in matters of national scope; encourages cost-containment practices; develops evaluation methods for new technology; provides research, marketing, and actuarial services; coordinates public relations, advertising, public education, and professional relations programs; and administers membership standards. In addition, the association coordinates the claim process for **nationwide plans,** which are large membership accounts with offices located throughout the country. It also administers Medicare and other federal and state health programs.

HIPAA Tip

For BCBS claims, enter the subscriber's group number as it appears on the membership card. When entering the name of the member plan, be sure to include the state or the geographic area, such as Blue Cross and Blue Shield of Illinois, if this is part of the plan name.

FEDERAL EMPLOYEE HEALTH BENEFITS PLAN

Employees of the federal government may select the BCBS **Federal Employee Health Benefits (FEHB) plan** as their health insurance plan. The FEHB plan, which began in 1960, is the largest privately underwritten health insurance contract in the world. Federal employees enroll in a fee-for-service program that operates as a PPO. Members may enroll in a Standard Option plan or a Basic Option plan. Under the Standard Option plan, members may choose to receive treatment from a physician within the PPO network (the most cost-effective option) or outside the network (at a higher cost). Under the Basic Option plan, members must use PPO providers in order to receive benefits. (Some exceptions apply, such as for emergency care.) Both plans require copayments and coinsurance. Under Standard Option, members must also pay applicable deductibles.

KEY FEATURES OF BLUE CROSS AND BLUE SHIELD PLANS

BCBS member plans cover their members' health care costs in much the same way as commercial insurance companies cover their policyholders' costs. Some different terms, however, are used. A patient enrolled in a BCBS plan, referred to as a subscriber, is issued a **certificate,** not a policy. This certificate lists the benefits and responsibilities of the plan. A subscriber receives coverage directly from a BCBS member plan, through a small or large private employer, or through the federal government or a state government.

The BCBS Association was founded by state hospital associations and medical societies in the 1930s to provide low-cost, basic insurance. Today, BCBS has one investor-owned company, WellPoint, and a number of nonprofit companies that still operate as charitable, or nonprofit, corporations. Unlike commercial insurers that distribute profits to stockholders, these BCBS plans pay out about ninety cents of every premium dollar as benefits to subscribers. The remaining 10 percent of their income is used for operating expenses and reserves. Reserves are required by law in case operating or claims expenses exceed expectations. BCBS member plans that operate as nonprofit organizations cannot raise rates without approval from state departments of insurance. The process often includes a public hearing. Note, however, that some states require all carriers to get approval for rate increases.

BCBS member plans often accept subscribers whom other carriers will not cover. Many small groups and individuals who are unable to get coverage elsewhere can join Blue Cross and Blue Shield. Some member plans offer coverage regardless of medical condition during special enrollment periods. This widespread availability means that more people have medical insurance, thus reducing the number of bad debts and charity cases that physicians and other health care providers must absorb.

> ✔ **Compliance Tip**
>
> BCBS member plans offer subscribers a variety of benefit packages that range from fee-for-service to managed care plans. Many plans require preauthorization and second opinions. Because each subscriber's package may have different rules and because the details of each plan are negotiated regularly, it is important to get complete and up-to-date information from the plan to ensure prompt payment of health care claims.

PHYSICIAN PARTICIPATION AND REIMBURSEMENT

Health care providers can sign participation contracts with BCBS member plans. Providers who sign these contracts agree to submit all claims on behalf of patients and to accept the BCBS allowed amounts as payment in full for covered services. Most plans determine payment amounts to participating providers based on the standard methods of establishing fee schedules. Participating providers may not engage in balance billing. Payment is made directly to all participating providers.

Participating providers may also choose to contract with BCBS's Preferred Provider Network (PPN). A PPN contract requires physicians to adhere to network regulations, including providing quality service, properly utilizing services and resources, and containing the cost of services. In addition, PPN members agree to accept fees that are slightly lower than those paid to participating providers who are not PPN members. There are several advantages to PPN membership: physicians are notified when new groups enroll in the PPN, and those groups are given a physician directory that lists all members.

At times, a patient may see a physician who is not a plan participant. When the physician is a nonparticipating (nonPAR) provider, payment is made directly to the patient, even if the nonparticipating provider files the claim. A nonparticipating provider can collect the entire fee from a member patient, even if the fee exceeds plan payment levels.

> **HIPAA Tip**
>
> BCBS claims often require a PAR provider identification number (PIN) that is assigned by the member plan in addition to the National Provider Identifier (NPI).

FILING CLAIMS FOR SPECIAL CASES AND NATIONAL GROUPS

The Blue Cross and Blue Shield Association administers the **BlueCard Program,** which is an **out-of-area program** that allows for reciprocal coverage while a subscriber is away from the local area. An out-of-area program covers specific services for a member who receives care at a **host plan** elsewhere. The **home plan,** the plan that the subscriber contracts with, usually keeps all information on membership and claims for the subscriber.

The BlueCard Program links participating health care providers and independent BCBS member plans across the United States through a single electronic network for claim processing and reimbursement. The program makes sure that subscribers have health care services while they are traveling or living in another member plan's service area. The subscribers have the same benefits as in their home plan and access to BlueCard providers.

When an out-of-area BCBS membership card is presented to a participating provider, the provider verifies the membership and coverage by contacting BlueCard Eligibility. The provider then files the claim with the local host plan, which sends the claim to the subscriber's home plan. The subscriber's home plan processes it and sends the approved claim back to the local host plan, which pays the provider. The home plan also sends the subscriber an explanation of benefits.

For example, Emma Block, a New York resident and a member of a New York BCBS member plan, has gallbladder surgery in Kansas City. Through the BlueCard Program, a Kansas City participating physician will perform the surgery and bill Blue Cross and Blue Shield of Kansas City. The physician will receive reimbursement according to the Kansas City plan's payment method.

BLUECARD WORLDWIDE

The BlueCard Program also contains an international component, called **BlueCard Worldwide.** This plan allows BCBS plan members traveling or living abroad to receive the benefits they would receive at home. As with the domestic BlueCard program, BlueCard Worldwide links a network of participating BCBS health care providers and hospitals outside the United States with independent BCBS member plans in the United States in an attempt to provide the same level of coverage abroad that members receive at home and to coordinate claim processing and reimbursement.

MEMBERSHIP CARD INFORMATION

A Blue Cross and Blue Shield plan membership card contains vital information needed to file claims for member patients. The front and back of the card should be photocopied and placed in the patient's medical record for easy reference. A new photocopy of the card should be made annually or whenever the patient receives a new card.

In addition to the subscriber's name, most BCBS cards have the following information: plan name; type of plan; subscriber identification number (a series of numbers with a three-letter alpha prefix); effective date of coverage; BCBS plan codes and coverage codes; participation in a reciprocity plan with other BCBS plans; copayments, coinsurance, and deductible amounts; information about additional coverage, such as prescription medication or mental-health care; information about preauthorization requirements; claim submission address; and contact phone numbers. Figure 8-1 shows the front and back of a typical card.

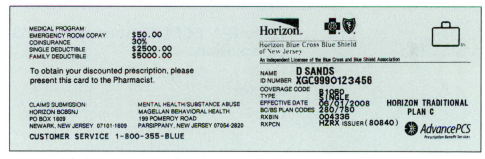

Front

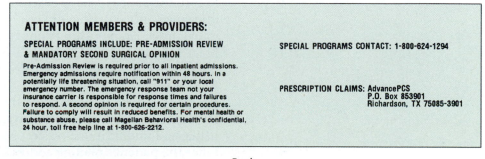

Back

Figure 8-1 Sample BCBS Identification Card

The BCBS plan identification cards for FEHB subscribers include the words *Government-wide Service Benefit Plan* and also specify the level of the plan. Individuals enrolled in low-option plans pay higher deductibles and copayments than do individuals in high-option plans. The coverage of the plans is similar.

FILING DEADLINES

As a matter of routine, most medical offices file insurance claims on a regular basis, usually within a thirty-day billing cycle. Timely filing means prompt reimbursement, especially for BCBS claims. However, that is not the only reason for efficient insurance claims procedures.

BCBS's contracts with participating providers specify timely filing guidelines, which are time limits for filing claims. Failure to submit claims to member plans within the contracted time frame results in refusal to pay. If this happens, the provider cannot bill the subscriber either; in other words, the physician cannot collect any fees for the services. Although exceptions can be made for special circumstances, every effort should be made to meet the contract's filing deadlines.

COMPLETING CLAIMS

General claim completion guidelines for CMS-1500 forms are shown in Table 8-1. Figure 8-2 (on page 178) shows a completed claim for a patient with an employer-sponsored group health plan from a Blue Cross and Blue Shield member plan.

Table 8-1 BCBS Summary of CMS-1500 Claim Completion

Form Locator	Content
1	Indicate Group if the patient is covered by an employer-sponsored plan; check Other if the patient is covered by an individual health plan.
1a	Enter the insurance identification number that appears on the patient's insurance card.
2	Record the patient's name *exactly* as it appears on the insurance card, entering it in last name, first name, middle initial order. Do not use any punctuation or abbreviations.
3	Enter the patient's date of birth in eight-digit format; make the appropriate selection for male or female.
4	If the insured and the patient are the same person, enter SAME. If not, enter the name of the person who holds the insurance policy (the insured/subscriber), in last name, first name, and middle initial order.
5	Enter the patient's mailing address, including the number and street, city, state, ZIP code, and the home telephone number.

(Table 8-1 Continued)

6	Select the appropriate box for the relationship: self, spouse, child, or other. *Self* means that the patient is the policyholder. *Other* includes an unmarried domestic partner.
7	If FL 4 is SAME, leave this blank. If FL 4 is completed and the insured's address is the same as the patient's, enter SAME. If the insured's address is different, enter the mailing address and telephone number of the person listed in FL 4.
8	Select the appropriate boxes for marital status and employment status. Select Other for patients who are unmarried domestic partners or who are covered under a child's plan. If the patient is neither employed nor a student, leave the employment status box blank.
9	Secondary claim: enter patient's name in last, first, and middle initial order.
9a	Secondary claim: enter the policy or group number of that insurance.
9b	Secondary claim: enter the patient's date of birth and gender.
9c	Secondary claim: enter employer's name, if applicable.
9d	Secondary claim: enter the name of the secondary plan.
10a–10c	Choose the appropriate box to indicate whether the patient's condition is the result of a work injury, an automobile accident, or another type of accident. If any Yes is selected, the claim should first be sent to the liable party (worker's compensation, auto insurance, or other), and then a secondary claim should be sent to the patient's plan. The state postal code must be shown if Yes is checked in FL 10b for Auto Accident.
10d	Varies with the insurance plan; complete if instructed.
11	Enter the group number if it appears on the insurance identification card.
11a	Enter the insured's date of birth and sex if the patient is not the same person as the insured.
11b	If the policy is under a group, enter the name of the employer, school, or entity.
11c	Enter the name of the HMO, PPO, or other private plan. Note that some payers require the payer identification number of the primary insurer in this field.
11d	Select Yes if the patient is covered by additional (secondary and/or tertiary) insurance. If yes, FL 9a–9d must be completed.
12	Enter Signature on File or SOF to indicate that there is a signature on file authorizing release of information necessary to process and/or adjudicate the claim. If not, a legal signature for the patient should be entered and dated.
13	Enter Signature on File or SOF to indicate that there is a signature on file assigning benefits to the provider. Note that many plans require assignment of benefits under their policies.
14	Enter the date documented in the medical record that symptoms first began for the current illness, injury, or pregnancy. For pregnancy, enter the first date of the last menstrual period (LMP). Previous pregnancies are not a similar illness. The date may be either before or on the current date of service. Leave blank if unknown.

(Table 8-1 Continued)

15	If the patient has consulted the provider for treatment of the same or a similar condition, enter the first date.
16	Enter the dates the patient is employed but unable to work in the current occupation (From: the first full day of disability; To: the last day of disability before returning to work).
17	Enter the name (first name, middle initial, last name) and credentials of the professional who referred or ordered the services or supplies on the claim.
17a, b	Enter the appropriate identifying number (either NPI or non-NPI, a payer-assigned unique identifier) for the referring physician.
18	If the services provided are needed because of a related inpatient hospitalization, the admission and discharge dates are entered. For patients still hospitalized, the admission date is listed in the From box, and the To box is left blank.
19	Complete according to the payer's instructions.
20	Complete if billing for outside lab services. Choosing No means that tests were performed by the billing physician or laboratory. Choosing Yes means that the test was done outside of the office of the physician's who is billing for it. When Yes is selected, enter the purchase charge and complete FL 32. When billing for multiple purchased lab services, each service should be submitted on a separate claim.
21	Enter up to four ICD-9-CM codes in priority order. At least one code must be reported. Relate lines 1, 2, 3, 4 to the lines of service in FL 24e by line number. Do not provide narrative description in this box. The codes used should specify the highest level of detail possible, including the use of a fifth digit when appropriate.
22	Leave blank; Medicaid-specific.
23	Some procedures and diagnostic tests require preauthorization. If required, enter the preauthorization number assigned by the payer.
24	The service line information section is used to report the procedures performed for the patient. Each item of service line information has a procedure code and a charge, with additional information as detailed below.
24A	Enter the date(s) of service, from and to: If there is only one date of service, enter that date under From. Leave To blank or reenter the From date. If grouping services, the place of service, procedure code, charges, and individual provider for each line must be identical for that service line. Grouping is allowed only for services on consecutive days. The number of days must correspond to the number of units in FL 24G.
24B	Enter the place of service (POS) code that describes the location at which the service was provided. If the service was provided to a hospitalized inpatient (POS 21). enter the hospital's provider information in FL 32.
24C	Check with the payer to determine whether this element (emergency indicator) is necessary. If it is required, enter Y (yes) or N (No) in the unshaded bottom portion of the field.

(Table 8-1 Continued)

24D	Enter the CPT/HCPCS codes, applicable modifiers, and/or anesthesia time in minutes for services provided. Do not use hyphens.
24E	Using the numbers (1, 2, 3, 4) listed to the left of the diagnosis codes in FL 21, enter the diagnosis for the each service listed in FL 24D.
24F	For each service listed in FL 24D, enter charges without dollar signs or decimals. If the claim reports an encounter with no charge, such as a capitated visit, a value of zero (0) may be used.
24G	Enter the number of days or units, as applicable. This field is most commonly used for multiple visits, units of supplies, anesthesia units or minutes, or oxygen volume. If only one service is performed, the numeral 1 must be entered.
24H	Leave blank; Medicaid-specific.
24I–24J	FL 24I and FL 24J work together. These boxes are used to enter an ID number for the rendering provider of the service. If the number is an NPI, it goes in FL 24J in the nonshaded area next to the 24I label NPI. If the number is a non-NPI (other ID number), the qualifier identifying the type of number goes in FL 24I next to the number in 24J.
25	Enter the physician's or supplier's federal tax identification number (either a Social Security number or an Employer Identification Number). Check the appropriate box for SSN or EIN.
26	Enter the patient account number used by the practice's accounting system.
27	If the physician accepts assignment, select Yes.
28	Enter the total of all charges in FL 24F. If the claim is to be submitted on paper and there are more services to be billed, put "continued" here and put the total charge on the last claim form page.
29	Amount of the payments received from the patient for the services listed on this claim. If no payment was made, enter none or 0.00.
30	Enter the balance resulting from subtracting the amount in FL 29 from the amount in FL 28.
31	Enter the provider's or supplier's signature, the date of the signature, and the provider's credentials (such as MD).
32	If IN 20 is completed, enter the name, address, state, the Zip code of the location where services were rendered. Enter the NPI in 32a.
33	Enter the billing provider's or supplier's name, address, ZIP code, telephone number, NPI, non-NPI number and appropriate qualifier. The NPI should be placed in FL 33a. Enter the identifying non-NPI number and qualifier of the billing provider in box 33b.

1500

HEALTH INSURANCE CLAIM FORM

APPROVED BY NATIONAL UNIFORM CLAIM COMMITTEE 08/05

PICA — PICA

CARRIER

PATIENT AND INSURED INFORMATION

1. MEDICARE (Medicare #) ☐ MEDICAID (Medicaid #) ☐ TRICARE CHAMPUS (Sponsor's SSN) ☐ CHAMPVA (Member ID#) ☐ GROUP HEALTH PLAN (SSN or ID) ☐ FECA BLK LUNG (SSN) ☐ OTHER (ID) ☒

1a. INSURED'S I.D. NUMBER (For Program in Item 1): XGC9990123456

2. PATIENT'S NAME (Last Name, First Name, Middle Initial): SANDS, GLORIA, T

3. PATIENT'S BIRTH DATE MM DD YY: 10 12 1983 — SEX M ☐ F ☒

4. INSURED'S NAME (Last Name, First Name, Middle Initial): SAME

5. PATIENT'S ADDRESS (No., Street): 26 PLANT AVE

6. PATIENT RELATIONSHIP TO INSURED: Self ☒ Spouse ☐ Child ☐ Other ☐

7. INSURED'S ADDRESS (No., Street):

CITY: RAYTOWN — STATE: CO

8. PATIENT STATUS: Single ☒ Married ☐ Other ☐; Employed ☒ Full-Time Student ☐ Part-Time Student ☐

CITY — STATE

ZIP CODE: 80033 — TELEPHONE (Include Area Code): (720)5551233

ZIP CODE — TELEPHONE (INCLUDE AREA CODE) ( )

9. OTHER INSURED'S NAME (Last Name, First Name, Middle Initial)

10. IS PATIENT'S CONDITION RELATED TO:

11. INSURED'S POLICY GROUP OR FECA NUMBER

a. OTHER INSURED'S POLICY OR GROUP NUMBER

a. EMPLOYMENT? (CURRENT OR PREVIOUS) ☐ YES ☒ NO

a. INSURED'S DATE OF BIRTH MM DD YY — SEX M ☐ F ☐

b. OTHER INSURED'S DATE OF BIRTH MM DD YY — SEX M ☐ F ☐

b. AUTO ACCIDENT? ☐ YES ☒ NO — PLACE (State)

b. EMPLOYER'S NAME OR SCHOOL NAME

c. EMPLOYER'S NAME OR SCHOOL NAME

c. OTHER ACCIDENT? ☐ YES ☒ NO

c. INSURANCE PLAN NAME OR PROGRAM NAME: ANTHEM BCBS PPO

d. INSURANCE PLAN NAME OR PROGRAM NAME

10d. RESERVED FOR LOCAL USE

d. IS THERE ANOTHER HEALTH BENEFIT PLAN? ☐ YES ☒ NO *If yes*, return to and complete item 9 a-d.

READ BACK OF FORM BEFORE COMPLETING & SIGNING THIS FORM.

12. PATIENT'S OR AUTHORIZED PERSON'S SIGNATURE I authorize the release of any medical or other information necessary to process this claim. I also request payment of government benefits either to myself or to the party who accepts assignment below.

SIGNED SOF DATE

13. INSURED'S OR AUTHORIZED PERSON'S SIGNATURE I authorize payment of medical benefits to the undersigned physician or supplier for services described below.

SIGNED SOF

PHYSICIAN OR SUPPLIER INFORMATION

14. DATE OF CURRENT: MM DD YY — ILLNESS (First symptom) OR INJURY (Accident) OR PREGNANCY(LMP)

15. IF PATIENT HAS HAD SAME OR SIMILAR ILLNESS. GIVE FIRST DATE MM DD YY

16. DATES PATIENT UNABLE TO WORK IN CURRENT OCCUPATION FROM MM DD YY TO MM DD YY

17. NAME OF REFERRING PHYSICIAN OR OTHER SOURCE: ROBERT S WETMORE MD

17a.

17b. NPI 7891234563

18. HOSPITALIZATION DATES RELATED TO CURRENT SERVICES FROM MM DD YY TO MM DD YY

19. RESERVED FOR LOCAL USE

20. OUTSIDE LAB? ☐ YES ☒ NO — $ CHARGES

21. DIAGNOSIS OR NATURE OF ILLNESS OR INJURY. (Relate Items 1,2,3 or 4 to Item 24e by Line)

1. 380 12
2. ___ . ___
3. ___ . ___
4. ___ . ___

22. MEDICAID RESUBMISSION CODE — ORIGINAL REF. NO.

23. PRIOR AUTHORIZATION NUMBER: R10S25

	24. A. DATE(S) OF SERVICE From MM DD YY	To MM DD YY	B. PLACE OF SERVICE	C. EMG	D. PROCEDURES, SERVICES, OR SUPPLIES (Explain Unusual Circumstances) CPT/HCPCS	MODIFIER	E. DIAGNOSIS POINTER	F. $ CHARGES	G. DAYS OR UNITS	H. EPSDT Family Plan	I. ID. QUAL.	J. RENDERING PROVIDER ID. #
1	04 19 2010		11		99212		1	80 10	1		NPI	1234567891
2											NPI	
3											NPI	
4											NPI	
5											NPI	
6											NPI	

25. FEDERAL TAX I.D. NUMBER: 52975321 — SSN ☐ EIN ☒

26. PATIENT'S ACCOUNT NO.: SAN0003

27. ACCEPT ASSIGNMENT? (For govt. claims, see back) ☒ YES ☐ NO

28. TOTAL CHARGE $ 80 10

29. AMOUNT PAID $ 0 00

30. BALANCE DUE $ 80 10

31. SIGNATURE OF PHYSICIAN OR SUPPLIER INCLUDING DEGREES OR CREDENTIALS (I certify that the statements on the reverse apply to this bill and are made a part thereof.)

SIGNED Ralph J Barton MD DATE 04/20/10

32. SERVICE FACILITY LOCATION INFORMATION

a. NPI b.

33. BILLING PROVIDER INFO & PHONE # (720) 5541222
CENTER CLINIC
3810 EXECUTIVE BLVD
RAYTOWN CO 80033

a. 4455667788 b.

NUCC Instruction Manual available at: www.nucc.org

Figure 8-2 Completed Claim Form for Blue Cross and Blue Shield

Explore the Internet

Visit the website for the national Blue Cross and Blue Shield Association. Enter your ZIP code, and look up information about the Blue Cross and Blue Shield affiliate for the state in which you live. What types of plans are offered?

Professional Focus

Blue Cross and Blue Shield

In the first decade of this century, the Blue Cross and Blue Shield Association's member plans are insuring more than 100 million—or one in three—U.S. citizens. BCBS member plans provide a variety of health care plans, including health maintenance organizations (HMOs), preferred provider organizations (PPOs), point-of-service (POS) programs, fee-for-service coverage, and consumer-driven health care. The member plans are the nation's largest provider of managed care services.

Chapter Summary

1. The Blue Cross and Blue Shield Association is a national group of local companies that offer prepaid coverage for health care. Blue Cross was founded in 1929 to cover hospital care. Blue Shield was founded in 1939 to cover physician services. Today, most local Blue Cross and Blue Shield member plans operate as joint corporations. The plans belong to the national Blue Cross and Blue Shield Association.

2. Four features of Blue Cross and Blue Shield member plans are that (a) they issue certificates to subscribers; (b) many are nonprofit, or charitable, organizations that cannot raise rates without state approval; (c) they offer unique contractual relationships with health care providers; and (d) they are widely available to individuals and small groups.

3. Participating providers must file all claims for their patients and must accept the BCBS fee schedule. Nonparticipating providers do not file claims directly with the BCBS plan; the patient pays the provider and then files a claim with the plan. NonPARs can charge their usual fees to BCBS patients.

4. The BlueCard Program allows host plans to process claims for services performed in their communities for patients covered by BCBS home plans in other areas.

5. The BlueCard Worldwide program allows plan members to receive the same level of coverage abroad that they would receive at home.

6. The information listed on a BCBS subscriber's identification card usually includes plan name; type of plan; subscriber identification number; effective date of coverage; BCBS plan codes and coverage codes; participation in a reciprocity plan with other BCBS plans; copayments, coinsurance, and deductible amounts; additional coverage; preauthorization requirements; claims submission address; and contact information.

7. Two reasons to complete BCBS claim forms within the timely filing guidelines are to ensure prompt payment and to prevent the member plan from refusing to honor the claim for payment.

Check Your Understanding

Part 1. In the space provided, write the word or phrase that best completes each sentence.

1. _____ was first established to cover physician services.

2. The Blue Cross and Blue Shield consumer-driven health plan is called _____.

3. The _____ pays the PAR provider under the BlueCard Program.

4. _____ was established to cover hospital expenses.

5. The _____ covers Blue Cross and Blue Shield plan subscribers who travel nationally.

6. The Blue Cross and Blue Shield Association does not provide _____.

7. Large Blue Cross and Blue Shield membership accounts with offices throughout the country are called _____.

8. Another name for a Blue Cross and Blue Shield plan member is _____.

9. The _____ covers Blue Cross and Blue Shield plan subscribers who travel abroad.

10. The BCBS _____ is a health insurance plan for employees of the federal government.

Part 2. Read the cases below and answer the questions.

A.

Physician Information:
Name: Mary Kant, MD
NPI: 5678901234
Blue Cross and Blue Shield Provider ID Number: 21-8554-56

Patient Information Form:
Name: William D. Degracia (New Patient)
Age: 26
Sex: Male
Birth Date: October 11, 1984
Marital Status: Single
Employer: Cone Plumbing and Air Conditioning
Insurance Carrier: Anthem Blue Cross and Blue Shield
Insured's ID Number: 088-09-7675
Insured's Group Number: G68063
Insured's Plan Name: BlueCare Plus Direct (HMO)

Patient's Encounter Form:

Date: 6-25-2010

T-99 BP 127/83

CC: Redness and swelling, right big toe.

Dx: Paronychia, right big toe.

Rx: Bacitracin to be applied.

List of Fees for Service:

Charges: Office visit, ten-minute exam, problem-focused, straightforward decision making, $45; office visit copayment charge, $20

Amount collected: $20, office visit copayment

Supply the following data elements:

Billing Provider _____

Billing Provider's Primary Identifier _____

Billing Provider's Secondary Identifier _____

Subscriber/Patient _____

Subscriber's Primary Identifier _____

Claim Filing Indicator Code _____

Payer Name /ID _____

Place of Service Code _____

Diagnosis Codes _____

Total Charge _____

Amount Collected _____

Service Line Information

Date of Service _____

Procedure Code/Charge _____

Diagnosis _____

Date of Service _____

Procedure Code/Charge_____

Diagnosis _____

B.

Physician Information:

Name: Michael A. Hardinsky, MD

NPI: 6789012345

Blue Cross and Blue Shield Provider ID Number: 0003480000-00

Patient Information Form:
Name: Susan A. Beeme (Established Patient)
Sex: Female
Birth Date: February 14, 1993
Responsible Person: Jennifer Beeme (mother)
Birth Date: May 12, 1963
Marital Status: Divorced
Employer: Runnymeade Court Realty
Insurance Carrier: Anthem Blue Cross and Blue Shield
Insured's ID Number: 24536574-02
Insured's Group Number: 00041
Insured's Plan Name: Blue Traditional (indemnity plan)

Patient Encounter Form:
Date: 6-25-2010
T-99 BP 127/83
CC: Patient's diabetes first diagnosed April 12, 2003; presents for diabetes recheck; lab workup shows acceptable range from about 78 to mid-100s with an occasional number over 200. Overall control is good.
Dx: Diabetes Mellitus, type II.

List of Fees for Service:
Office visit with problem-focused history and examination; straightforward decision making, $65
    Lab: Urinalysis by dip stick ($6); quantitative glucose analysis, blood ($9)
    Amount collected: 20% copayment, $16.00

Supply the following data elements:
Billing Provider _____

Billing Provider's Primary Identifier _____

Billing Provider's Secondary Identifier _____

Subscriber _____

Patient _____

Relationship _____

Subscriber's Primary Identifier _____

Claim Filing Indicator Code _____

Payer Name/ID _____

Place of Service Code _____

Diagnosis Codes _____

Total Charge _____

Amount Collected _____

Service Line Information

Date of Service _____

Procedure Code/Charge _____

Diagnosis _____

Date of Service _____

Procedure Code/Charge _____

Diagnosis _____

Date of Service _____

Procedure Code/Charge _____

Diagnosis _____

CHAPTER 9 Medicare

Learning Outcomes

After completing this chapter, you will be able to define the key terms and:

9-1 Identify two parts of Medicare coverage.

9-2 Discuss the fees that Medicare participating and nonparticipating physicians are allowed to charge.

9-3 Explain the difference between an excluded service and a medically unnecessary service.

9-4 Name four situations in which Medicare is the secondary payer.

Key Terms

advance beneficiary notice of noncoverage (ABN)

carriers

Correct Coding Initiative (CCI)

crossover claim

fiscal intermediary

formulary

hospice

limiting charge

local coverage determination (LCD)

Medical Savings Account (MSA)

medically unlikely edits (MUEs)

Medicare

Medicare administrative contractor (MAC)

Medicare Advantage

Medicare beneficiary

Medicare Fee Schedule (MFS)

Medicare Modernization Act (MMA)

Medicare Part A

Medicare Part B

Medicare Part C

Medicare Part D

Medicare Remittance Notice (MRN)

Medicare Summary Notice (MSN)

Medigap insurance

Medi-Medi beneficiary

national coverage determination (NCD)

Original Medicare Plan

Physician Quality Reporting Initiative (PQRI)

primary payer

secondary payer

timely filing

Why This Chapter Is Important to You

The information in this chapter will enable you to:

- Become familiar with the federal health insurance plan for older Americans and some people with disabilities.
- Explain Medicare coverage to patients.
- File Medicare claims correctly.

What Do You Think?

Two factors, demographics and politics, are large influences on Medicare. First, the portion of the country's population that is elderly and eligible for Medicare is increasing rapidly. The 65 million members of the baby boom generation (people born between 1946 and 1964) will turn sixty-five between 2011 and 2030. This group will make up 21 percent of the population. Over the past forty years, the number of people over eighty-five has grown at a much faster rate than has the overall population. At the start of this century, more than 4 million people—1.6 percent of the population—are over eighty-five years of age. Second, with more people on Medicare's rolls and a new prescription drug benefit, the costs of the program add up to a significant share of the federal budget. To offset these costs, the Centers for Medicare and Medicaid Services (CMS), which runs Medicare, has put a number of cost controls and billing regulations in place. Since CMS mandates that a physician who treats a Medicare patient must also complete the claim for the patient, medical insurance specialists often handle many Medicare claims. What resources can be used to stay up to date about changes in this important system?

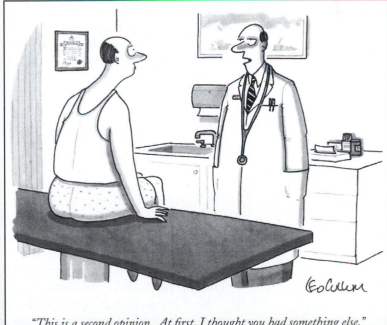

"*This is a second opinion. At first, I thought you had something else.*"

MEDICARE OVERVIEW

The federal health insurance program for people who are sixty-five or older is known as **Medicare.** Medicare also provides benefits to people with some disabilities and end-stage renal disease (ESRD), which is permanent kidney failure. A person covered by Medicare is called a **Medicare beneficiary.** Some beneficiaries qualify through the Social Security Administration. Others are eligible through the Railroad Retirement System. Medicare has two major parts, one for care given by institutions and the other for services by physicians.

The federal government does not pay Medicare claims directly. Instead, it contracts with insurance organizations to process claims on its behalf. Insurance companies that process claims for hospitals, skilled nursing facilities, intermediate care facilities, long-term care facilities, and home health care agencies are known as **fiscal intermediaries.** Insurance companies that process claims for physicians, providers, and suppliers are referred to as **carriers.** In 2003, Medicare passed legislation requiring the Part A fiscal intermediaries and the Part B contractors to be replaced with **Medicare administrative contractors (MACs),** which handle claims and related functions for both Parts A and B. (These entities are also called *A/B MACs.*) CMS has until 2011 to fully implement the changeover to the nineteen regional MACs.

Providers are assigned to a MAC based on the state in which they are physically located. DME MACs handle claims for durable medical equipment, supplies, and drugs billed by physicians.

Medicare Part A

Medicare Part A helps pay for inpatient hospital services, care in a skilled nursing facility, home health care, and hospice care. A **hospice** is a public or private organization that provides services for terminally ill patients and their families. Hospice care extends beyond medical services to include psychological and spiritual care.

Fees paid by Medicare Part A for inpatient hospital services are based on groupings of diagnoses. Hospital cases across the country have been analyzed to arrive at the fixed fees Medicare pays for hospital services. The payment is based on the principal diagnosis.

People who are eligible for Social Security benefits are automatically enrolled in Medicare Part A. They do not have to pay insurance premiums. Although people age sixty-five or older who do not qualify for Social Security benefits have the option of enrolling in Part A, they must pay premiums to get benefits.

Medicare Part B

Medicare Part B helps pay for physician services, outpatient hospital services, durable medical equipment, and other services and supplies. All Medicare providers must file claims on behalf of patients at no cost to the patients. Medical office insurance specialists file claims under Part B for physician services, even if the services are performed in hospital settings. They do not usually file claims for Part A benefits.

Part B coverage is optional. Everyone who is eligible for Part A may choose to enroll in Part B by paying monthly premiums (usually deducted automatically from Social Security retirement benefit payments). Therefore, the medical insurance specialist should check the patient's Medicare identification card for coverage information each visit, since coverage may be renewed monthly in some states and might expire between office visits.

Medicare Part C

In 1997, **Medicare Part C** (originally called Medicare + Choice) became available to individuals who are eligible for Part A and enrolled in Part B. Under Part C, private health insurance companies can contract with CMS to offer Medicare benefits through their own policies.

In 2003, under the Medicare Prescription Drug, Improvement, and Modernization Act (commonly called the **Medicare Modernization Act,** or **MMA**), **Medicare Advantage** became the new name for Medicare + Choice plans, and certain rules were changed to give Part C enrollees better benefits and lower costs.

Medicare Part D

Medicare Part D, authorized under the MMA, provides voluntary Medicare prescription drug plans that are open to people who are eligible for Medicare. All Medicare prescription drug plans are private insurance plans, and most participants pay monthly premiums to access discounted prices. A prescription drug plan has a list of drugs it covers, called a **formulary,** often structured in payment tiers.

Medicare Insurance Card

Each Medicare enrollee receives a health insurance card (see Figure 9-1). This card lists the beneficiary's name, sex, and Medicare number and the effective dates for Part A and Part B coverage. The Medicare number is assigned by CMS and usually consists of the Social Security number followed by a numeric or alphanumeric ending. The letter at the end provides additional information about the patient. For example, *A* stands for wage earner, *B* for spouse's number, and *D* for widow or widower.

Medicare Part B Plans

Medicare beneficiaries can choose from among a number of insurance plans.

Medicare beneficiaries who enroll in the Medicare fee-for-service plan (referred to by Medicare as the **Original Medicare Plan**) can choose any licensed physician certified by Medicare. They must pay the premium, the

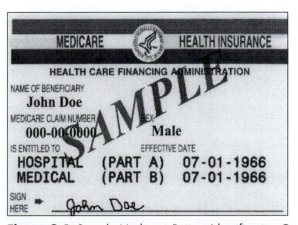

Figure 9-1 Sample Medicare Patient Identification Card

coinsurance (which is 20 percent), and the annual deductible specified each year by the Medicare law, which is voted on by Congress. How much of a patient's medical bills has been applied to the annual deductible is shown on the **Medicare Remittance Notice (MRN)** that the office receives and also on the **Medicare Summary Notice (MSN)** that the patient receives. Each time a beneficiary receives services, a fee is billable. Most offices bill the patient for any balance due after the MRN is received, rather than at the time of the appointment.

Medicare also offers Medicare Advantage plans. Beneficiaries can choose to enroll in one of the following types of plans instead of in the Original Medicare Plan:

- Medicare managed care plans.
- Medicare preferred provider organization plans (PPOs).
- Medicare private fee-for-service plans.
- Medical Savings Accounts.

Medicare Managed Care Plans

Some beneficiaries choose to join managed care plans such as HMOs. Most managed care plans charge monthly premiums and small copayments for office visits, but not deductibles. Medicare managed care plans, like other managed care plans, often require patients to use a specific network of physicians, hospitals, and facilities. Some plans offer patients the option of seeing providers outside the network for a higher fee. On the other hand, they offer coverage for services not reimbursed in fee-for-service plans, such as routine physical examinations and additional days in the hospital.

Managed care plans offer beneficiaries a number of advantages:

- Low copayment when receiving treatment.
- Minimal paperwork.
- Coverage for additional services.
- No need for a supplemental Medigap policy (covered below).

Disadvantages of Medicare managed care plans include the following:

- Physician choices limited to those in the particular plan.
- Prior approval from the primary care physician (PCP) typically needed before seeing a specialist, undergoing elective surgery, or receiving other services.

Preferred Provider Organization (PPO)

In the Medicare preferred provider organization plan (PPO), patients are given a financial incentive to use doctors within a network, but they may choose to go outside the network. Visits outside the network incur additional costs, which may include higher copayments or higher coinsurance. A PPO contracts with a certain group of providers to offer health care services to patients. Unlike HMOs, many PPOs do not require patients to select PCPs.

Private Fee-for-Service (PFFS)

Under a private fee-for-service plan, patients receive services from any Medicare-approved provider or facility they choose. The plan is operated by a private insurance company that contracts with Medicare to provide

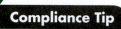

Compliance Tip

The Original Medicare Plan is administered by the Center for Medicare Management, a department of CMS.

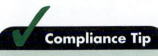
services to beneficiaries. The plan sets its own rates for services, and physicians are allowed to bill patients the amount of the charge not covered by the plan as long as it does not exceed 15 percent. A copayment may or may not be required. Under a private fee-for-service plan, patients may pay rates that are higher or lower than the rates on the Medicare Fee Schedule, but they cannot be balance billed.

Medical Savings Accounts

The Medicare Modernization Act created a new plan for Medicare called a **Medical Savings Account (MSA)**. Similar to private medical savings accounts, this plan combines a high-deductible fee-for-service plan with a tax-exempt trust to pay for qualified medical expenses. CMS will pay premiums for the insurance policies and make a contribution to the MSA. The only beneficiary premium is for supplemental benefits that may be offered by the plan. Beneficiaries use the money in their MSAs to pay for their health care before the high deductible is reached. At that point, the Medicare Advantage plan offering the MSA pays for all expenses for covered services. The maximum annual deductible is set by federal law.

MEDICARE CHARGES

The **Medicare Fee Schedule (MFS)** is the basis for payments for all Original Medicare Plan services. This national system is based on the Resource-Based Relative Value Scale (RBRVS) system using cost factors that represent the physician's time and how much it costs to run a practice (see Chapter 5).

Participation

Annually, physicians choose whether they want to participate in the Medicare program. Participating physicians agree to accept assignment for all Medicare claims and to accept Medicare's allowed charge according to the Medicare Fee Schedule as payment in full for services. A PAR physician may bill the patient for coinsurance and deductibles but may not collect amounts higher than the Medicare amount allowed by the fee schedule. Medicare is responsible for paying 80 percent of this allowed charge (after patients have met their annual deductibles). Patients are responsible for the other 20 percent. The physician may bill the patient for services not covered by Medicare.

Example

A Medicare PAR provider has a usual charge of $200 for a diagnostic flexible sigmoidoscopy (CPT 45330), and the Medicare-allowed charge is $84. The provider must write off the difference between the two charges. The patient is responsible for 20 percent of the allowed charge, not of the provider's usual charge:

Provider's usual fee:	$200.00
Medicare allowed charge:	$ 84.00
Medicare pays 80 percent	$ 67.20
Patient pays 20 percent	$ 16.80

The total the provider can collect is $84. The provider must write off the $116 difference between the usual fee and the allowed charge.

Nonparticipation

Nonparticipating physicians decide whether to accept assignment on a claim-by-claim basis. Providers who elect not to participate in the Medicare program but who accept assignment on a claim are paid 5 percent less for their services than PAR providers. For example, if the Medicare-allowed amount for a service is $100, the PAR provider receives $80 (80 percent of $100), and the nonPAR provider receives $76 ($80 minus 5 percent). NonPAR providers who do not accept assignment are subject to Medicare's charge limits. They may not charge a Medicare patient more than 115 percent of the amount listed in the Medicare nonparticipating fee schedule. This amount—115 percent of the fee listed in the nonPAR MFS—is called the **limiting charge**.

For a claim that is not assigned, the provider can collect the full payment of the limiting charge from the patient at the time of the visit. The claim is then submitted to Medicare. If approved, Medicare will pay 80 percent of the allowed amount on the nonPAR fee schedule—not the limiting amount. Medicare sends this payment directly to the patient, since the physician has already been paid.

Example

The following example illustrates the different fee structures for PARs, nonPARs who accept assignment, and nonPARs who do not accept assignment.

Participating Provider	
Physician's standard fee	$120.00
Medicare fee	$60.00
Medicare pays 80% ($60.00 × 80%)	$48.00
Patient or supplemental plan pays 20% ($60.00 × 20%)	$12.00
Provider adjustment (write-off) ($120.00 − $60.00)	$60.00
Nonparticipating Provider (Accepts Assignment)	
Physician's standard fee	$120.00
Medicare nonPAR fee ($60.00 − 5%)	$57.00
Medicare pays 80% ($57.00 × 80%)	$45.60
Patient or supplemental plan pays 20% ($57.00 × 20%)	$11.40
Provider adjustment (write-off) ($120.00 − $57.00)	$63.00
Nonparticipating Provider (Does Not Accept Assignment)	
Physician's standard fee	$120.00
Medicare nonPAR fee ($60.00 − 5%)	$57.00
Limiting charge (115% × $57.00)	$65.55
Patient billed	$65.55
Medicare pays patient (80% × $57.00)	$45.60
Total provider can collect	$65.55
Patient out-of-pocket expense ($65.55 − $45.60)	$19.95

✓ Compliance Tip

Physicians must accept assignment for clinical diagnostic laboratory services (generally, procedures with CPT codes in the 80000s). A physician may not bill Medicare patients for these services. If the physician does not accept Medicare assignment for them, the right to bill the patient is forfeited. The physician may accept assignment for laboratory services only and refuse to accept assignment for other services. In this case, two separate claims may be filed. One claim accepts assignment for laboratory services, and the other refuses assignment for other services.

Physicians who treat Medicare beneficiaries must file claims for their patients even if they do not participate and do not accept assignment on the claims. CMS mandates electronic transmission of Medicare claims using the HIPAA 837 format, except by very small practices.

Filing Medicare claims is similar to filing claims for other plans, with one main exception. Procedure codes for Medicare claims come from the Healthcare Common Procedure Coding System (HCPCS). As covered in Chapter 4, this coding system is made up of CPT codes and national codes. As with CPT codes, HCPCS codes may use modifiers. These modifiers are different from CPT modifiers. The medical insurance specialist must be careful to use CPT modifiers with CPT codes and HCPCS modifiers with HCPCS codes.

Professional Focus

Medicare's Correct Coding Initiative and Medically Unlikely Edits

Medicare's National Correct Coding Council develops correct coding guidelines in order to control improper procedural coding in Part B claims. This council issues policies, called the **Correct Coding Initiative (CCI),** to correct two types of errors: (1) unintentional coding errors resulting from a misunderstanding of coding, and (2) intentionally incorrect coding done to increase payments. CCI guidelines are part of the automatic edits for electronic claims.

Since CCI has been in place, Medicare claim rejections have multiplied. The most common cause for rejection is unbundling, a term for breaking out and separately reporting procedures that should be reported under a single procedure code. Under CCI, when services are provided to a beneficiary by a single physician on a single day, the coder must double-check for any bundled codes (see Chapter 4)

that may apply. Entering the correct codes on claims saves the medical office time and money in resubmitting rejected claims.

In 2007, CMS established units of service edits, referred to as **medically unlikely edits (MUEs),** in order to lower the Medicare fee-for-service paid claims error rate. MUEs are intended to reduce the number of health care claims that are sent back simply because of clerical or practice management program (PMP) errors.

MUEs are edits that test a claim for the same beneficiary, CPT code, date of service, and billing provider against Medicare's rule. The initial set of MUEs is based on anatomical considerations. An example is an MUEs edit that rejects a claim for a hysterectomy on a male patient. MUEs also automatically reject claim items containing units of service billed in excess of Medicare allowances.

Timely Filing

Medicare law sets specific guidelines for **timely filing** of claims for benefits. Claims should be filed no later than the end of the calendar year following the year in which the service was furnished, except as follows:

- The time limit on filing claims for service furnished in the last three months of a year is the same as if the services had been furnished in the subsequent year. Thus, the time limit on filing claims for services

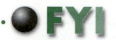
furnished in the last three months of the year is December 31 of the second year following the year in which the services were rendered.

- When the last day for timely filing of a claim falls on a Saturday, Sunday, or federal non-workday or legal holiday, the filing will be considered timely if the claim is filed on the next workday.

For example, a patient received surgery in August 2009. The claim for payment must be filed on or before December 31, 2010. A service provided in October 2009 must be filed on or before December 31, 2011. A claim received by a carrier more than one year after the service has been rendered is subject to a 10 percent reduction.

Not Medically Necessary Services and Excluded Services

Medicare does not provide coverage for certain services and procedures. Claims will be denied for services that are not considered reasonable and necessary for the patient and for services that are excluded by Medicare.

Advance Beneficiary Notice

Participating physicians agree to not bill patients for services that Medicare declares as being not reasonable and necessary unless the patients were informed ahead of time in writing and agreed to pay for the services. **Local coverage determinations (LCDs)** and **national coverage determinations (NCDs)** issued by Medicare help sort out medical necessity issues. LCDs (formerly called Local Medicare Review Policies, or LMRPs) and NCDs contain detailed and updated information about the coding and medical necessity of specific services, including:

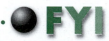
- A description of the service.
- A list of indications (instances in which the service is deemed medically necessary).
- The appropriate CPT/HCPCS code.
- The appropriate ICD-9-CM code.
- A bibliography containing recent clinical articles to support the Medicare policy.

If a provider thinks that a procedure will not be covered by Medicare because it is not reasonable and necessary, the patient is notified of this before the treatment by means of a standard **advance beneficiary notice of noncoverage (ABN)** from CMS (see Figure 9-2). A filled-in form is given to the patient for signature. The ABN form is designed to:

- Identify the service or item that Medicare is unlikely to pay for.
- State the reason Medicare is unlikely to pay.
- Show the patient an estimate of how much the service or item will cost the beneficiary if Medicare does not pay.

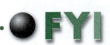
The purpose of the ABN is to help the beneficiary make an informed decision about services that might have to be paid out-of-pocket. A provider who could have been expected (by Medicare) to know that a service would

(B) Patient Name:	(C) Identification Number:

ADVANCE BENEFICIARY NOTICE OF NONCOVERAGE (ABN)

NOTE: If Medicare doesn't pay for **(D)**_____ below, you may have to pay.

Medicare does not pay for everything, even some care that you or your health care provider have good reason to think you need. We expect Medicare may not pay for the **(D)**_____ below.

(D)_____	(E) Reason Medicare May Not Pay:	(F) Estimated Cost:

WHAT YOU NEED TO DO NOW:

- Read this notice, so you can make an informed decision about your care.
- Ask us any questions that you may have after you finish reading.
- Choose an option below about whether to receive the **(D)**_____listed above.
  Note: If you choose Option 1 or 2, we may help you to use any other insurance that you might have, but Medicare cannot require us to do this.

(G) OPTIONS:	Check only one box. We cannot choose a box for you.

❑ **OPTION 1.** I want the **(D)**_____ listed above. You may ask to be paid now, but I also want Medicare billed for an official decision on payment, which is sent to me on a Medicare Summary Notice (MSN). I understand that if Medicare doesn't pay, I am responsible for payment, but **I can appeal to Medicare** by following the directions on the MSN. If Medicare does pay, you will refund any payments I made to you, less co-pays or deductibles.

❑ **OPTION 2.** I want the **(D)**_____ listed above, but do not bill Medicare. You may ask to be paid now as I am responsible for payment. **I cannot appeal if Medicare is not billed.**

❑ **OPTION 3.** I don't want the **(D)**_____listed above. I understand with this choice I am **not** responsible for payment, and **I cannot appeal to see if Medicare would pay.**

(H) Additional Information:

This notice gives our opinion, not an official Medicare decision. If you have other questions on this notice or Medicare billing, call **1-800-MEDICARE** (1-800-633-4227/**TTY**: 1-877-486-2048).

Signing below means that you have received and understand this notice. You also receive a copy.

(I) Signature:	(J) Date:

According to the Paperwork Reduction Act of 1995, no persons are required to respond to a collection of information unless it displays a valid OMB control number. The valid OMB control number for this information collection is 0938-0566. The time required to complete this information collection is estimated to average 7 minutes per response, including the time to review instructions, search existing data resources, gather the data needed, and complete and review the information collection. If you have comments concerning the accuracy of the time estimate or suggestions for improving this form, please write to: CMS, 7500 Security Boulevard, Attn: PRA Reports Clearance Officer, Baltimore, Maryland 21244-1850.

Form CMS-R-131 (03/08)   Form Approved OMB No. 0938-0566

Figure 9-2 Advance Beneficiary Notice of Noncoverage

not be covered and who performed the service without informing the patient could be liable for the charges.

When provided, the ABN must be verbally reviewed with the beneficiary or his/her representative and questions posed during that discussion must be answered before the form is signed. The form must be provided in advance to allow the beneficiary or representative time to consider options and make an informed choice. The ABN may be delivered by employees or subcontractors of the provider, and is not required in an emergency situation. After the form has been completely filled in and signed, a copy is given to the beneficiary or his or her representative. In all cases, the provider must retain the original notice on file.

Excluded Services

Participating providers may bill patients for services that are not covered by the Medicare program, such as routine physicals and many screening tests. Giving a patient written notification that Medicare will not pay for a service before providing it is a good policy, although it is not required. When patients are notified ahead of time, they understand their financial responsibility to pay for the service. The ABN form may be used for this type of voluntary notification. In this case, the purpose of the ABN is to advise beneficiaries, before they receive services that are not Medicare benefits, that Medicare will not pay for them and to provide beneficiaries with an estimate of how much they may have to pay.

Physician Quality Reporting Initiative (PQRI)

The **Physician Quality Reporting Initiative (PQRI)** is a voluntary quality reporting program established by CMS in which physicians or other eligible professionals collect and report their practice data in relation to a set of patient-care performance measures that are established annually. The program's goal is to determine best practices, define measures, support improvement, and improve systems. For example, the 2008 PQRI program had 119 possible measurements.

Physicians who successfully report are eligible for an additional 1.5 percent payment from CMS. The PQRI incentive is an all-or-nothing lump-sum payment. The provider must meet the basic requirement of reporting at least 80 percent of the time on up to three measures applicable to the professionals' practice. If more than three quality measures are applicable, the professional need only report on three.

Not every medical specialty has performance measures that apply. To implement the program, practices identify the measures that affect the greatest number of their patients. Once the measures are chosen, coders are trained to assign the applicable quality codes. These codes include CPT Category II codes (see Chapter 5), which are supplemental codes that can be used to facilitate data collection relating to certain quality of care indicators, such as prenatal care, tobacco use cessation, and assessment of hydration status. PQRI also requires using some HCPCS G codes to allow reporting of certain clinical topics that do not have CPT Category II codes assigned as yet.

To assist physicians and other eligible professionals who elect to participate in this program, the American Medical Association (along with CMS, Mathematica Policy Research, Inc., and the National Committee for Quality Assurance) has developed participation tools. The tools are designed to:

- Aid physicians wishing to participate in the program to identify measures relevant to their practice.
- Facilitate the data collection required to report clinical performance data.

These worksheets, located on the AMA website (www.AMA-assn.org), contain these items, which can be printed out:

1. Measure description: An informational sheet is available for each measure in the PQRI program.
2. Data collection sheet: For each measure in the PQRI program, the data collection sheet provides a step-by-step tool for clinical use and office/billing staff use, allowing the physician to record the clinical information required for the measure by checking the

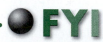

FYI

The PQRI establishes a *structural* quality measure that rewards physicians who use electronic health records and electronic prescribing.

FYI

PQRI codes are reported on claims even though they have no direct monetary value. Depending on the contractor, either $0.00 or $0.01 is used because claim processing systems require some value to be attached to codes.

appropriate box, and the coder to subsequently select the corresponding billing code.

3. Code specifications: A complete list of ICD-9 (International Classification of Diseases, Ninth Revision) and CPT® (Current Procedural Terminology) codes to identify patients eligible for the measure. A list of the quality codes for each measure is also included. The coding specifications document is to be used in conjunction with the data collection sheet to determine the appropriate code or combination of codes to be reported.

WHO PAYS FIRST?

Many beneficiaries choose to buy **Medigap insurance** policies from federally approved private insurance carriers to fill gaps in Medicare coverage. Generally, the plan pays the beneficiary's deductibles and coinsurance. Some policies also cover services Medicare does not.

Note that Medicare beneficiaries enrolled in managed care plans usually do not need Medigap insurance. Their plans have the same benefits that Medigap policies offer without an additional premium.

If a beneficiary has Medigap insurance, Medicare is the **primary payer.** That means that Medicare pays first, and then the Medigap carrier determines its obligations. File the claim with Medicare first. Some individuals are eligible for both Medicaid and Medicare (**Medi-Medi beneficiary**). Claims for these patients are first submitted to Medicare. Then they are sent to Medicaid along with the Medicare Remittance Notice. Most Medicare carriers transmit these **crossover claims** to the state Medicaid payer automatically.

In some situations, Medicare is the **secondary payer.** Generally, these situations are related to accidents or job-related illnesses or injuries. Medicare is a secondary payer when:

- The patient is covered through an employer's group health plan or the spouse's employer's group health plan.
- The services are for treatment of a work-related illness or injury covered by workers' compensation or federal black lung benefits.
- No-fault insurance or liability insurance covers the services, such as those for illness or injury resulting from an automobile accident.
- A patient with end-stage renal disease is covered by an employer's group health plan. In this case, Medicare is the secondary payer for the first eighteen months.

For Medicare patients in these situations, file first with the other insurance plan and then with Medicare. When completing the Medicare claim, indicate the type of insurance that is primary, using the claim filing indicator code as specified in the HIPAA 837 claim guidelines. The primary remittance advice is sent with the claim to Medicare. Sometimes the CMS-1500 is used to send secondary claims to Medicare. If required, the paper form should be completed as shown in Table 9-1 (on page 196–198) and illustrated in Figure 9-3 (on page 199).

Table 9-1 Medicare Summary of CMS-1500 Claim Completion

Form Locator	Content
1	Indicate Medicare; if the patient has other primary insurance and Medicare is the secondary payer (MSP), select Medicare along with the Group Health Plan or Other box.
1a	Enter the Medicare health insurance claim number that appears on the patient's Medicare card.
2	Record the patient's name *exactly* as it appears on the Medicare card, entering it in last name, first name, middle initial order. Do not use any punctuation or abbreviations. Do not put any spaces within the last name; for example, Joan A. Van Doren is entered as Vandoren Joan A.
3	Enter the patient's date of birth in eight-digit format; make the appropriate selection for male or female.
4	Enter the name of the individual whose other insurance may pay primary to Medicare. If the insured and the patient are the same person, enter SAME.
5	Enter the patient's mailing address, including the number and street, city, state, ZIP code, and the home telephone number.
6	Select the appropriate box for the relationship: self, spouse, child, or other. *Self* means that the patient is the policyholder. *Other* includes an unmarried domestic partner.
7	If FL 4 is SAME, leave this blank. If FL 4 is completed and the insured's address is the same as the patient's, enter SAME. If the insured's address is different, enter the mailing address and telephone number of the person listed in FL 4.
8	Select the appropriate boxes for marital status and employment status. Select Other for patients who are unmarried domestic partners or who are covered under a child's plan. If the patient is neither employed nor a student, leave the employment status box blank.
9	FLs 9–9D refer to Medigap policies. Form locator 9 is completed when a Medicare patient agrees to assign benefits of a Medigap policy to a Medicare participating provider. If the policyholder of the Medigap coverage is not the patient, enter the insured's name. If a Medicare patient has a secondary insurance plan that is not Medigap, form locator 9 should be left blank. Medicare forwards claims for these policies directly to the secondary carriers, as long as the carrier has a contract with Medicare. If the supplemental carrier does not have a contract with Medicare, the patient is responsible for submitting the claim to the supplemental carrier once a MSN is received.
9A	Medigap, Mgap, or MG followed by the policy number.
9B	Medigap policyholder's date of birth.
9C	Claims processing address for the Medigap insurer, which is usually found on the enrollee's Medigap identification card.
9D	Medigap insurance plan name or the Medigap insurer's identifier.
10a–10c	Choose the appropriate box to indicate whether the patient's condition is the result of a work injury, an automobile accident, or another type of accident. If any Yes is selected, the claim should be sent first to the liable party (workers' compensation, auto insurance, or other) and then a secondary claim sent to the Medicare. The state postal code must be shown if Yes is checked in FL 10b for Auto Accident.
10d	Varies with the insurance plan; complete if instructed.
11	FL 11 indicates whether the patient has any insurance primary to Medicare. If there is no plan primary to Medicare, enter None. If there is coverage primary to Medicare, the insured's policy identification number is entered, and FLs 11a–11c must also be completed.
11a	For MSP, enter the policyholder's date of birth and sex if they differ from the information in FL 3.

11b	If the policy is obtained through an employer or a school, enter the name in FL 11b; otherwise leave it blank. If the patient's employment status has changed—for example, if the patient has retired—enter Retired followed by the retirement date.
11c	Name and address of the primary carrier.
11d	Leave blank.
12	Enter Signature on File or SOF to indicate that there is a signature on file authorizing release of information of any medical or other information necessary to process and/or adjudicate the claim. If not, a legal signature for the patient should be entered and dated.
13	Blank or enter Signature on File or SOF to indicate that there is a signature on file assigning benefits to the provider if another plan is primary.
14	Enter the date documented in the medical record that symptoms first began for the current illness, injury, or pregnancy. For pregnancy, enter the first date of the last menstrual period (LMP). Previous pregnancies are not a similar illness. If a Medicare patient is receiving chiropractic services, enter the date that this course of treatment began.
15	Leave blank.
16	Enter the dates the patient is employed but unable to work in the current occupation (From: the first full day of disability; To: the last day of disability before returning to work).
17	Enter the name (first name, middle initial, last name) and credentials of the professional who referred or ordered the services or supplies on the claim.
17a	Enter the appropriate identifying number(s) (either NPI or non-NPI, a payer-assigned unique identifier) for the referring physician.
18	If the services provided are needed because of a related inpatient hospitalization, the admission and discharge dates are entered. For patients still hospitalized, the admission date is listed in the From box, and the To box is left blank.
19	Complete according to the MAC's instructions.
20	Complete if billing for outside lab services. Choosing No means that tests were performed by the billing physician or laboratory. Choosing Yes means that the test was done outside of the office of the physician who is billing for it. When Yes is selected, enter the purchase charge and complete FL 32. When billing for multiple purchased lab services, each service should be submitted on a separate claim.
21	Enter up to eight ICD-9-CM codes in priority order. At least one code must be reported. Relate lines 1, 2, 3, 4 to the lines of service in FL 24e by line number. Do not provide narrative description in this box. The codes used should specify the highest level of detail possible, including the use of a fifth digit when appropriate.
22	Leave blank; Medicaid-specific.
23	Enter the preauthorization number assigned by the payer or a CLIA (clinical laboratory) number.
24	The service line information section is used to report the procedures performed for the patient. Each item of service line information has a procedure code and a charge, with additional information as detailed below.
24A	Enter the from and to date(s) of service. If there is only one date of service, enter that date under From, and leave To blank or reenter the From date. If grouping services, the place of service, procedure code, charges, and individual provider for each line must be identical for that service line. Grouping is allowed only for services on consecutive days. The number of days must correspond to the number of units in FL 24G.
24B	Enter the place of service (POS) code that describes the location at which the service was provided. If the service was provided to a hospitalized inpatient (POS 21), enter the hospital's provider information in FL 32.
24C	Check with the payer to determine whether this element (emergency indicator) is necessary. If required, enter Y (yes) or N (No) in the unshaded bottom portion of the field.
24D	Enter the CPT and/or HCPCS codes and applicable modifiers for services provided. Do not use hyphens.

24E	Using the numbers (1, 2, 3, 4) listed to the left of the diagnosis codes in FL 21, enter the diagnosis for the each service listed in FL 24D.
24F	For each service listed in FL 24D, enter charges without dollar signs or decimals. If the claim reports an encounter with no charge, such as a capitated visit, a value of zero (0) may be used.
24G	Enter the number of days or units, as applicable. This field is most commonly used for multiple visits, units of supplies, anesthesia units or minutes, or oxygen volume. If only one service is performed, the numeral 1 must be entered.
24H	Leave blank; Medicaid-specific.
24I–24J	FL 24I and FL 24J work together. These boxes are used to enter an ID number for the rendering provider of the service. If the number is an NPI, it goes in FL 24J in the nonshaded area next to the 24I NPI label. If the number is a non-NPI (other ID number), the qualifier identifying the type of number goes in FL 24I next to the number in 24J.
25	Enter the physician's or supplier's federal tax identification number (either a Social Security number or an Employer Identification Number). Check the appropriate box for SSN or EIN.
26	Enter the patient account number used by the practice's accounting system.
27	If the physician accepts assignment, select Yes. If the patient is also covered by a Medigap plan and the patient has authorized payment directly to the provider, the provider must also be a Medicare participating physician and must accept assignment.
28	Enter the total of all charges in FL 24F. If the claim is to be submitted on paper and there are more services to be billed, put *continued* here, and put the total charge on the last claim form page.
29	Amount of the payments received for the services listed on this claim. If no payment was made, enter none or 0.00.
30	Enter the balance resulting from subtracting the amount in FL 29 from the amount in FL 28.
31	Enter the provider's or supplier's signature (or "Signature on File" or SOF), the date of the signature, and the provider's credentials (such as MD).
32	Enter the name, address, city, state, and ZIP code of the location where the services were rendered if not the physician's office or the patient's home. Physicians billing for purchased diagnostic tests must identify the supplier's name, address, ZIP code, and NPI in FL 32a. FL 32b is left blank.
33	Enter the billing provider's or supplier's name, address, ZIP code, telephone number, and NPI in FL 33a. FL 33b is left blank.

1500

HEALTH INSURANCE CLAIM FORM

APPROVED BY NATIONAL UNIFORM CLAIM COMMITTEE 08/05

PICA		PICA

1. MEDICARE [X] (Medicare #)   **MEDICAID** [ ] (Medicaid #)   **TRICARE CHAMPUS** [ ] (Sponsor's SSN)   **CHAMPVA** [ ] (Member ID#)   **GROUP HEALTH PLAN** [ ] (SSN or ID)   **FECA BLK LUNG** [ ] (SSN)   **OTHER** [ ] (ID)

1a. INSURED'S I.D. NUMBER (For Program in Item 1)
456221234A

2. PATIENT'S NAME (Last Name, First Name, Middle Initial)
NAPJER, JOHN, D

3. PATIENT'S BIRTH DATE MM DD YY **05 05 1938** SEX M [X] F [ ]

4. INSURED'S NAME (Last Name, First Name, Middle Initial)
SAME

5. PATIENT'S ADDRESS (No., Street)
47 CARRIAGE DR

6. PATIENT RELATIONSHIP TO INSURED
Self [X] Spouse [ ] Child [ ] Other [ ]

7. INSURED'S ADDRESS (No., Street)

CITY CHESHIRE   **STATE** CO

8. PATIENT STATUS
Single [ ] Married [X] Other [ ]
Employed [ ] Full-Time Student [ ] Part-Time Student [ ]

CITY   **STATE**

ZIP CODE 80034   **TELEPHONE (Include Area Code)** (720)1235555

ZIP CODE   **TELEPHONE (INCLUDE AREA CODE)** ( )

9. OTHER INSURED'S NAME (Last Name, First Name, Middle Initial)

10. IS PATIENT'S CONDITION RELATED TO:

11. INSURED'S POLICY GROUP OR FECA NUMBER

a. OTHER INSURED'S POLICY OR GROUP NUMBER

a. EMPLOYMENT? (CURRENT OR PREVIOUS) [ ] YES [X] NO

a. INSURED'S DATE OF BIRTH MM DD YY SEX M [ ] F [ ]

b. OTHER INSURED'S DATE OF BIRTH MM DD YY SEX M [ ] F [ ]

b. AUTO ACCIDENT? [ ] YES [X] NO PLACE (State)

b. EMPLOYER'S NAME OR SCHOOL NAME

c. EMPLOYER'S NAME OR SCHOOL NAME

c. OTHER ACCIDENT? [ ] YES [X] NO

c. INSURANCE PLAN NAME OR PROGRAM NAME

d. INSURANCE PLAN NAME OR PROGRAM NAME

10d. RESERVED FOR LOCAL USE

d. IS THERE ANOTHER HEALTH BENEFIT PLAN? [ ] YES [ ] NO **If yes**, return to and complete item 9 a-d.

READ BACK OF FORM BEFORE COMPLETING & SIGNING THIS FORM.
12. PATIENT'S OR AUTHORIZED PERSON'S SIGNATURE I authorize the release of any medical or other information necessary to process this claim. I also request payment of government benefits either to myself or to the party who accepts assignment below.

SIGNED **SOF**   DATE

13. INSURED'S OR AUTHORIZED PERSON'S SIGNATURE I authorize payment of medical benefits to the undersigned physician or supplier for services described below.

SIGNED

14. DATE OF CURRENT: MM DD YY **10 01 2010** ◄ ILLNESS (First symptom) OR INJURY (Accident) OR PREGNANCY(LMP)

15. IF PATIENT HAS HAD SAME OR SIMILAR ILLNESS. GIVE FIRST DATE MM DD YY

16. DATES PATIENT UNABLE TO WORK IN CURRENT OCCUPATION FROM MM DD YY TO MM DD YY

17. NAME OF REFERRING PHYSICIAN OR OTHER SOURCE
17a.
17b. NPI

18. HOSPITALIZATION DATES RELATED TO CURRENT SERVICES FROM MM DD YY TO MM DD YY

19. RESERVED FOR LOCAL USE

20. OUTSIDE LAB? [ ] YES [X] NO $ CHARGES

21. DIAGNOSIS OR NATURE OF ILLNESS OR INJURY. (Relate Items 1,2,3 or 4 to Item 24e by Line)
1. **78.06**   3.
2. **78.56**   4.

22. MEDICAID RESUBMISSION CODE   ORIGINAL REF. NO.

23. PRIOR AUTHORIZATION NUMBER

24. A. DATE(S) OF SERVICE From MM DD YY	To MM DD YY	B. PLACE OF SERVICE	C. EMG	D. PROCEDURES, SERVICES, OR SUPPLIES (Explain Unusual Circumstances) CPT/HCPCS	MODIFIER	E. DIAGNOSIS POINTER	F. $ CHARGES	G. DAYS OR UNITS	H. EPSDT Family Plan	I. ID. QUAL.	J. RENDERING PROVIDER ID.#
1	10 02 2010		11		99203		1,2	95 00	1		NPI	8221238999
2											NPI	
3											NPI	
4											NPI	
5											NPI	
6											NPI	

25. FEDERAL TAX I.D. NUMBER SSN [ ] EIN [X]
123459666

26. PATIENT'S ACCOUNT NO.
NAP0123

27. ACCEPT ASSIGNMENT? (For govt. claims, see back) [X] YES [ ] NO

28. TOTAL CHARGE $ **95 00**

29. AMOUNT PAID $ **0 00**

30. BALANCE DUE $ **95 00**

31. SIGNATURE OF PHYSICIAN OR SUPPLIER INCLUDING DEGREES OR CREDENTIALS (I certify that the statements on the reverse apply to this bill and are made a part thereof.)

SIGNED **SOF** DATE

32. SERVICE FACILITY LOCATION INFORMATION
a. NPI   b.

33. BILLING PROVIDER INFO & PHONE # (720) 5541222
CENTER CLINIC
3810 EXECUTIVE BLVD
RAYTOWN CO 80033
a. **4455667788** b.

NUCC Instruction Manual available at: www.nucc.org

Figure 9-3 Example of CMS-1500 for Medicare

Chapter Summary

1. The two major parts of Medicare coverage are Part A, which helps pay for inpatient hospital services, care in a skilled nursing facility, home health care, and hospice care; and Part B, which helps pay for physician services, outpatient hospital services, durable medical equipment, and other services and supplies.

2. Medicare fees are developed from the RBRVS system and are listed in the Medicare Fee Schedule. A participating physician accepts the Medicare Fee Schedule as the allowed charge. A nonPAR physician who accepts assignment is paid from the nonparticipating fee schedule, which is 5 percent lower than the PAR fee. A nonPAR who does not accept assignment is subject to Medicare's charge limits and may not charge a Medicare patient more than 115 percent of the amount listed in the Medicare nonparticipating fee schedule.

3. An excluded service is one that is never covered by Medicare, while a medically unnecessary service may be covered in the appropriate circumstances. Physicians are required to use the advance beneficiary notice of noncoverage (ABN) to inform patients about planned services that Medicare considers medically unnecessary.

4. Medicare is the secondary payer when services are covered by (a) the patient's or spouse's employer's group health plan, (b) workers' compensation or federal black lung benefits, (c) no-fault or liability insurance, or (d) an employer's group health plan for a patient with end-stage renal disease.

Part 1. Write "T" or "F" in the blank to indicate whether you think the statement is true or false.

_____ **1.** A claim for physician services performed in a hospital setting should be filed under Medicare Part A.

_____ **2.** A Medicare participating physician accepts assignment on all Medicare claims.

_____ **3.** The National Provider Identifier is used for Medicare.

_____ **4.** Organizations that handle Medicare Part B claims and payments are known as intermediaries.

_____ **5.** The Correct Coding Initiative provides guidelines for correct coding of procedures.

_____ **6.** Medigap plans are secondary payers.

_____ **7.** Nonparticipating physicians can decide whether to accept assignment on claims on a case-by-case basis.

_____ **8.** Medicare Advantage is another name for the Medicare Prescription Drug, Improvement, and Modernization Act of 2003 that includes a prescription drug benefit.

_____ **9.** Participating and nonparticipating physicians are paid using the same fee schedule.

_____ **10.** Advance beneficiary notices (ABNs) may be used for excluded services as well as for services that may not be deemed reasonable and necessary by Medicare.

Part 2. Choose the best answer.

_____ **1.** Medicare is the federal health care plan for:
    a. mothers with preschool-aged children
    b. people age sixty-five or older and some disabled people
    c. disadvantaged youth

_____ **2.** A Medicare beneficiary enrolled in an HMO does not need:
    a. Medicaid
    b. a Medigap policy
    c. a MediCal policy

_____ **3.** HCPCS is a system to identify:
    a. diagnoses
    b. procedures
    c. both a and b

_____ **4.** A Medicare participating physician may bill a Medicare patient for:
    a. coinsurance
    b. excess charges
    c. neither a nor b

_____ **5.** Medicare is a secondary payer when:
    a. services for the treatment of automobile accident injuries are covered by liability insurance
    b. the patient qualifies for Medicaid
    c. the patient subscribes to a Medicare supplemental health insurance plan

_____ **6.** The payment for a physician's service under Medicare is based on:
    a. the amount set by government mandate
    b. an amount based on what the physician usually charges for the service
    c. an amount based on what area physicians usually charge for the service

_____ **7.** If a Medicare beneficiary is covered by an employer's group health plan, Medicare is:
   a. a primary payer
   b. a secondary payer
   c. not in force

_____ **8.** The Medicare fee-for-service plan is known as:
   a. the Original Medicare Plan
   b. the HMO
   c. Medicare Advantage

_____ **9.** The Medicare Modernization Act provides for:
   a. prescription drug coverage
   b. higher coinsurance
   c. more Medigap plans

_____ **10.** Under Medicare Advantage, beneficiaries can choose to enroll in:
   a. Medical Savings Accounts
   b. Medicare preferred provider organization plans (PPOs)
   c. both a and b

Part 3. Read the cases below and answer the questions.

A.

Physician Information:
Name: Ralph L. Markarian, MD
NPI: 1234567890
Accepts assignment for Medicare patients

Patient Information Form:
Name: Bonita S. Chavez (Established Patient)
Age: 86
Sex: Female
Birth Date: April 16, 1924
Marital Status: Widowed
Employer: Retired
Medicare ID Number: 221-54-3376C
Additional Insurance Carrier: None

Patient's Encounter Form:
Date: 5-20-2010
T-98   BP 140/98
CC: Patient visit for diabetes recheck. Off medications for blood pressure and diabetes. Has lost eight pounds since last visit due to change in diet. Discussed diabetes monitoring and lifestyle changes to maintain weight control.
Dx: Type II diabetes. Elevated blood pressure.

List of Fees for Service:
Charges: Level III office visit, $75
No payment collected.
Note: Deductible has been met for 2010.

Supply the following data elements:

Billing Provider _____

Billing Provider's Primary Identifier _____

Subscriber/Patient _____

Subscriber's Primary Identifier _____

Claim Filing Indicator Code _____

Medicare Assignment Code (A) Assigned C (Not Assigned)

Place of Service Code _____

Diagnosis Codes _____

Total Charge _____

Amount Collected _____

Service Line Information

Date of Service _____

Procedure Code/Charge_____

Diagnosis _____

B.

Physician Information:

Name: William B. Rheingold, MD

NPI: 2345678901

Accepts assignment for Medicare patients

Patient Information Form:

Name: Clair Gibbons (Established Patient)

Sex: Female

Birth Date: July 31, 1935

Marital Status: Single

Employer: Retired

Medicare ID Number: 455-03-7722A

Additional Insurance Carrier: None

Patient's Encounter Form:

Date: October 12, 2010

T-98 BP 120/85

CC: Patient has history of breast cancer; presents with shortness of breath. Ordered chest X-ray in the office, which showed a small pleural effusion on the left. Performed a thoracentesis, drew off fluid; sent for cytology and chemistry analysis.

Dx: Unspecified pleural effusion; personal history of malignant neoplasm of breast.

List of Fees for Service:

Services and Charges:

　Level III office visit, $80

　Thoracentesis, $65

　Radiologic examination, chest, two views, frontal and lateral, $15

No payment collected.

Note: Deductible has been met for 2010.

Supply the following data elements:

Billing Provider _____

Billing Provider's Primary Identifier _____

Subscriber/Patient _____

Subscriber's Primary Identifier _____

Claim Filing Indicator Code _____

Medicare Assignment Code __ (A) Assigned __ C (Not Assigned)

Place of Service Code _____

Diagnosis Codes _____

Total Charge _____

Amount Collected _____

Service Line Information

Date of Service _____

Procedure Code/Charge_____

Diagnosis _____

Date of Service _____

Procedure Code/Charge_____

Diagnosis _____

Date of Service _____

Procedure Code/Charge_____

Diagnosis _____

Part 4. The following information is presented on a patient's Medicare MSN. What does the patient owe?_____

BILL SUBMITTED BY: Dr. Anthony B. Starpish
29 Washington Square North
New York, NY 10011

Date	Services and Service Code	Medicare Charges	Approved
2-10-2010	1 Destruction of hemorrhoids (46934-78)	$325.00	$194.78*

(Note: *The approved amount is based on the fee schedule.)

Explanation:

Of the total charges, Medicare approved	$194.78	(The provider agreed to accept this amount.)
Your 20 percent	− $38.96	
The 80 percent Medicare pays	$155.82	

You have already met the deductible for 2010.

Part 5. Fill in the blanks in the following payment situations.

Participating Provider

Physician's standard fee	$210.00
Medicare fee	$115.00
Medicare pays 80%	$_____
Patient or supplemental plan pays 20%	$_____
Provider adjustment (write-off)	$_____

Nonparticipating Provider (Accepts Assignment)

Physician's standard fee	$210.00
Medicare nonPAR fee	$109.25
Medicare pays 80%	$_____
Patient/supplemental plan pays 20%	$_____
Provider adjustment (write-off)	$_____

Nonparticipating Provider (Does Not Accept Assignment)

Physician's standard fee	$210.00
Medicare nonPAR fee	$109.25
Limiting charge	$_____
Patient billed	$_____
Medicare pays patient	$_____
Total provider can collect	$_____
Patient out-of-pocket expense	$_____

CHAPTER 10 Medicaid

Learning Outcomes

After completing this chapter, you will be able to define the key terms and:

10-1 Identify two ways Medicaid programs vary from state to state.

10-2 List the primary kinds of Medicaid benefits determined by federal law, and give examples of additional benefits that states may authorize.

10-3 Explain two broad classifications of people who are eligible for Medicaid assistance.

10-4 Explain four areas a medical insurance specialist should pay special attention to when filing Medicaid claims.

Key Terms

categorically needy

Early and Periodic Screening, Diagnosis, and Treatment (EPSDT)

Federal Medicaid Assistance Percentage (FMAP)

fiscal agent

Medicaid

MediCal

medically indigent

medically needy

payer of last resort

State Children's Health Insurance Program (SCHIP)

Temporary Assistance for Needy Families (TANF)

third-party liability

Welfare Reform Act

Why This Chapter Is Important to You

The information in this chapter will enable you to:

- Learn who qualifies for Medicaid assistance.
- Become familiar with the kinds of medical services covered by Medicaid programs.
- Learn important procedures for filing claims for Medicaid patients.

What Do You Think?

As an assistance program, Medicaid is federally mandated. However, each state has its own rules and regulations. How can the medical insurance specialist research the state rules that apply? What types of routine or health maintenance services are generally covered by Medicaid?

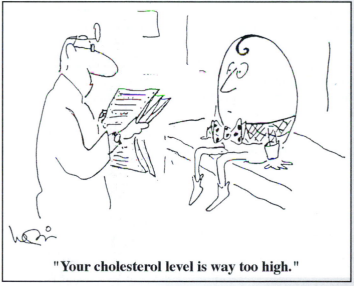

"Your cholesterol level is way too high."

INTRODUCTION TO MEDICAID

M̲ost of the claims that medical insurance specialists file are for benefits due under health insurance plans. However, one government program that pays for health care services is actually an assistance program, not an insurance program.

Medicaid pays for health care services for people with incomes below the national poverty level. Both federal and state governments pay for the program, and in some areas local taxes support it as well. The federal government makes payments to states under the **Federal Medicaid Assistance Percentage (FMAP).** The amount of the payment is based on the state's average per capita income in relation to the national income average. States with high per capita incomes receive less federal funding than do states with low per capita incomes. In each state, Medicaid is administered by a **fiscal agent,** an organization that processes claims for a government program. The Center for Medicaid and State Operations, a department of the Centers for Medicare and Medicaid Services (CMS), oversees the programs that are administered by the states.

The first Medicaid programs were required by federal law as part of the Social Security Act of 1965. Under the legislation, the federal government determines which kinds of medical services are covered and paid for by the federal portion of the program. States participate in their Medicaid programs in two ways: (1) they may authorize additional kinds of services or make additional groups eligible, and (2) they determine eligibility within federal guidelines. Because of this participation by state governments, Medicaid programs change often and vary widely from state to state. Thus, this chapter gives only general information about Medicaid.

A physician may choose to participate in the Medicaid program or not to accept Medicaid patients. Participating in the Medicaid program means agreeing to accept Medicaid reimbursement for covered services as payment in full. The physician must write off the difference, if any, between fees charged for services and the amount reimbursed. The physician may not bill the patient for the difference. However, the physician may bill the patient for services not covered by Medicaid.

> **HIPAA Tip**
>
> **HIPAA Rules Apply**
> The HIPAA Privacy Rule, Electronic Health Care Transaction and Code Sets standards, and Security Rule apply to physicians who are treating Medicaid patients.

MEDICAID COVERAGE

According to federal guidelines, Medicaid pays for the following types of health care:

- Physician services.
- Laboratory and X-ray services.
- Inpatient hospital services.
- Outpatient hospital services.
- Rural health clinic services.
- Home health care.
- Family planning services.
- Federally qualified health-center (FQHC) services.
- Skilled care at a public nursing facility.

- Prenatal and nurse-midwife services.
- Early and Periodic Screening, Diagnosis, and Treatment (EPSDT) services.
- Emergency care.

Family planning services include counseling, diagnosis, treatment, drugs, and supplies related to planning the number and spacing of children. **Early and Periodic Screening, Diagnosis, and Treatment (EPSDT)** is a prevention, early-detection, and treatment program for children under the age of twenty-one who are enrolled in Medicaid. Covered services include medical history; physical exam; assessment of development and immunization status; and screening for anemia, lead absorption, tuberculosis, sickle cell trait and disease, and dental, hearing, and vision problems. States must pay for all services identified in an EPSDT exam, even if they do not pay for the services for other eligible individuals.

The **State Children's Health Insurance Program (SCHIP),** part of the Balanced Budget Act of 1997, requires states to develop and implement plans for health insurance coverage for uninsured children. The more than 5 million children served by SCHIP come from low-income families whose incomes are not low enough to qualify for Medicaid. The program is funded jointly by the federal government and the states. It provides coverage for many preventive services and covers children up to age nineteen.

The Ticket to Work and Work Incentives Improvement Act of 1999 (TWWIIA) expands the availability of health care services for workers with disabilities. Previously, persons with disabilities often had to choose between health care and work. TWWIIA gives states the option of allowing individuals with disabilities to purchase Medicaid coverage that is necessary to enable them to maintain employment.

The state portion of a Medicaid program often includes a number of additional services under its federally funded Medicaid program. Some examples of extra assistance enacted by individual states include:

- Clinic services.
- Emergency room care.
- Ambulance services.
- Chiropractic services.
- Mental-health services.
- Certain cosmetic procedures.
- Allergy services.
- Dermatology services.
- Dental care.
- Home and community-based are to certain persons with chronic impairments.
- Podiatry services.
- Eyeglasses and eye refraction.
- Prescription drugs.
- Prosthetic devices.
- Private-duty nursing.
- Other diagnostic, screening, preventive, and rehabilitative services.

In recent years, however, because of large state budget deficits, state laws have cut back on some of these benefits—for example, prescription drug benefits and hearing, vision, and dental benefits for adults. Many states have also had to restrict eligibility for Medicaid and to reduce Medicaid payments to doctors, hospitals, nursing homes, and other providers.

In each state, the Medicaid and/or social services agency can provide a list of services and any limits or preauthorization requirements for those services. Any additional services, such as those just listed, are paid entirely from state funds.

Professional Focus

Medicaid Fraud and Abuse

The Medicaid Alliance for Program Safeguards is committed to fighting fraud and abuse, which divert dollars that should be spent to safeguard the health and welfare of Medicaid clients. Although states are primarily responsible for policing fraud in the Medicaid program, CMS provides technical assistance, guidance, and oversight in these efforts. Fraud schemes often cross state lines, and CMS strives to improve information sharing among the Medicaid programs and other stakeholders.

Medicaid fraud can take many forms. Here are some of the more common schemes:

- Billing for "phantom patients" who did not really receive services
- Billing for medical services or goods that were not provided
- Billing for old items as if they were new
- Billing for more hours than there are in a day
- Billing for tests that the patient did not need
- Paying kickbacks in exchange for referrals for medical services or goods
- Charging Medicaid for personal expenses not related to caring for a Medicaid client
- Overcharging for health care services or goods that were provided
- Concealing ownership in a related company
- Using false credentials
- Double-billing for health care services or goods that were provided

MEDICAID ELIGIBILITY

Generally, Medicaid recipients are people with low incomes who have children or are over the age of sixty-five, are blind, or have permanent disabilities. Within federal guidelines, states determine income levels and other qualifications for eligibility.

One group of Medicaid recipients is known as **categorically needy.** Their needs are addressed under the Personal Responsibility and Work Opportunity Reconciliation Act of 1996 (P.L. 104-193), commonly known as the **Welfare Reform Act,** which created **Temporary Assistance for Needy Families (TANF).** Eligibility for TANF is determined at the county level. This program helps with living, as opposed to medical, expenses.

Some states extend Medicaid eligibility to include another group of people classified as **medically needy** or **medically indigent.** These

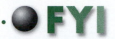

About half of Medicaid beneficiaries are enrolled in HMOs that restrict patients to a network of physicians, hospitals, and clinics. Individuals enrolled in managed care plans must obtain all services and referrals through their primary care physicians (PCPs). The PCP is responsible for coordinating and monitoring the patient's care. If the patient needs to see a specialist, the PCP must provide a referral. Without a referral, Medicaid will not pay for the service.

individuals earn enough money to pay for basic living expenses, but they cannot afford high medical bills. In some cases, Medicaid recipients in the medically needy classification must pay deductibles before they receive benefits. Some Medicaid recipients in this category must pay coinsurance for medical services. States choose their own names for the programs. For example, California calls its program **MediCal.**

Once Medicaid eligibility is determined, the recipient gets an identification card or coupon explaining effective dates and additional information such as a coinsurance requirement, if any. Different states authorize coverage for different lengths of time. Some states issue cards twice a month, some once a month, and others every two months or every six months. Most states, however, are moving to electronic verification of eligibility under the Electronic Medicaid Eligibility Verification System (EMEVS). Eligibility should be checked each time a patient makes an appointment and before the patient sees the physician. Many states provide both online and telephone verification systems.

FILING MEDICAID CLAIMS

Medicaid claims are filed in the patient's home state. Because Medicaid is covered by HIPAA, Medicaid claims are usually submitted using the HIPAA 837 claim (see Chapter 6). In some situations, however, a paper claim using the CMS-1500 format may be used, or a state-specific form may be requested. If the CMS-1500 is required, follow the guidelines in Table 10-1 and complete the form as shown in Figure 10-1 (page 213). HCPCS codes (level I and II) are used for the procedures. In each state, the fiscal agent provides the rules for submitting claims. The website for each state is shown in Table 10-2 (on page 214).

Table 10-1 Medicaid CMS-1500 Claim Completion Form

Locator	Data
1	Choose Medicaid
1a	Medicaid ID number
2	Patient's name
3	Patient's eight-digit date of birth and gender
4	Blank
5	Patient's address
6	Blank
7	Blank
8	Blank
9	Blank
9a	Blank
9b	Blank
9c	Blank
9d	Blank
10a–10c	Choose Appropriate Box
10d	Blank

(Table 10-1 Continued)

11	Blank
11a	Blank
11b	Blank
11c	Blank
11d	Blank
12	Blank; signature not required
13	Blank; signature not required
14	Blank
15	Blank
16	Blank
17	Name/credentials of referring/ordering physician
17a	Provider's NPI/Medicaid ID number
18	Complete as appropriate
19	Complete according to state guidelines
20	Choose No
21	Appropriate ICD codes
22	Complete for resubmissions
23	Preauthorization/precertification number
24A	Dates of service (eight-digit format); no consecutive dates permitted
24B	Appropriate POS code
24C	Emergency indicator, if required
24D	Appropriate CPT/HCPCS codes with up to three modifiers
24E	Diagnosis key number for CPT/HCPCS codes
24F	Amount charged
24G	Appropriate days/units reported; use "1" if a single service
24H	Enter appropriate codes if services provided under EPSDT (varies by state)
24I–24J	NPI/other ID number for rendering provider
25	State guidelines.
26	Patient's account number
27	Choose Yes
28	Total of charges in FL 24F
29	Blank or $0.00
30	State guidelines
31	Provider's signature/date or "Signature on file" or SOF
32	Appropriate name/address of facility where services where rendered if other than provider's office or patient's home.
33	Billing provider's name, address, and NPI/Medicaid ID number

HEALTH INSURANCE CLAIM FORM

APPROVED BY NATIONAL UNIFORM CLAIM COMMITTEE 08/05

CARRIER

| | | PICA | | | | | | PICA | |

1. MEDICARE (Medicare #) □ **MEDICAID** (Medicaid #) ☒ **TRICARE CHAMPUS** (Sponsor's SSN) □ **CHAMPVA** (Member ID#) □ **GROUP HEALTH PLAN** (SSN or ID) □ **FECA BLK LUNG** (SSN) □ **OTHER** (ID) □   **1a. INSURED'S I.D. NUMBER** (For Program in Item 1)
80512D

2. PATIENT'S NAME (Last Name, First Name, Middle Initial)
JONES, SAMANTHA

3. PATIENT'S BIRTH DATE MM 11 DD 20 YY 1950 **SEX** M □ F ☒

4. INSURED'S NAME (Last Name, First Name, Middle Initial)

5. PATIENT'S ADDRESS (No., Street)
1124 BEST ST

6. PATIENT RELATIONSHIP TO INSURED
Self □ Spouse □ Child □ Other □

7. INSURED'S ADDRESS (No., Street)

CITY RAYTOWN **STATE** CO

8. PATIENT STATUS
Single □ Married □ Other □
Employed □ Full-Time Student □ Part-Time Student □

CITY **STATE**

ZIP CODE 80034 **TELEPHONE (Include Area Code)** (720) 1045555

ZIP CODE **TELEPHONE (INCLUDE AREA CODE)** ( )

9. OTHER INSURED'S NAME (Last Name, First Name, Middle Initial)

10. IS PATIENT'S CONDITION RELATED TO:

11. INSURED'S POLICY GROUP OR FECA NUMBER

a. OTHER INSURED'S POLICY OR GROUP NUMBER

a. EMPLOYMENT? (CURRENT OR PREVIOUS)
YES □ NO ☒

a. INSURED'S DATE OF BIRTH MM DD YY **SEX** M □ F □

b. OTHER INSURED'S DATE OF BIRTH MM DD YY **SEX** M □ F □

b. AUTO ACCIDENT? PLACE (State)
YES □ NO ☒

b. EMPLOYER'S NAME OR SCHOOL NAME

c. EMPLOYER'S NAME OR SCHOOL NAME

c. OTHER ACCIDENT?
YES □ NO ☒

c. INSURANCE PLAN NAME OR PROGRAM NAME

d. INSURANCE PLAN NAME OR PROGRAM NAME

10d. RESERVED FOR LOCAL USE

d. IS THERE ANOTHER HEALTH BENEFIT PLAN?
YES □ NO □ *If yes*, return to and complete item 9 a-d.

READ BACK OF FORM BEFORE COMPLETING & SIGNING THIS FORM.
12. PATIENT'S OR AUTHORIZED PERSON'S SIGNATURE I authorize the release of any medical or other information necessary to process this claim. I also request payment of government benefits either to myself or to the party who accepts assignment below.

SIGNED _____ DATE _____

13. INSURED'S OR AUTHORIZED PERSON'S SIGNATURE I authorize payment of medical benefits to the undersigned physician or supplier for services described below.

SIGNED _____

PATIENT AND INSURED INFORMATION

14. DATE OF CURRENT: MM DD YY ◄ ILLNESS (First symptom) OR INJURY (Accident) OR PREGNANCY(LMP)

15. IF PATIENT HAS HAD SAME OR SIMILAR ILLNESS. GIVE FIRST DATE MM DD YY

16. DATES PATIENT UNABLE TO WORK IN CURRENT OCCUPATION FROM MM DD YY TO MM DD YY

17. NAME OF REFERRING PHYSICIAN OR OTHER SOURCE
17a.
17b. NPI

18. HOSPITALIZATION DATES RELATED TO CURRENT SERVICES FROM MM DD YY TO MM DD YY

19. RESERVED FOR LOCAL USE

20. OUTSIDE LAB? $ CHARGES
YES □ NO ☒

21. DIAGNOSIS OR NATURE OF ILLNESS OR INJURY. (Relate Items 1,2,3 or 4 to Item 24e by Line)
1. 84.31
2.
3.
4.

22. MEDICAID RESUBMISSION CODE ORIGINAL REF. NO.

23. PRIOR AUTHORIZATION NUMBER

24. A. DATE(S) OF SERVICE From MM DD YY	To MM DD YY	B. PLACE OF SERVICE	C. EMG	D. PROCEDURES, SERVICES, OR SUPPLIES (Explain Unusual Circumstances) CPT/HCPCS	MODIFIER	E. DIAGNOSIS POINTER	F. $ CHARGES	G. DAYS OR UNITS	H. EPSDT Family Plan	I. ID. QUAL.	J. RENDERING PROVIDER ID.#
1	12 10 2010		11		99213		1	90 00	1		NPI	2121000899
2											NPI	
3											NPI	
4											NPI	
5											NPI	
6											NPI	

PHYSICIAN OR SUPPLIER INFORMATION

25. FEDERAL TAX I.D. NUMBER SSN □ EIN □

26. PATIENT'S ACCOUNT NO.
JON0010

27. ACCEPT ASSIGNMENT? (For govt. claims, see back)
YES ☒ NO □

28. TOTAL CHARGE $

29. AMOUNT PAID $

30. BALANCE DUE $

31. SIGNATURE OF PHYSICIAN OR SUPPLIER INCLUDING DEGREES OR CREDENTIALS (I certify that the statements on the reverse apply to this bill and are made a part thereof.)
Julie Groat MD
SIGNED 12/12/2010 DATE

32. SERVICE FACILITY LOCATION INFORMATION
a. NPI b.

33. BILLING PROVIDER INFO & PHONE # (720) 5541222
CENTER CLINIC
3810 EXECUTIVE BLVD
RAYTOWN CO 80033
a. 4455667788 b.

NUCC Instruction Manual available at: www.nucc.org

Figure 10-1 Sample Medicaid CMS-1500 Claim

Table 10-2 Medicaid Websites by State

State	Abbr.	Website
ALABAMA	AL	*http://www.medicaid.state.al.us/*
ALASKA	AK	*http://www.hss.state.ak.us/dhcs/Medicaid/*
ARIZONA	AZ	*http://www.ahcccs.state.az.us/site/*
ARKANSAS	AR	*http://www.medicaid.state.ar.us/*
CALIFORNIA	CA	*http://www.dhs.ca.gov/mcs/*
COLORADO	CO	*http://www.chcpf.state.co.us/default.asp*
CONNECTICUT	CT	*http://www.ct.gov/dss/*
DELAWARE	DE	*http://www.dhss.delaware.gov/*
DISTRICT OF COLUMBIA	DC	*http://doh.dc.gov/doh/site/default.asp*
FLORIDA	FL	*http://www.fdhc.state.fl.us/Medicaid/*
GEORGIA	GA	*http://dch.georgia.gov*
HAWAII	HI	*http://med-quest.us/*
IDAHO	ID	*http://www.healthandwelfare.idaho.gov/*
ILLINOIS	IL	*http://www.hfs.illinois.gov/medical/*
INDIANA	IN	*http://www.state.in.us/*
IOWA	IA	*http://www.dhs.state.ia.us/*
KANSAS	KS	*http://da.state.ks.us/hpf/*
KENTUCKY	KY	*http://chfs.ky.gov*
LOUISIANA	LA	*http://www.dhh.state.la.us/*
MAINE	ME	*http://www.maine.gov/*
MARYLAND	MD	*http://www.dhmh.state.md.us/*
MASSACHUSETTS	MA	*http://www.mass.gov/*
MICHIGAN	MI	*http://www.Michigan.gov/mdch*
MINNESOTA	MN	*http://www.dhs.state.mn.us/*
MISSISSIPPI	MS	*http://www.medicaid.state.ms.us/*
MISSOURI	MO	*http://www.dss.mo.gov/*
MONTANA	MT	*http://www.dphhs.mt.gov*
NEBRASKA	NE	*http://hhs.state.ne.us/*
NEVADA	NV	*http://dhcfp.state.nv.us/*
NEW HAMPSHIRE	NH	*http://www.dhhs.state.nh.us/*
NEW JERSEY	NJ	*http://www.state.nj.us/*
NEW MEXICO	NM	*http://www.state.nm.us/*
NEW YORK	NY	*http://www.health.state.ny.us/*
NORTH CAROLINA	NC	*http://www.dhhs.state.nc.us/*
NORTH DAKOTA	ND	*http://www.nd.gov/humanservices/*
OHIO	OH	*http://jfs.ohio.gov/ohp/*
OKLAHOMA	OK	*http://www.ohca.state.ok.us/*
OREGON	OR	*http://www.oregon.gov/DHS/*
PENNSYLVANIA	PA	*http://www.dpw.state.pa.us/*
RHODE ISLAND	RI	*http://www.dhs.state.ri.us/*
SOUTH CAROLINA	SC	*http://www.dhhs.state.sc.us/*
SOUTH DAKOTA	SD	*http://www.state.sd.us/*
TENNESSEE	TN	*http://www.state.tn.us/tenncare/*
TEXAS	TX	*http://www.hhsc.state.tx.us/Medicaid/*
UTAH	UT	*http://health.utah.gov/medicaid/*
VERMONT	VT	*http://www.ovha.state.vt.us/medicaid.cfm*
VIRGINIA	VA	*http://www.dmas.virginia.gov/*
WASHINGTON	WA	*http://fortress.wa.gov/dshs/maa/*
WEST VIRGINIA	WV	*http://www.wvdhhr.org/bms/*
WISCONSIN	WI	*http://www.dhfs.state.wi.us/medicaid/*
WYOMING	WY	*http://wyequalitycare.acs-inc.com/*

Medicaid managed care claims are filed differently than other Medicaid claims. Claims are sent to the managed care organization instead of to the state Medicaid department. Participating providers agree to the guidelines of the managed care organization, provided that they are in compliance with federal requirements.

Sometimes a physician in one state treats a patient who lives in another state, either because the patient is traveling or because the patient lives near a state boundary and has easier access to physicians in the neighboring state. Since Medicaid is administered on a state-by-state basis, the Medicaid claim must be filed in the patient's home state. Nevertheless, most Medicaid programs have state-to-state agreements to cover each other's Medicaid patients. The fiscal agent in the patient's home state may be contacted to get forms and claim processing information.

When filing Medicaid claims for any state, the medical insurance specialist should pay special attention to:

- *Eligibility*—Medicaid eligibility varies from month to month if the recipient's income fluctuates. Comply with the state's requirements for verifying eligibility. Check the patient's Medicaid identification card or coupon, and photocopy the front and back on each visit. Date the photocopy. Some states require this photocopy to be attached to the submitted claim form. An example of a Medicaid card is shown in Figure 10-2.

- *Preauthorization*—Most states require preauthorization for specified services. Check with the state's fiscal agent to find out how to get preauthorization by telephone and whether a written confirmation form must also be filed. If the state requires preauthorization, charges for services that did not get prior approval will not be paid. In emergencies, such as emergency room situations, authorization may be obtained after the treatment.

- *Filing Deadline*—The time line for filing a Medicaid claim ranges from two months to one year from the date of service. Find out the state's requirements, and file claims promptly.

- *Third-Party Liability*—**Third-party liability** is the obligation of a government program or insurance plan to pay all or part of a patient's medical costs. Before filing a claim with Medicaid, it is important to determine whether the patient has other insurance coverage.

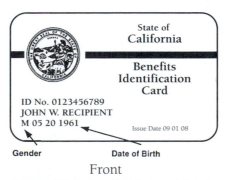

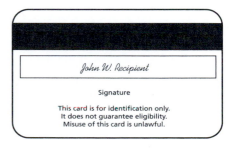

Front   Back

Figure 10-2 Sample Medicaid Card

If a patient who is eligible for Medicaid has additional health care coverage through an insurance plan or another government program such as Medicare, the patient's Medicaid eligibility does not relieve the other program or plan of its responsibility. In fact, the other program or insurance carrier is the primary carrier in these cases. Medicaid is the secondary carrier. File the claim first with the primary carrier, and file for Medicaid benefits last. Because of this sequence, Medicaid is referred to as the **payer of last resort.**

Chapter Summary

1. Medicaid programs differ among states in the services covered and the way eligibility is determined.

2. The federal government requires all states, as participants in the Medicaid program, to provide at least the following services to the categorically needy: (a) physician services, (b) laboratory and X-ray services, (c) inpatient hospital services, (d) outpatient hospital services, (e) rural health clinic services, (f) home health care, (g) family planning services, (h) federally qualified health-center (FQHC) services, (i) skilled care at a public nursing facility, (j) prenatal and nurse-midwife services, (k) Early and Periodic Screening, Diagnosis, and Treatment (EPSDT) services, and (l) emergency care. A state may fund additional services for the categorically needy and may choose to pay for services to the medically needy. Some states may also have medical general assistance programs that provide services to individuals not eligible for the federal Medicaid program.

3. Two broad classifications of people who are eligible for Medicaid are the categorically needy and the medically needy or medically indigent.

4. The four areas a medical insurance specialist should pay particular attention to when filing Medicaid claims are eligibility, preauthorization, filing deadline, and third-party liability.

Part 1. Fill in the answer to each question. Some answers have more than one word.

1. A government program that helps pay living expenses for low-income families and children is known as _____ _____ _____ _____ _____.

2. People who qualify for federal government programs for living expenses are classified as _____ needy.

3. The longest time limit for filing Medicaid claims is one _____ from the date of service.

4. The obligation of a government program or insurance plan to pay all or part of a patient's medical costs is _____ liability.

5. EPSDT services are for children _____ than the age of twenty-one.

6. One of the services authorized for payment with EPSDT funds is a physical _____.

7. In California the Medicaid program is called _____.

8. Medicaid is an assistance program for people with a _____ who are aged, blind, disabled, or pregnant and for members of their families.

9. EPSDT stands for _____ Screening, Diagnosis, and Treatment.

10. Some Medicaid recipients must pay deductibles and _____.

11. Medicaid programs must pay for both outpatient and _____ hospital care for the categorically needy.

12. Within federal guidelines, states determine who is _____ for Medicaid.

13. The federal government revised the rules covering Medicaid eligibility in the _____ Reform Act.

14. SCHIP stands for the _____ Health Insurance Program.

15. FMAP is a _____ program that determines how Medicaid payments are made to the states.

16. If the patient is eligible for Medicaid but has additional health coverage, the other program is the _____ payer.

17. Medicaid is called the _____ of last resort.

18. The _____ coding system is used to report procedures on Medicaid claims.

19. Because Medicaid is under HIPAA, Medicaid claims are usually submitted using the _____ claim.

20. The _____ program covers recipients under age twenty-one who need screening and diagnostic services.

Part 2. Read the cases below and answer the questions.

A.

Physician Information:
Name: Selena R. Rodez, MD
NPI: 8901234567
Medicaid PIN: HC29004

Patient Information Form:
Name: Grace B. Chin (New Patient)
Age: 47
Sex: Female
Birth Date: November 7, 1963
Social Security Number: 056-99-0034

Medicaid Eligibility: June 1-30, 2010 (Note: Copayment of $10 per office visit required.)
Medicaid Number: 056990034
Insurance Carrier: None

Patient''s Encounter Form:
Date: 6-20-2010
T-98 BP 135/80
CC: Patient has cut in the white part of her eye, cause unknown. No visual problems. Reports some pain.
Dx: Eyeball abrasion, left eye.
Rx: Ophthalmic solution, 2 drops to left eye X 10 days.

List of Fees for Service:
Charges: Office visit, Level I, $35
Copayment collected

Supply the following data elements:
Billing Provider _____
Billing Provider's Primary Identifier _____
Billing Provider's Secondary Identifier _____
Subscriber/Patient _____
Subscriber's Primary Identifier _____
Claim Filing Indicator Code _____

Place of Service Code _____
Diagnosis Codes _____
Total Charge _____
Amount Collected _____

Service Line Information
Date of Service _____
Procedure Code/Charge _____
Diagnosis _____

B.

Physician Information:
Name: Gloria A. Poyner, MD
NPI: 9012345678
Medicaid PIN: DC55289

Patient Information Form:
Name: George Eustis Kador (New Patient)
Sex: Male
Birth Date: November 27, 1948
Social Security Number: 033-45-7034
Medicaid Eligibility: July 1–31, 2010 (Note: Copayment of $7.50 per office visit required.)
Medicaid Number: 046971134
Insurance Carrier: None

Patient''s Encounter Form:

Date: 7-7-2010

T-98 BP 135/80

CC: Patient presents with complaint of recent onset of palpitations. Reviewed social and medical history and records. Performed detailed system review and prescribed a twenty-four-hour electrocardiographic monitoring (a continuous original ECG waveform), supplying the monitor with hookup and recording; scanning analysis with report; reviewed and interpreted the analysis and report.

Dx: Palpitations

Date: 7-8-2010

Follow-up Office Visit: Diagnosed ectopic auricular beats. Discussed therapy with patient in this follow-up visit.

Dx: Supraventricular premature beats

List of Fees for Services

7-7-2010

Services and Charges: Office visit, comprehensive history, comprehensive examination, moderately complex medical decision making, $65

ECG monitoring for twenty-four hours—recording, analysis/report, physician analysis and interpretation, $125

Copayment collected

7-8-2010

Services and Charges: Office visit, expanded history and examination, fifteen minutes with patient, $45

Copayment collected

Supply the following data elements:

Billing Provider _____

Billing Provider's Primary Identifier _____

Billing Provider's Secondary Identifier _____

Subscriber/Patient _____

Subscriber's Primary Identifier _____

Claim Filing Indicator Code _____

Place of Service Code _____

Diagnosis Codes _____

Total Charge _____

Amount Collected _____

Service Line Information

Date of Service _____

Procedure Code/Charge _____

Diagnosis _____

Date of Service _____

Procedure Code/Charge _____

Diagnosis _____

Date of Service _____

Procedure Code/Charge _____

Diagnosis _____

CHAPTER 11

TRICARE and CHAMPVA

Learning Outcomes

After completing this chapter, you will be able to define the key terms and:

11-1 Explain who is eligible for TRICARE and CHAMPVA and how to verify eligibility.

11-2 Discuss the programs offered to TRICARE beneficiaries.

11-3 Describe the use of a nonavailability statement in the TRICARE program.

11-4 Explain where to file claims first when TRICARE and CHAMPVA beneficiaries are also covered by other insurance programs.

11-5 Identify filing deadlines and time limits for responses to requests for additional information.

Key Terms

catastrophic cap
CHAMPVA
CHAMPVA for Life
cost-share
Defense Enrollment Eligibility Reporting System (DEERS)

military treatment facility (MTF)
nonavailability statement (NAS)
Primary Care Manager (PCM)
sponsor

TRICARE
TRICARE Extra
TRICARE for Life
TRICARE Prime
TRICARE Prime Remote
TRICARE Reserve Select (TRS)
TRICARE Standard

Why This Chapter Is Important to You

The information in this chapter will enable you to:

- Know who qualifies for military health care programs.
- Know where to send beneficiaries for answers to insurance coverage and claim questions.
- File TRICARE and CHAMPVA claims.

What Do You Think?

TRICARE and CHAMPVA are government medical insurance plans primarily for families of members of the U.S. uniformed services. Special regulations apply to situations in which beneficiaries seek medical services outside of military treatment facilities. What are the best ways to find out about the rules and regulations pertaining to these patients?

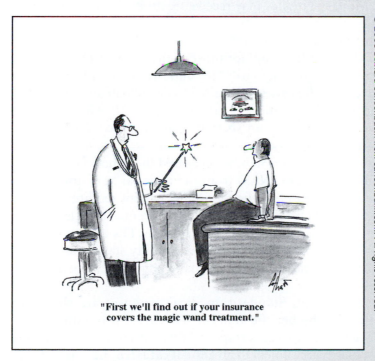

"First we'll find out if your insurance covers the magic wand treatment."

TRICARE is the Department of Defense's health insurance plan for military personnel and their families. TRICARE offers three different health care plans to its beneficiaries in the Army, Navy, Air Force, Marine Corps, Coast Guard, Public Health Service, and National Oceanic and Atmospheric Administration. TRICARE replaced the program known as CHAMPUS (Civilian Health and Medical Program of the Uniformed Services).

TRICARE benefits spouses and children of active-duty service members, who are called **sponsors.** The health care for the service members themselves is automatically provided or paid for by their branch of service. TRICARE also serves military retirees and their families, some former spouses, and survivors of deceased military members.

A TRICARE beneficiary must be listed in the Department of Defense's **Defense Enrollment Eligibility Reporting System (DEERS).** DEERS is a worldwide database of people covered by TRICARE. DEERS helps the Department of Defense track the use of medical services to better plan for beneficiaries' needs. It also helps eliminate fraudulent use of military benefits.

TRICARE Standard

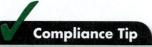

Compliance Tip

Most high-cost procedures require preauthorization. Medical information specialists should contact their TRICARE contractor for specific information.

TRICARE Standard is a fee-for-service program that covers medical services provided by a civilian physician or a **military treatment facility (MTF).** Military families may receive treatment at an MTF, but the services offered vary by facility, and first priority is given to active-duty service members.

TRICARE Standard pays for most of the costs of medically necessary services received from any TRICARE-authorized provider. The TRICARE-authorized providers are not required to participate in the TRICARE network but must be certified by the program. TRICARE Standard allows beneficiaries to self-refer for specialty care, meaning that a referral is not needed from a primary care provider.

Previously, TRICARE Standard required the beneficiary to have a **nonavailability statement (NAS)** from the regional MTF for most services. This document states that the service the patient requires is not available at the nearby military treatment facility. Current, a NAS is not needed for most outpatient services. However, some MTFs are exempt from this change. Also, in many cases the nonavailability statement is required for civilian inpatient care. Best practice is to advise the beneficiary to check with TRICARE.

Under TRICARE Standard, medical expenses are shared between TRICARE and the beneficiary. The TRICARE program uses the term **cost-share** for the patient's responsibility for coinsurance. Patient cost-share payments are subject to an annual **catastrophic cap,** a limit on the total medical expenses that the patient must pay in one year. Once this cap has been met, TRICARE pays 100 percent of additional charges for that coverage year.

TRICARE Prime

TRICARE Prime is a managed care plan similar to an HMO. After enrolling in the plan, each individual is assigned a **Primary Care Manager (PCM)** who coordinates and manages that patient's medical care. The PCM may be a single military or civilian provider or a group of providers. In addition to most of the benefits offered by TRICARE Standard, the program offers preventive care, including routine physical examinations. Active-duty service members are automatically enrolled in TRICARE Prime. TRICARE Prime enrollees receive the majority of their health care services from military treatment facilities, and they receive priority at these facilities.

An individual must pay an annual enrollment fee to join the TRICARE Prime program. Under TRICARE Prime, there is no deductible, and no payment is required for outpatient treatment at a military facility. For active-duty family members, no payment is required for visits to civilian network providers, but different copayments apply for other beneficiaries, depending on the type of visit. For example, for retirees and their family members, an outpatient visit with a civilian provider requires a $12 copayment.

TRICARE Prime Remote

TRICARE Prime Remote provides no-cost health care through civilian providers for service members and their families who are on remote assignment. Participants must live and work more than 50 miles (approximately one hour's drive time) from the nearest Military Treatment Facility. Their residence address must be registered with DEERS for eligibility, which is based on their Zip code.

TRICARE Extra

TRICARE Extra is an alternative managed care plan for individuals who want to receive services primarily from civilian facilities and physicians rather than from military facilities. Since it is a managed care plan, individuals must receive health care services from a select network of health care professionals. They may also seek treatment at military facilities, but active-duty personnel and other TRICARE Prime enrollees receive priority at those facilities, so care may not always be available. TRICARE Extra is more expensive than TRICARE Prime but less costly than TRICARE Standard. There is no enrollment fee, but there is an annual deductible.

TRICARE Reserve Select

Due to the large number of military reservists who have been called up for active duty, the Department of Defense implemented **TRICARE Reserve Select (TRS).** This program is a premium-based health plan available for purchase by certain members of the National Guard and Reserve activated on or after September 11, 2001. TRS provides members and their covered family members with comprehensive health care coverage similar to TRICARE Standard and TRICARE Extra.

TRICARE and the HIPAA Privacy Rule

The Military Health System (MHS) and the TRICARE health plan are required to comply with the HIPAA privacy policies and procedures for the use and disclosure of PHI. The MHS's Notice of Privacy Practices, which describes how a patient's medical information may be used and disclosed and how a patient can access the information, is posted at the TRICARE website. The HIPAA Electronic Health Care Transaction and Code Sets requirements, as well as the Security Rule, must also be followed.

CHAMPVA

CHAMPVA is the Civilian Health and Medical Program of the Veterans Administration, which is now known as the Department of Veterans Affairs. This government program helps pay health care costs for families of veterans who are totally and permanently disabled because of service-related injuries. It also covers the surviving spouse and children of a veteran who died from a service-related disability. Some surviving spouses of service members who died on active duty may be eligible for CHAMPVA.

The Veterans Health Care Eligibility Reform Act of 1996 requires veterans with a 100 percent disability to be enrolled in the program to receive benefits. Prior to this legislation, enrollment was not required. The Department of Veterans Affairs determines eligibility. CHAMPVA enrollees do not need to obtain nonavailability statements, as they are not eligible to receive service in military treatment facilities. A VA hospital is not considered a military treatment facility.

BENEFICIARY IDENTIFICATION

People who qualify for TRICARE or CHAMPVA are called beneficiaries. Beneficiaries get identification cards that contain information needed for claim forms (see Figure 11-1). When a patient qualifies for one of these programs, the medical insurance specialist checks the effective and expiration dates to be sure that the card authorizes civilian medical care. Then a photocopy of the front and back of the identification card is filed in the patient's medical record. If a patient is a child under the age of ten, the parent's card is checked; beneficiaries under the age of ten usually do not get identification cards.

Although the claim processor needs eligibility information from the DEERS system, there are times when a beneficiary is not listed. For example, even though military sponsors must enroll their families in DEERS, sometimes the sponsors do not keep up with changes in family status or location. Also, new service members may not have had time to enroll their families.

The medical insurance specialist should ask all TRICARE and CHAMPVA patients whether they are enrolled in DEERS. Patients can

HIPAA Tip

Sponsors may telephone DEERS to verify eligibility; providers may not contact DEERS directly because the information is protected by the HIPAA Privacy Rule.

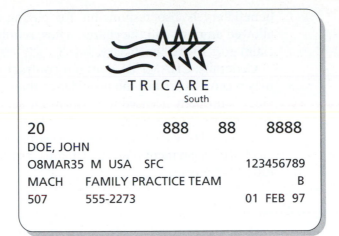

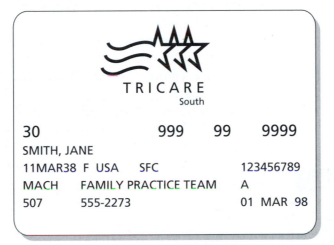

Figure 11-1 Sample Military Health Insurance Identification Card

check their status through the nearest personnel office of any branch of service or through the toll-free number of the DEERS center.

BILLING BENEFICIARIES

TRICARE pays only for services rendered by authorized providers. Authorized providers are certified by TRICARE regional contractors as having met specific requirements, and each is assigned a PIN. Providers then must decide whether to participate.

Participating physicians must accept assignment—that is, patients may not be billed for more than the allowed charges for covered services. Participating physicians must also file the claims for patients. Payments on assigned claims are made directly to physicians by the regional TRICARE contractor.

A physician who does not participate has the option to accept assignment on a case-by-case basis. When the physician does not accept assignment, the TRICARE beneficiary is billed for the total actual charge. In this case, the beneficiary is responsible for filing the claim. The beneficiary is also responsible for paying any difference between the allowed amount and the charge. Thus, reimbursement for a nonassigned claim goes to the beneficiary.

Generally, CHAMPVA does not contract with providers. Beneficiaries may receive care from the provider of their choosing as long as that provider is properly licensed to perform the services being delivered. Providers who treat CHAMPVA patients are prohibited from charging more than the CHAMPVA allowable amounts. Providers agree to accept the CHAMPVA payment and the patient's cost-share payment as payment in full for services.

Filing for TRICARE Benefits

Participating providers file claims on behalf of patients. Claims are filed with the contractor for their region. Claims are submitted to the regional contractor based on the patient's home address, not the location of the facility providing the service. Contact information for regional contractors is available on the TRICARE Web site. The three administrative regions (see Figure 11-2) are TRICARE North, TRICARE South, and TRICARE West.

When services are received from a nonparticipating provider, individuals use DD Form 2642, Patient's Request for Medical Payment, to file their own claims. A copy of the itemized bill from the provider must be attached to the form. This bill must include the following information:

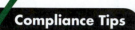

Compliance Tips

- TRICARE contractors encourage the use of electronic claims, in particular the HIPAA-compliant 837 claim.
- In some cases, paper forms, such as the paper CMS-1500 claim form, are used.

- Physician's name.
- Physician's address.
- Physician's identification number.
- Beneficiary/patient's name.
- Date of service.
- Procedure code(s) or clear description of service(s).
- Number of services provided.
- Diagnosis.
- Place of service.
- Charge for each service.
- Sponsor's Social Security number.

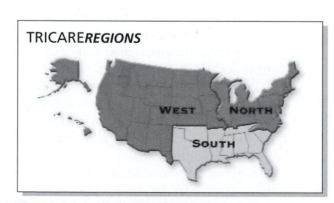

Figure 11-2 TRICARE Regions Map

If a CMS-1500 paper claim is needed, follow the guidelines in Table 11-1. A completed example is shown in Figure 11-3 (on page 229).

Table 11-1 TRICARE CMS-1500 Claim Form Completion

Form Locator	Data
1	Select TRICARE.
1a	Sponsor's Social Security number.
2	Patient's name.
3	Patient's eight-digit date of birth and gender.
4	Sponsor's full name, unless the sponsor is also the patient, in which case enter *Same*.
5	Patient's address and phone number.
6	Patient's relationship to the sponsor.
7	If the sponsor is on active duty, enter the duty address; if retired, the home address.
8	Patient's marital and employment status.
9	Enter None.
10a–10c	If any of the boxes in 10a–10c are selected, it may be necessary to file DD Form 2527, Statement of Personal Injury—Possible Third Party Liability. If the patient was treated at a hospital for an injury possibly due to a third party, or if the patient was treated in a physician's office for a possible third-party liability injury and the charges are $500 or more, the form must be filed.
11	Enter None.
11a–11c	Blank.
11d	Choose Yes or No.
12	Yes, unless there is no patient contact at the time of service—for example, if laboratory tests are conducted by an outside laboratory. In these cases, enter Patient not present.
13–16	Blank.
17–17a	Name and identification number of the referring provider or institution.
18	Hospital admission and discharge dates in eight-digit format. If the patient has been admitted but not yet discharged, enter the admission date in From, and leave To blank.
19	Blank.
20	Yes or No.
21	Appropriate ICD codes.
22	Not required.
23	If a preauthorization other than a nonavailability indicator is required, attach a copy of the form.
24A	Date of service (eight-digit format)
24B	Place of service code.
24C	**EMG:** Check TRICARE contractor for information.

24D	Appropriate CPT/HCPCS codes and any modifiers.
24E	Diagnosis key number for CPT/HCPCS codes.
24F	Amount charged.
24G	Appropriate days/units reported.
24H	Blank.
24I–24J	ID Qualifier/ID numbers.
25	Make the appropriate selection, and enter the tax ID.
26	Optional; patient account number.
27	Choose Yes or No.
28	Total charges.
29–30	Blank.
31	Check with the carrier to see if an actual signature is required.
32	If the services on this claim were performed at a location other than the provider's office or the patient's home, enter the name and address of the facility where services were performed.
33	Billing provider's name, address, phone number, provider identification number, and group number.

When TRICARE is the secondary payer, six form locators on a paper claim are filled in differently than when TRICARE is the primary payer:

11	Policy number of the primary insurance plan.
11a	Birth date and gender of the primary plan policyholder.
11b	Employer of the primary plan policyholder if the plan is a group plan through an employer.
11c	Name of the primary insurance plan.
11d	Select Yes or No as appropriate.
29	Enter all payments made by other insurance carriers. Do not include payments made by the patient.

Filing for CHAMPVA Benefits

Most CHAMPVA claims are filed by the provider and submitted to the centralized CHAMPVA claims processing center in Denver, Colorado. The information required on a claim is the same as the information required for TRICARE. As with TRICARE, the CHAMPVA program is covered by HIPAA regulations.

When beneficiaries are filing their own claims, the CHAMPVA Claim Form (VA Form 10-7959A) must be used. The claim must always be accompanied by an itemized bill from the provider.

HEALTH INSURANCE CLAIM FORM

APPROVED BY NATIONAL UNIFORM CLAIM COMMITTEE 08/05

☐☐ PICA · · · PICA ☐☐☐

| 1. MEDICARE (Medicare #) | MEDICAID (Medicaid #) | TRICARE CHAMPUS [X] (Sponsor's SSN) | CHAMPVA (Member ID#) | GROUP HEALTH PLAN (SSN or ID) | FECA BLK LUNG (SSN) | OTHER (ID) | 1a. INSURED'S I.D. NUMBER (For Program in Item 1) **301694218** |

2. PATIENT'S NAME (Last Name, First Name, Middle Initial)
RODRIGUEZ, MARIE, P

3. PATIENT'S BIRTH DATE MM 01 DD 14 YY 1969 · SEX M ☐ F [X]

4. INSURED'S NAME (Last Name, First Name, Middle Initial)
RODRIGUEZ, JESUS, I

5. PATIENT'S ADDRESS (No., Street)
316 WASHINGTON AVE

6. PATIENT RELATIONSHIP TO INSURED Self ☐ Spouse [X] Child ☐ Other ☐

7. INSURED'S ADDRESS (No., Street)
SAME

CITY CLEVELAND **STATE** OH

8. PATIENT STATUS Single ☐ Married [X] Other ☐

CITY · **STATE**

ZIP CODE 44101-3164 **TELEPHONE (Include Area Code)** (555) 3216179

Employed ☐ Full-Time Student ☐ Part-Time Student ☐

ZIP CODE · **TELEPHONE (INCLUDE AREA CODE)** ( )

9. OTHER INSURED'S NAME (Last Name, First Name, Middle Initial)

10. IS PATIENT'S CONDITION RELATED TO:

11. INSURED'S POLICY GROUP OR FECA NUMBER
NONE

a. OTHER INSURED'S POLICY OR GROUP NUMBER

a. EMPLOYMENT? (CURRENT OR PREVIOUS) YES ☐ NO [X]

a. INSURED'S DATE OF BIRTH MM DD YY · SEX M ☐ F ☐

b. OTHER INSURED'S DATE OF BIRTH MM DD YY SEX M ☐ F ☐

b. AUTO ACCIDENT? YES ☐ NO [X] PLACE (State)

b. EMPLOYER'S NAME OR SCHOOL NAME

c. EMPLOYER'S NAME OR SCHOOL NAME

c. OTHER ACCIDENT? YES ☐ NO [X]

c. INSURANCE PLAN NAME OR PROGRAM NAME

d. INSURANCE PLAN NAME OR PROGRAM NAME

10d. RESERVED FOR LOCAL USE

d. IS THERE ANOTHER HEALTH BENEFIT PLAN? YES ☐ NO [X] If yes, return to and complete item 9 a-d.

READ BACK OF FORM BEFORE COMPLETING & SIGNING THIS FORM.
12. PATIENT'S OR AUTHORIZED PERSON'S SIGNATURE I authorize the release of any medical or other information necessary to process this claim. I also request payment of government benefits either to myself or to the party who accepts assignment below.

SIGNED *SIGNATURE ON FILE* DATE

13. INSURED'S OR AUTHORIZED PERSON'S SIGNATURE I authorize payment of medical benefits to the undersigned physician or supplier for services described below.

SIGNED

14. DATE OF CURRENT: MM DD YY ILLNESS (First symptom) OR INJURY (Accident) OR PREGNANCY(LMP)

15. IF PATIENT HAS HAD SAME OR SIMILAR ILLNESS. GIVE FIRST DATE MM DD YY

16. DATES PATIENT UNABLE TO WORK IN CURRENT OCCUPATION FROM MM DD YY TO MM DD YY

17. NAME OF REFERRING PHYSICIAN OR OTHER SOURCE

17a. · 17b. NPI

18. HOSPITALIZATION DATES RELATED TO CURRENT SERVICES FROM MM DD YY TO MM DD YY

19. RESERVED FOR LOCAL USE

20. OUTSIDE LAB? YES ☐ NO [X] $ CHARGES

21. DIAGNOSIS OR NATURE OF ILLNESS OR INJURY. (Relate Items 1,2,3 or 4 to Item 24e by Line)
1. 401.1
2. 427.41
3. ____.____
4. ____.____

22. MEDICAID RESUBMISSION CODE · ORIGINAL REF. NO.

23. PRIOR AUTHORIZATION NUMBER

24. A. DATE(S) OF SERVICE From MM DD YY	To MM DD YY	B. PLACE OF SERVICE	C. EMG	D. PROCEDURES, SERVICES, OR SUPPLIES (Explain Unusual Circumstances) CPT/HCPCS MODIFIER	E. DIAGNOSIS POINTER	F. $ CHARGES	G. DAYS OR UNITS	H. EPSDT Family Plan	I. ID. QUAL.	J. RENDERING PROVIDER ID.#
1	10 06 2010		11		99212	1	46 00	1		NPI	
2	10 06 2010		11		93000	1, 2	70 00	1		NPI	
3										NPI	
4										NPI	
5										NPI	
6										NPI	

25. FEDERAL TAX I.D. NUMBER SSN ☐ EIN [X] 161246791

26. PATIENT'S ACCOUNT NO. RUD210

27. ACCEPT ASSIGNMENT? (For govt. claims, see back) YES [X] NO ☐

28. TOTAL CHARGE $ 116 00

29. AMOUNT PAID $

30. BALANCE DUE $ 80 10

31. SIGNATURE OF PHYSICIAN OR SUPPLIER INCLUDING DEGREES OR CREDENTIALS (I certify that the statements on the reverse apply to this bill and are made a part thereof.)
David Rosenberg MD
SIGNED 10/06/2010 DATE

32. SERVICE FACILITY LOCATION INFORMATION
a. NPI b.

33. BILLING PROVIDER INFO & PHONE # ( )
DAVID ROSENBERG MD
1400 WEST CENTER ST
TOLEDO OH 43601
a. 128099081 b.

NUCC Instruction Manual available at: www.nucc.org

Figure 11-3 Sample TRICARE CMS-1500 Claim

TRICARE and CHAMPVA do not duplicate benefits from another insurance program or health plan. The medical insurance specialist must know where to file claims when a beneficiary has additional coverage from Medicaid, supplemental insurance, another health plan, workers' compensation, or Medicare.

If a beneficiary qualifies for Medicaid or has coverage from a supplemental insurance policy (similar to Medigap policies discussed in Chapter 9), TRICARE or CHAMPVA is the primary payer. File with TRICARE or CHAMPVA first. On the other hand, TRICARE and CHAMPVA are secondary payers when the patient has coverage from another primary health plan. For example, a CHAMPVA member (but not a TRICARE member) may be enrolled in Medicare Parts A and B. In this case, Medicare receives the claim first. Then a copy of the Medicare Remittance Notice or other remittance advice is attached to the CHAMPVA claim.

TRICARE and CHAMPVA do not pay for illnesses or injuries covered by workers' compensation unless compensation benefits have been exhausted. File a workers' compensation claim first (see Chapter 12).

TRICARE and Medicare

The **TRICARE for Life** plan offers health care at a military treatment facility to individuals age sixty-five and over who are eligible for both Medicare and TRICARE. TRICARE for Life acts as a secondary payer to Medicare; Medicare pays first, and the remaining out-of-pocket expenses are paid by TRICARE. Claims are filed automatically.

Benefits are similar to those of a Medicare HMO, with an emphasis on preventive and wellness services. Prescription drug benefits are also included. All enrollees in TRICARE for Life must be enrolled in Medicare Parts A and B and must have Part B premiums deducted from their Social Security checks. (Individuals already enrolled in a Medicare HMO may not participate in TRICARE for Life.) Other than Medicare costs, TRICARE for Life beneficiaries pay no enrollment fees and no cost-share fees for inpatient or outpatient care at a military facility. Treatment at a civilian network facility requires a copay.

CHAMPVA and Medicare

CHAMPVA for Life extends CHAMPVA benefits to spouses or dependents who are age sixty-five and over. Similar to TRICARE for Life, CHAMPVA for Life benefits are payable after payment by Medicare or other third-party payers. Eligible beneficiaries must be sixty-five or older and enrolled in Medicare Parts A and B. For services not covered by Medicare, such as outpatient prescription medications, CHAMPVA acts as the primary payer.

Filing Forms on Time

Explore the Internet

Use a search engine such as Yahoo or Google to access the official government website for TRICARE. Locate the TRICARE Beneficiaries information section. From the list of options, select TRICARE Resources and then TRICARE Handbook. From the list of Browse subjects, read about the topic Medicare and TRICARE in the TRICARE Handbook. Then return to the TRICARE Beneficiaries information section, and study eligibility requirements and covered services.

TRICARE and CHAMPVA claims must be filed within one year from the date services were provided. For example, a claim for services performed on December 31, 2010, must be filed by December 31, 2011. Of course, medical insurance claims are usually filed more promptly. If an unusual situation occurs, the medical insurance specialist should contact the fiscal intermediary for the area to be sure of complying with this deadline. If additional information is requested, the claim must be resubmitted either within ninety days of the notice or by the regular filing deadline, whichever is later.

Chapter Summary

1. TRICARE serves active duty personnel, their spouses and children, military retirees and their families, some former spouses, and survivors of deceased military members. CHAMPVA covers families of veterans who have service-related 100 percent disabilities and the surviving spouses and children of veterans who have died from service-related injuries. A medical insurance specialist determines eligibility by checking the beneficiary's identification card and verifying that the beneficiary is enrolled in the Defense Enrollment Eligibility Reporting System (DEERS).

2. TRICARE Standard is a fee-for-service plan in which medical expenses are shared between TRICARE and the beneficiary. The enrollee typically pays an annual deductible and a cost-share percentage. TRICARE Prime is a managed care plan. After enrolling in the plan, each individual is assigned a Primary Care Manager (PCM) who coordinates and manages that patient's medical care. TRICARE Extra is also a managed care plan, but instead of services being provided primarily from military facilities, civilian facilities and physicians provide the majority of care. TRICARE Reserve Select is available for reservists (and their families) called up for active duty.

3. When an individual lives within a certain distance from a military hospital, a nonavailability statement (NAS) may be required by the local military hospital before the patient enters the civilian hospital for nonemergency inpatient care.

4. File first with TRICARE or CHAMPVA when a beneficiary is also covered by Medicaid or supplemental insurance. File a secondary claim with TRICARE or CHAMPVA when the beneficiary has another health plan or when workers' compensation benefits are exhausted.

5. The filing deadline for TRICARE and CHAMPVA claims is one year from the date of service. Requested additional information must be resubmitted within ninety days of the claim processor's request or by the original filing deadline, whichever is later.

Check Your Understanding

Part 1. Write short answers to the following questions.

1. What is the difference between TRICARE and CHAMPVA?

2. What are two benefits of DEERS?

3. What are the main programs of TRICARE?

4. The physician who employs you is a participating physician with TRICARE. Elaine Dempsey is a new patient in the medical office. She is covered by Blue Cross and Blue Shield through her employer. However, her husband is in the Navy, stationed at Mystic, Connecticut. How should Elaine's claim be filed?

Part 2. In the space provided, write the word or phrase that best completes each sentence.

1. The maximum amount a TRICARE beneficiary must pay for deductible and cost-share each year is called the _____.

2. The worldwide database of TRICARE beneficiaries is called _____.

3. TRICARE Standard is a _____ plan.

4. The name for the uniformed service member in a family qualified for TRICARE or CHAMPVA is _____.

5. The two TRICARE managed care plans are _____ and _____.

6. Coinsurance for a TRICARE or CHAMPVA beneficiary is called the _____.

7. The health care program for active-duty service members, spouses and children of active-duty service members, military retirees and their families, some former spouses, and survivors of deceased military members is called _____.

8. The filing deadline for TRICARE and CHAMPVA claims is _____.

9. TRICARE Prime requires a _____ to be assigned to patients.

10. The DEERS system is administered by _____.

Part 3. Read the cases below and answer the questions.

A.

Physician Information:
Name: Asha Gupta, MD
NPI: 5432109876
TRICARE PAR
CHAMPUS (TRICARE) ID: HL59004

Patient Information Form:
Name: Mary Amy Piotrowska (Established Patient)
Sex: Female
Birth Date: 7-5-83
Marital Status: Married
Social Security Number: 031-10-7944

Insurance Information:
Primary Insurance Carrier: TRICARE Standard
Insurance ID Number: 565-97-9087
Insurance Group Number: 565-97-9087 (N4441514)
Secondary Carrier: None
ID Card: EFF 10-10-2009 EXP 10-10-2010

Policyholder Information:
Primary Policyholder: Alfred R. Piotrowska
Employer: U.S. Navy
Address: USS Newport, Box 39
                     Sarasota, Florida 33580
Active Duty, Captain
Social Security Number: 565-97-9087
Sex: Male
Birth Date: 6-10-81

Patient's Encounter Form:
Date: 6-25-2010
T-99.7   BP 130/90
CC: Patient reports stuffy nose, sore throat, and low-grade fever.
Dx: Sinusitis.

List of Fees for Service:
Charges: Office visit, Level II (total time, ten minutes), $45
No payment collected.

Supply the following data elements:
Billing Provider _____
Billing Provider's Primary Identifier _____
Billing Provider's Secondary Identifier _____
Subscriber _____
Patient _____
Subscriber's Primary Identifier _____
Relationship _____
Claim Filing Indicator Code _____

Payer Name/ID _____
Place of Service Code _____
Diagnosis Codes _____
Total Charge _____
Amount Collected _____

Service Line Information
Date of Service _____
Procedure Code/Charge _____
Diagnosis _____

B.

Physician Information:
Name: Rory Mancinni, MD
NPI: 3210987654
TRICARE PAR
CHAMPUS (TRICARE) ID: LR33205

Patient Information:
Name: Mary Beth Carteret (Established Patient)
Sex: Female
Birth Date: 12-3-2009
Marital Status: Single
Social Security Number: 066-15-6664

Insurance Information:
Primary Insurance Carrier: TRICARE Prime
Insurance ID Number: 230-77-9987
Insurance Group Number: 230-77-9987 (AF2233)
Secondary Carrier: None
ID Card: EFF 11-10-2009 EXP 11-10-2010

Policyholder Information:
Primary Policyholder: Alice Carteret
Employer: U.S. Air Force
Address: Culver Air Force Base
Carson, North Carolina 27560
Active Duty, Major
Social Security Number: 230-77-9987
Sex: Female
Birth Date: 4-17-76

Patient''s Encounter Form:

Date: 6-25-2010

T-99.7 BP 130/90

CC: Ms. Carteret presents her child for a routine health check and a scheduled DPT + polio immunization.

Dx: Routine infant health check. Need for prophylactic vaccination with diphtheria-tetanus-pertussis with poliomyelitis vaccine.

List of Fees for Services:

Services and Charges: Office visit (periodic preventive medicine reevaluation),
   $45
   DPT, immunization, active, $7
   Poliomyelitis vaccine, immunization, active, $5
No payment collected

Supply the following data elements:

Billing Provider _____

Billing Provider's Primary Identifier _____

Billing Provider's Secondary Identifier _____

Subscriber _____

Patient _____

Subscriber's Primary Identifier _____

Relationship _____

Claim Filing Indicator Code _____

Payer Name/ID _____

Place of Service Code _____

Diagnosis Codes _____

Total Charge _____

Amount Collected _____

Service Line Information

Date of Service _____

Procedure Code/Charge _____

Diagnosis_____

Date of Service _____

Procedure Code/Charge _____

Diagnosis _____

Date of Service _____

Procedure Code/Charge _____

Diagnosis _____

Learning Outcomes

After completing this chapter, you will be able to define the key terms and:

12-1 Discuss what workers' compensation insurance covers and which federal and state agencies administer the programs.

12-2 List the five types of compensation that employees may receive for work-related illnesses and injuries.

12-3 List five questions to ask the state compensation board about workers' compensation regulations.

12-4 Explain why medical information that pertains to a workers' compensation case should be separated from the patient's chart for diseases and disorders that are not work-related.

Key Terms

Federal Employees'
   Compensation Act (FECA)
final report
first report of injury or illness
nontraumatic injury

occupational disease/
   illness
Office of Workers'
   Compensation Programs
   (OWCP)
progress report

state compensation
   board/commission
supplemental report
traumatic injury
workers' compensation
   insurance

Why This Chapter Is Important to You

The information in this chapter will enable you to:

- Know what to do if a patient with a work-related injury or illness comes to your medical office.
- Know where to call for more information about state or federal workers' compensation insurance.
- Understand the importance of filing claim forms and other medical information for patients with work-related injuries or illnesses.

What Do You Think?

Workers' compensation coverage provides important medical insurance benefits to people who experience work-related injuries or illnesses. Unfortunately, many instances of abuse of workers' compensation have been uncovered. In a significant number of these situations, court cases have found workers' claims for temporary or permanent disability to be untruthful. Are medical office staff members responsible for questioning or reporting information they suspect to be fraudulent?

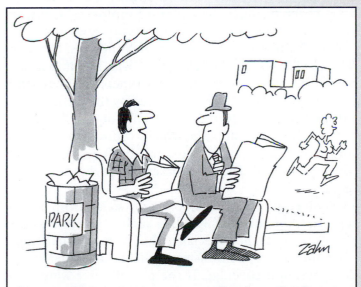

"I'm getting worker's compensation from the Street Department. The shovel I was leaning on broke."

WHEN EMPLOYEES ARE HURT AT WORK

When someone is injured accidentally in the course of performing work or a work-related duty or becomes ill as a result of the employment environment, the cost of medical care for the injury or illness is covered by federal or state plans known as **workers' compensation insurance.** These plans also provide benefits for lost wages and permanent disabilities.

Workers' compensation covers two kinds of situations that require medical care. A **traumatic injury** is caused by a specific event or series of events within a single workday or shift. An example is a broken leg caused by a fall from a catwalk in a warehouse. **Occupational disease/illness** (also known as **nontraumatic injury**) is caused by the work environment over a longer period of time. An example of an occupational disease is a lung condition caused by repeated exposure to fumes in the workplace.

Compensation for work-related illnesses and injuries may be one of five types:

1. Medical treatment.
2. Lost wages (temporary disability).
3. Permanent disability payments (either partial or full disability).
4. Compensation for dependents of employees who are fatally injured.
5. Vocational rehabilitation.

FEDERAL PROGRAMS, FORMS, AND PROCEDURES

Work-related illnesses or injuries suffered by civilian employees of federal agencies, including volunteers in the Peace Corps and AmeriCorps programs, are covered under the **Federal Employees' Compensation Act (FECA).** Other federal workers' compensation laws include the Federal Coal Mine Health and Safety Act (which includes the Black Lung Benefits Act), the Longshore and Harbor Workers' Compensation Act, and the Energy Employees Occupational Illness Compensation Program Act. All of these plans are administered by the **Office of Workers' Compensation Programs (OWCP),** except for the Longshore and Harbor Workers' Compensation Act, which is administered by the Division of Longshore and Harbor Workers. Both the OWCP and the Division of Longshore and Harbor Workers are part of the U.S. Department of Labor.

Injured federal employees can choose a physician from among those who are authorized by the OWCP. When such a patient requests treatment, the medical insurance specialist should verify that the selected physician is authorized to administer medical care under the patient's workers' compensation coverage. If the patient later wants to change physicians, the OWCP must approve the change. If a patient seeks care from an unauthorized physician, the medical insurance specialist should remind the patient that he or she may be responsible for the cost of that treatment.

The medical insurance specialist should verify a patient's coverage under workers' compensation by contacting the patient's employer and asking for the name of the insurance carrier. Then the carrier should be contacted to find out whether the selected physician is authorized and what information the carrier will need in order to process the claim.

As with other federal health care programs, payment to physicians and other health care providers under FECA is based on the Medicare Fee Schedule. The physician may not bill the patient for more than the allowed charge.

Deadlines for completing the various forms involved in workers' compensation cases are determined by federal law. Bills for medical services must be sent to the OWCP by December 31 of the year following the year in which services were provided, or by December 31 of the year following the year when the condition was first accepted as covered by the workers' compensation program, whichever is later. Generally, of course, bills are submitted promptly by the medical office.

Professional Focus

Workers' Compensation Terminology

Physicians' reports in workers' compensation cases use specific terms to describe the job-related effects of certain injuries and disabilities. These terms have been agreed to by state compensation commissions and carriers to create a common understanding of the patient's condition. Here are some examples:

- Levels of pain are described as minimal, slight, moderate, or severe.
- Disability due to heart disease, pulmonary dysfunction, abdominal weakness, or spinal injuries is described in terms of one of the following levels:
  —Limitation to light work.
  —Precluding heavy work.
  —Precluding heavy lifting, repeated bending, and stooping.
  —Precluding heavy lifting.
  —Precluding very heavy work.
  —Precluding very heavy lifting.
- Disability due to lower-extremity injuries are described as:
  —Limitation to sedentary work.
  —Limitation to semisedentary work.

STATE PROGRAMS, FORMS, AND PROCEDURES

State programs cover traumatic and nontraumatic injuries to state and private business employees within each state, although there are some exceptions. Eligibility and exceptions vary from state to state. A **state compensation board/commission** administers workers' compensation laws for employees eligible under state laws. These boards or commissions handle employee appeals and provide information to employers and health care providers about regulations.

Determining State Regulations

Compliance with state laws is important in workers' compensation cases. Medical insurance specialists should become familiar with the regulations that apply in their states. To learn the law, ask these five important questions of the state compensation board:

1. What forms and records are required from the medical office, and where can the office get blank forms?

Each state has its own system of claim forms and required medical records that must be provided by the physician who treats a person with a job-related injury or illness. The practice should secure the correct forms and comply with filing instructions, deadlines, and rules concerning photocopies and signatures. For example, some states do not accept photocopied signatures, so the physician must sign all photocopies as well as the original.

2. What organizations and agencies should receive the claim forms, and what are their addresses?

Forms and records must be sent to the correct address. Sending information to the wrong place delays processing and reimbursement.

3. How is reimbursement determined, and can the physician bill the patient or employer for charges in excess of state-determined fees?

Reimbursement methods vary from state to state. The state program may use a system of allowed charges or a fee schedule that designates a flat fee for each medical service. It is important to know which method applies and whether excess charges may be billed to the patient or the patient's employer. The physician may be prohibited by law from billing the patient for excess charges.

4. Who chooses the physician?

States may regulate who can choose the treating physician in workers' compensation cases. In some states, the patient may choose the physician. In others, the physician must be approved by the employer, the insurance carrier, or the state regulatory agency. State programs may not pay for treatment by an unauthorized physician.

The workers' compensation policies of many insurance carriers require the employer to be in a managed care plan. In this case, the injured employee's claim is overseen by the patient's primary care physician. This physician is responsible for authorizing the appropriate care and for overseeing the employee's claim.

5. What are the filing deadlines?

Filing deadlines must be known and carefully followed. Failure to do so may result in loss of benefits.

General Guidelines for Claims

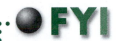

When a patient is covered by workers' compensation insurance, other insurance plans and programs do not cover the charges or will cover charges only after workers' compensation benefits are exhausted. The medical office specialist files for the patient's workers' compensation benefits through the appropriate insurance carrier. State forms and regulations vary.

Generally, the physician must complete narrative reports and a claim form. There are no universal rules for completing a claim form. Some plans use the HIPAA 837 or the CMS-1500, while others have their own claim forms. Although the specific procedures vary depending on the state and on the insurance carrier, the following are some general guidelines:

- Payment from the insurance carrier must be accepted as payment in full. Patients or employers may not be billed for any of the medical expenses.
- A separate file must be established when a provider treats an individual who is already a patient of the practice. Information in the patient's regular medical record (information not related to workers' compensation) must not be released to the insurance carrier.
- The patient's signature is not required on any billing forms.
- The workers' compensation claim number should be included on all forms and correspondence.
- Use the eight-digit format when reporting dates such as the date last worked.

Employees who become sick or injured due to a work-related incident or environment must report the illness or accident to their employer right away. When this happens, the employer sends a report of occupational illness or injury to the appropriate state office. The employer also typically completes a form that authorizes medical treatment. This form guarantees payment to the treating physician. The injured or ill employee brings it to the physician's office.

After the office visit, the physician prepares a **first report of injury or illness.** This report must include the following information:

- Dates of examination and treatment.
- Patient's history and description of the injury and/or illness as told to the physician.
- Name and address of the employer and name of the employee's supervisor.
- Detailed description of the physician's findings.
- Results of X-rays and other diagnostic tests.
- Diagnosis.
- Clinical treatment.
- The physician's opinion of the relationship between the work environment and the injury and/or illness and an explanation of how the physician arrived at that opinion.

The first report of injury or illness should be submitted as soon as possible after the office visit. In contrast to usual procedure, this report does not require the patient's signature. The medical insurance specialist sends

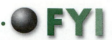

copies of the report to the state compensation board or commission, the carrier, and the employer; a copy is also filed in a separate work-related medical record for the patient.

When a patient's workers' compensation claim for temporary or permanent disability is accepted by the carrier, the physician continues to monitor the patient's medical condition or disability. The physician is asked to file **progress reports** (also known as **supplemental reports**) to explain changes, such as when an employee with a temporary disability can resume work. In some cases, the patient may receive temporary disability benefits while he or she is unable to return to work. Progress reports should include the patient's work status, anticipated additional required treatment, an estimate of future ability to perform occupational tasks, and the extent of permanent loss or disability.

Some states also require a **final report** from a physician who has completed treatment of a patient covered by workers' compensation.

KEEPING SEPARATE RECORDS

HIPAA Tip

Workers' Compensation and the HIPAA Privacy Rule

Workers' compensation cases provide one of the few situations in which a health care provider may disclose a patient's protected health information to an employer without the patient's authorization. Workers' compensation claim information is not subject to the same confidentiality rules as other medical information.

Workers' compensation cases are subject to review and court hearings. They usually require medical records in addition to the attending physician's reports and the health care claims. Handling the case and the claim requires information about medical care only for the work-related injury or illness. Records about treatment for other conditions are not needed. In fact, according to law, compensation boards and insurance carriers can review history and treatment information that pertains to the work-related injury or illness only.

When the physician treats a patient with a work-related illness or injury, the medical insurance specialist should set up a separate medical record for the case. This makes pertinent notes and records for the workers' compensation claim easy to find. A signed authorization to release information for the workers' compensation claim should be filed in this separate medical record.

For example, suppose Rachel Goldmeir is seeing Dr. Littlejohn for a back injury she suffered while rearranging office furniture during work as an interior designer for Dayton's Interiors. While still in the care of the physician, Ms. Goldmeir seeks care from Dr. Littlejohn for strep throat. The strep throat is not work-related. While the medical office must keep records about the illness, the workers' compensation claims processors do not need these records, nor are they entitled to review them. Therefore, a separate record and ledger for treatment of the back injury must be created. Information about medical care for the strep throat should go in Ms. Goldmeir's regular patient record.

Explore the Internet

Using your favorite search engine, search for the Workers Compensation website for your state. What are your state's requirements for workers' compensation coverage? Try to locate a sample claim form for your state. Then locate online newsletters. According to the newsletters, what are some current topics in workers' compensation?

Chapter Summary

1. Workers' compensation insurance covers medical costs, lost wages, and disability benefits for employees with work-related injuries or illnesses. The Office of Workers' Compensation Programs of the U.S. Department of Labor administers the program for civilian federal employees. State compensation boards or commissions administer state programs.

2. Five types of compensation that may be received as workers' compensation benefits are medical treatment, lost wages (temporary disability), permanent disability payments (either partial or full disability), compensation for dependents of employees who are fatally injured, and vocational rehabilitation.

3. Five questions to ask the state compensation board about workers' compensation regulations are:

   • What forms and records are required from the medical office, and where can the office get the blank forms?

   • What organizations and agencies receive information and claim forms, and what are their addresses?

   • How is reimbursement determined, and can the physician bill the patient or employer for charges in excess of state-determined fees?

   • Who chooses the physician?

   • What are the filing deadlines?

4. Medical information related to a workers' compensation case should be filed separately from the patient's regular medical record. Workers' compensation cases are subject to review and court hearings. According to law, organizations and agencies that process the claims may review only history and treatment information that pertains to the work-related injury or illness.

Check Your Understanding

Part 1. Match each term below with its correct definition.

A. FECA

B. final report

C. first report of injury or illness

D. occupational illness

E. OWCP

F. progress report

G. traumatic injury

_____ **1.** A federal law that provides workers' compensation insurance for civilian employees of the federal government.

_____ **2.** A report filed that includes the employer's name and address, the employee's supervisor's name, the dates of examination and treatment, the patient's history and description of what happened, and the physician's diagnosis and opinion of its work-relatedness.

_____ **3.** An injury caused by a specific event or series of events within a single workday or shift.

_____ **4.** The office that administers the Federal Employees' Compensation Act.

_____ **5.** A condition caused by the work environment over a period longer than one workday or shift.

_____ **6.** A report filed by the physician in a workers' compensation case when treatment of the patient's job-related case is finished.

_____ **7.** A report filed by the physician in a workers' compensation case when a patient's medical condition or disability changes.

Part 2. Read the cases below and answer the questions.

A.

Stephen C. Yu hurt his knee while at work. Assume that a first report of injury has been filed and case number RB67443 has been issued.

Physician Information:
Name: Lorraine Rutigliano, MD
Employer ID Number: 45-7659871

Patient Information Form:
Name: Stephen C. Yu (New Patient)
Sex: Male
Birth Date: 12-20-69
Address: 12 Baker Road
       Springfield, Missouri 65804
Social Security Number: 998-20-8761
Employer: Conrad's Body Shop
       70 Bradford Street
       Kansas City, Missouri 64590
Phone: 417-660-9988

Insurance Carrier: CIGNA KC (indemnity plan)
Insurance Carrier Address: 60 Twentieth Street
                               Kansas City, Missouri 64200
Insurance Group Number: G68063

Patient's Encounter Form:
Date: 3-21-2010
Account Number: None
WORKERS' COMPENSATION CASE
PATIENT RECORD NUMBER 665
CC: Patient twisted his knee on Thursday, 3-20-10. Pain is worse on the lateral and inferior aspect of the left
     knee. No tenderness with active or passive range of motion of the knee.
Dx: Right lateral collateral ligament sprain.

List of Fees for Service:
Charges: Office visit, Level II, $60

Supply the following data elements:
Billing Provider _____
Billing Provider's Primary Identifier _____
Subscriber _____
Patient _____
Relationship _____
Claim Filing Indicator Code _____

Place of Service Code _____
WC Claim Number _____
Payer's Name _____
Payer's ID _____
Diagnosis Codes _____
Total Charge _____
Amount Collected _____

Claim Information
Accident Cause (check one)
     Auto Accident ___ Another Party Responsible ___
     Employment Related ___ Other Accident ___
Date of Accident _____

Service Line Information
Date of Service _____
Procedure Code/Charge _____
Diagnosis Code _____

B.

In the following workers' compensation case, assume that a first report of injury has been filed and that case number CA9988 has been issued.

Physician Information:
Name: Dennis L. Pulaski, MD
Employer ID Number: 22-9872767

Patient Information Form:
Name: Myrna Branch Estephan (New Patient)
Sex: Female
Birth Date: April 25, 1947
Address: 346 Austin Boulevard
       San Antonio, Texas 78289
Social Security Number: 968-44-9876
Employer: Consuela's Nail Shop
       644 San Juan Street
       San Antonio, Texas 78299
Phone: 512-681-8674
Insurance Carrier: AETNA TX (PPO)
Insurance Carrier Address: 20 Forester Avenue
          San Antonio, Texas 78287
Insurance Group Number: AR 187267-T

Patient's Encounter Form:
Date: April 22, 2010
Account Number: None
WORKERS' COMPENSATION CASE
PATIENT RECORD NUMBER 56-D
CC: Patient presents for evaluation of left hand numbness that happened today. Nerve conduction studies confirm a left median nerve entrapment at the wrist (carpal tunnel).
Dx: Carpal tunnel syndrome.

List of Fees for Service:
Charges: Office visit; problem-focused history and examination, straightforward decision making (ten-minute appointment), $60

Nerve conduction, amplitude and latency/velocity study, each nerve, all sites along the nerve; sensory, $60

Supply the following data elements:

Billing Provider _____

Billing Provider's Primary Identifier _____

Subscriber _____

Patient _____

Relationship _____

Claim Filing Indicator Code _____

Place of Service Code _____

WC Claim Number _____

Payer's Name _____

Payer's ID _____

Diagnosis Codes _____

Total Charge _____

Amount Collected _____

Claim Information

Accident Cause (check one)

        Auto Accident ___ Another Party Responsible ___

        Employment Related ___ Other Accident ___

Date of Accident _____

Service Line Information

Date of Service _____

Procedure Code/Charge _____

Diagnosis Code _____

Date of Service _____

Procedure Code/Charge _____

Diagnosis Code _____

13 Disability

Learning Outcomes

After completing this chapter, you will be able to define the key terms and:

13-1 Discuss the purpose of disability compensation.

13-2 Name the six major federal disability programs, and describe who is eligible for program benefits.

13-3 Compare government and private disability plans.

13-4 List eight types of information the physician should include in a medical report for the claims department of a disability compensation program.

Key Terms

Civil Service Retirement
  System (CSRS)
disability compensation
  programs
Federal Employees
  Retirement System (FERS)
Federal Insurance
  Contribution Act (FICA)

Notice of Claim Filed
permanent disability
private disability insurance
prognosis
Social Security Disability
  Insurance (SSDI)
State Disability Insurance
  (SDI)

Supplemental Security
  Income (SSI)
temporary disability
Veteran's Compensation
  Program
Veteran's Pension Program

Why This Chapter Is Important to You

The information in this chapter will enable you to:

- Be aware of various types of government and private disability compensation programs.
- Know what to do when you receive a Notice of Claim Filed from the Social Security Administration.
- Help the physician complete requests for medical information for patients who qualify for disability insurance.

What Do You Think?

Disability coverage is designed to help people whose ability to work is affected by illness or injury. Many people are covered by their employers' plans or by state disability plans. Other people may purchase private disability coverage. What types of information must the medical office report in disability cases?

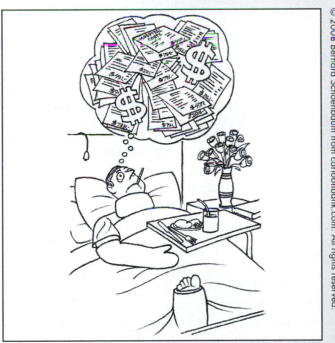

REPLACING LOST INCOME

M ost of the insurance and compensation plans handled by medical insurance specialists are designed to pay for health care costs resulting from illnesses or injuries. By comparison, **disability compensation programs** pay benefits for lost income when an illness or injury prevents a person from working. Unlike workers' compensation programs, which also include compensation for lost income, the illness or injury does not have to be work-related.

For example, suppose Mark Davidson, who works as a furniture mover, falls down the basement stairs at home and fractures a vertebra in his back. Mark's injury makes it impossible for him to do his job. The amount of cash benefits depends on the extent of Mark's injury and the provisions of the disability compensation program that covers him. The main purpose of most disability compensation programs is to replace wages lost while the person is unable to work.

The federal government, some states, and many private insurance companies offer disability compensation programs and policies. Eligibility and benefits vary. However, they all require the insured to provide convincing medical evidence that the condition resulting from the illness or injury satisfies the criteria of the program or policy.

Government Disability Programs

There are six major federal disability programs:

1. Social Security Disability Insurance (SSDI).
2. Supplemental Security Income (SSI).
3. Civil Service Retirement System (CSRS).
4. Federal Employees Retirement System (FERS).
5. Veteran's Compensation Program.
6. Veteran's Pension Program.

People who become disabled may qualify for **Social Security Disability Insurance (SSDI)** benefits if one of the following applies:

- They are salaried or hourly wage employees whose payroll deductions included those for the **Federal Insurance Contribution Act (FICA).**
- They are self-employed and paid Social Security taxes for the required minimum number of quarters.
- They are widows, widowers, or minor children of deceased workers who would be qualified for Social Security benefits if they were still alive.

Disability under the SSDI program is defined as a condition that prevents the worker from doing any work and that is expected to last at least twelve consecutive months or can be expected to result in the worker's death. Part of the review process includes an assessment of whether the worker can perform a different job or learn new skills that the condition will allow him or her to use.

The **Supplemental Security Income (SSI)** program is a welfare program, not an entitlement program. SSI provides payments to individuals in need, including aged, blind, and disabled individuals. Eligibility is determined using nationwide standards.

The **Federal Employees Retirement System (FERS)** provides disability coverage to federal workers hired after 1984. Employees hired before 1984 enrolled in the **Civil Service Retirement System (CSRS).** The FERS program consists of a federal disability program and the Social Security disability program. The two parts of the program have different eligibility rules, and some workers qualify for FERS benefits but not for SSDI benefits. If a worker is eligible for both, the amount of the SSDI payment is reduced based on the amount of the FERS payment.

Veterans of the uniformed services are covered by two federal plans, the **Veteran's Compensation Program** and the **Veteran's Pension Program.** Certain veterans may qualify to receive benefits from both VA programs. The Veteran's Compensation Program provides coverage for individuals with permanent and total disabilities that resulted from service-related illnesses or injuries. In order for a veteran to be eligible for benefits, the disability must affect his or her earning capacity. The Veteran's Pension Program provides benefits for service-related permanent disabilities to those who are unable to obtain gainful employment.

In states with disability programs, **State Disability Insurance (SDI)** covers most workers in the state, although in some states employees of the state and federal government, school district employees, and employees of churches are ineligible. As with Social Security Disability Insurance, SDI is usually paid for through payroll deductions.

Private Disability Policies

Individuals can purchase **private disability insurance** from insurance companies, or policies may be available to employees through employer-sponsored programs. These plans usually supplement benefits from government programs.

Private plans provide reimbursement for lost income when a disability prevents the injured person from working. They generally recognize two kinds of disabilities. Workers with **temporary disabilities** cannot do their regular jobs for a short time but are expected to recover completely and return to work. A **permanent disability** is a condition that prevents the insured worker from returning to the job held before the illness or injury.

FILING FOR DISABILITY BENEFITS

Although medical insurance specialists do not fill out claim forms for disability compensation programs, they may be asked to provide a physician's medical report and accompanying medical records. The physician will need help gathering the information for the report and assembling copies of pertinent records.

Inadequate medical information can result in denial of benefits. When a **Notice of Claim Filed** is received from Social Security or when another request for medical information is received, the medical insurance specialist works with the physician to document the worker's case.

The medical information provided should include evidence of the severity of the illness or injury and how long the physician expects the disability to last. When in doubt, provide more information than appears to be needed rather than not enough.

The disability compensation program may ask the physician to complete a form. Alternatively, the physician may be asked to provide a narrative with the facts and medical opinions that the claim examiner requires. The narrative should include:

- Medical history.
- Clinical signs and symptoms.
- Diagnosis.
- Treatment plan.
- **Prognosis,** that is, the physician's prediction of the outcome of the illness or injury and the likelihood of recovery.
- The patient's ability to perform various employment-related functions.
- Results of laboratory tests, with copies of laboratory reports.
- Other reports as applicable, including hospital history and discharge; audiograms; radiograms; blood tests; biopsies; range-of-motion tests; nuclear medicine tests; pulmonary function tests; and reports from psychologists, social workers, or social service agents.

If the medical narrative prepared for the claim examiner is incomplete, does not contain enough detail, or has errors, the patient may be denied benefits. Therefore, it is very important for the medical insurance specialist to proofread the report for mistakes or missing information before releasing it. In addition, the patient must sign a form to authorize release of information.

Explore the Internet

Visit the government disability website and research topics under the Health tab. Check particularly for information about professional health care resources and managed care.

Consulting and Educational Career Opportunities

Many new job opportunities are offered in nontraditional environments. The following list describes positions in some of these settings.

- *Pharmaceutical Companies*—The drugs that are tested in clinical trials must be coded for reporting test results to regulatory agencies.
- *Software Development Companies*—A firm that produces a software program for the health care industry requires people who understand claim processing and coding procedures. These employees write the specifications for the program and then test its performance using sample data.
- *Accounting Firms*—Many accounting firms have provider organizations as their clients. The accountants prepare these clients' tax returns and audit their financial records. To assist in this process, they employ professional coders who understand the reimbursement process.
- *Law Firms*—Because of the growing number of lawsuits resulting from fraud and abuse

initiatives, many law firms employ—or hire as consultants—both clinical advisers, such as registered nurses, and professional coders and billing specialists who can assist with compliance issues.

- *Independent Consultants*—There are many opportunities for consulting work with provider groups on issues such as compliance plans, preparation of correct forms, and audit procedures.
- *Seminar or Training and Education*—There are numerous opportunities for work as an educator, whether as college faculty or workshop or seminar faculty members training physicians and office staff.
- *Contract Work*—Contract work may involve working for a consulting company and being assigned to various client companies (such as on-site coding), or it may involve self-employment as a consultant. Jobs in education may also be as employees or as independent contractors.

Chapter Summary

1. Disability compensation is a government program or an insurance policy designed to reimburse the insured for lost wages caused by an illness or injury.

2. The six major federal disability programs are (a) Social Security Disability Insurance (SSDI), (b) Supplemental Security Income (SSI), (c) Civil Service Retirement System (CSRS), (d) Federal Employees Retirement System (FERS), (e) Veteran's Compensation Program, and (f) Veteran's Pension Program.

   The three categories of eligibility for SSDI are (a) salaried or hourly-wage employees whose payroll deductions included those for FICA; (b) self-employed individuals who paid a special Social Security tax; and (c) widows, widowers, or minor children with disabilities whose deceased spouses or parents would qualify for Social Security benefits if they were still alive.

   SSI provides cash payments to elderly, blind, and disabled people with incomes below the federal

poverty level. CSRS and FERS cover employees of the federal government. The two veteran's programs listed above benefit veterans of the uniformed services.

3. Some government disability programs, such as Social Security Disability Insurance and State Disability Insurance, are funded through employee payroll deductions. Other plans, such as Supplemental Security Income, are welfare programs. Private disability insurance can be purchased or may be available through an employer's plan.

4. Eight types of information the physician should include in a medical report for a disability compensation program are (a) medical history, (b) clinical signs and symptoms, (c) diagnosis, (d) treatment plan, (e) prognosis, (f) the patient's ability to perform various employment-related functions, (g) results of laboratory tests with copies of laboratory reports, and (h) other reports as applicable.

Check Your Understanding

Part 1. Answer the following questions.

1. What does disability compensation insurance pay for?

_____

2. What are the six major federal disability programs?

_____

3. Which federal disability program is a welfare program?

_____

4. What is the designation of the payroll deduction that pays for the Social Security Disability Insurance program?

_____

5. What is the term used by private disability compensation programs for a condition that prevents a worker from doing a regular job for a short time, but from which the worker is expected to recover?

_____

6. What is the term used by private disability compensation programs for a condition that prevents the insured from returning to the job?

_____

7. What can happen if the claims examiner for a disability compensation program does not have enough medical information?

_____

8. What does the Social Security Administration send the physician when a patient files a claim for disability compensation benefits?

_____

9. What term describes the physician's prediction of the outcome of the illness or injury and the likelihood of recovery?

_____

10. What must a patient sign before medical information can be sent to a claims examiner for a disability compensation program?

_____

Part 2. Analyze the following medical report for a disability compensation program, and identify the major types of information it contains. Select your answers from the following list: clinical signs and symptoms, diagnosis, medical history, prognosis, and treatment plan.

Medical Report on Barry Finestine

Date of Birth: 10-11-50

Date of Examination: 5-07-10

Employer: Marty's Movers, Randolph Road, Forester, NJ 07652

Mr. Finestine came in with a one-month history of back pain with sudden onset from lifting heavy furniture during an office relocation. He complained of pain radiating to his lower left leg to the level of the ankle. Flexion exercises made the condition worse.

Examination of the thoracic lumbar spine reveals flexion to 90 degrees; backward bending is 0 degrees; side bending bilaterally is 30 degrees; rotation bilaterally is 45 degrees. Range of motion of the lumbar spine is full for flexion, extension, lateral bending, and rotation, with some discomfort on extension. Muscle strength, bulk, tone, and light touch are intact. Deep tendon reflexes are two plus over four and symmetric. Toes are down going. Patrick's test is negative bilaterally. There is mild joint tenderness and mild left sciatic notch tenderness. Spring test is negative.

(1) Thoracic lumbar strain.

(2) Acute low-back pain with radicular pain into the left leg without neurologic evidence of radiculopathy.

(3) Probable chronic lumbar myositis.

(1) Bed rest with local heat for twenty-four hours.

(2) Flexion exercises, adding extension exercises as he improves.

(3) Prednisone two milligrams TID with meals and Tylenol #3 if needed for pain control.

Patient follow-up scheduled for one week.

Discussed with the patient need to avoid heavy lifting for the next three months.

Part 3. Study the following draft of a letter from a physician in response to a Notice of Claim Filed. Assume the role of the medical insurance specialist in this situation. In your opinion, are any elements missing from this letter that should be included?

re: ROGER MONTOYA

At home on the basement stairs, Mr. Montoya fell and injured his right wrist and right knee on January 2, 2010. The right wrist is swollen and has an obvious deformity. There is normal sensation and normal motion of fingers. He reports pain with movement of the wrist. Right knee patella is tender to palpitation. There is joint effusion of the knee.

An X-ray of the right wrist shows distal radial fracture. Right knee X-ray shows a fracture of the patella with no displacement of the fragments.

My diagnosis is: Colles fracture, right wrist, and patellar fracture, right knee.

I have immobilized the right leg. Mr. Montoya has been supplied with one crutch and instructed in crutch walking. He has been told to put as little weight as possible on the knee. He should not perform his normal work at Majors' Delicatessen.

Learning Outcomes

After completing this chapter, you will be able to define the key terms and:

14-1 Locate and describe the parts of the mouth and the teeth.

14-2 Recognize key words, conditions, and treatments related to dentistry.

14-3 Describe six types of benefits offered by dental insurance plans.

14-4 Discuss the claim form and coding methods commonly used to submit dental insurance claims.

Key Terms

ADA Dental Claim Form

canines

Current Dental Terminology (CDT)

dentin

Dentist's Pretreatment Estimate

Dentist's Statement of Actual Services

enamel

gingivae (*sing.,* gingiva)

incisors

mandible

maxilla

maxillofacial surgery

molars

occlusion

oral cavity

oral surgery

palate

premolars

prophylaxes (*sing.,* prophylaxis)

prostheses (*sing.,* prosthesis)

pulp

uvula

Why This Chapter Is Important to You

The information in this chapter will enable you to:

- Understand the language that dentists use to describe diagnoses and procedures.
- Help patients with dental insurance claims.

What Do You Think?

Some insurance specialists work in dental practices rather than in medical practices. How might the tasks or surroundings of a dental insurance specialist differ from those of a medical insurance specialist?

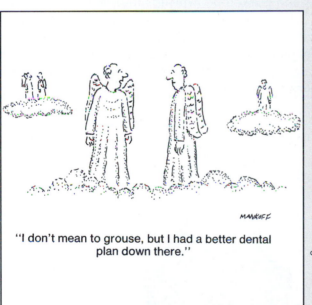

"I don't mean to grouse, but I had a better dental plan down there."

INTRODUCTION TO DENTAL TERMS

Medical terminology is used to describe oral (related to the mouth) anatomy, diagnoses, and treatments. In dentistry, the word elements of roots, combining vowels, prefixes, and suffixes are put together to describe the specific parts of the mouth and teeth as well as the procedures performed.

Overview of the Parts of the Mouth and the Teeth

The mouth, shown in Figure 14-1, is at the beginning of the digestive system. It has an outer part, made up of the lips and cheeks, and an inner section, or **oral cavity** leading to the throat. The oral cavity contains the gums, called **gingivae**; the teeth; the tongue; and the tonsils.

The mouth's underlying bone structure also has two major parts. The **mandible,** the U-shaped lower jawbone, has tooth sockets to hold the lower teeth. The upper jawbone is the **maxilla.** It houses the upper teeth and the **palate,** which is the roof of the mouth. The hard palate is a bony structure that separates the oral cavity from the inner nose, or nasal cavity. The soft palate, made up of muscle tissue, is located behind the hard palate. The soft palate extends downward toward the throat, ending in the cone-shaped **uvula.** The upper and lower jawbones are connected by a joint. When the jaws close, the contact between the upper and lower teeth is referred to as **occlusion.**

The teeth tear and grind food, which is moistened by saliva from the salivary glands. Saliva not only helps to soften food; it also contains an enzyme that begins the breakdown, or digestion, of food. When a person swallows, muscles pull the soft palate and uvula upward, closing the opening between the nasal cavity and the pharynx. This keeps food from entering the nasal cavity.

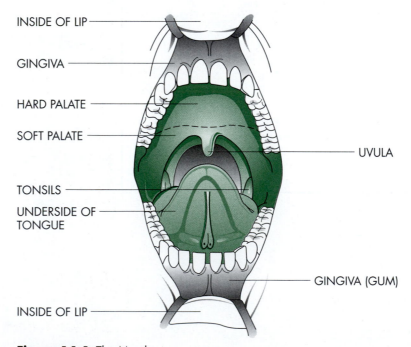

Figure 14-1 The Mouth

The thirty-two permanent teeth that adults have are set in two arches, one in the mandible and the other in the maxilla. Each of the jaws holds four **incisors,** which are the cutting teeth; two **canines;** four **premolars;** and six **molars.** In dental insurance claims, the teeth are numbered from a person's right to left, upper to lower, as shown in Figure 14-2.

Figure 14-3 shows the structure of a tooth. The teeth are held in their sockets by periodontal ligaments. Each tooth is covered by an outer coating, the **enamel.** A hard material called **dentin** fills up 80 to 90 percent of the tooth, covering the soft core, or **pulp,** which contains nerves and blood vessels.

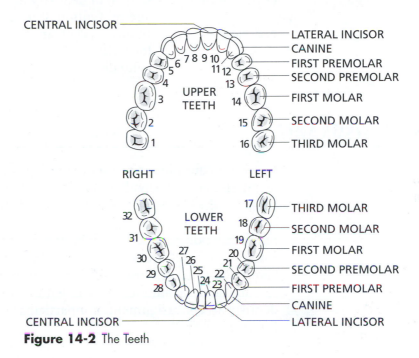

Figure 14-2 The Teeth

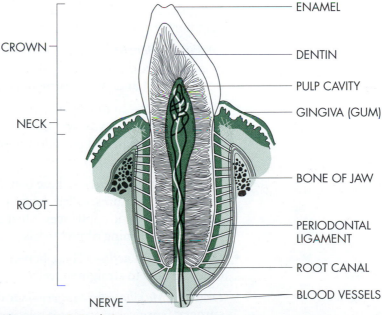

Figure 14-3 Tooth Structure

A tooth has three main sections: the crown, the neck, and the root. The cavity that contains the pulp is called the root canal. The part that is covered with enamel is the crown. The neck is the section where the tooth meets the gum. The section below the gum line is the root.

Following are examples of dental terms used in dental practices:

Term	Meaning
Endodontics	Branch of dentistry dealing with tooth pulp
Gingivitis	Inflammation of the gingiva(e)
Malocclusion	Poor alignment of upper and lower teeth
Orthodontics	Branch of dentistry dealing with the correction and prevention of irregular teeth and malocclusion
Periodontics	Branch of dentistry that studies the tissues around the teeth
Periodontitis	Gum disease

DENTAL INSURANCE

As with medical insurance, a broad range of dental insurance plans can be purchased by individuals and by employers. More than 188 million people in the United States have access to dental insurance through group health plans or under Medicaid. Most insurance carriers' dental plans reimburse policyholders, or subscribers, for dental expenses. However, some carriers offer managed care plans for dental benefits. Currently, about one-third of those insured are covered by some form of managed care for dental insurance. Also, as with medical insurance, participating dentists accept assignment; nonparticipating dentists are paid specific listed fees.

Dental benefits vary. Some of the plans include:

- *Preventive Benefits*—These benefits cover **prophylaxes,** or cleanings, at regular intervals and the application of fluoride treatments to coat the teeth of children.

- *Diagnostic Benefits*—Diagnostic procedures, such as X-rays and laboratory work, are used by the dentist to evaluate conditions and determine what dental treatment is needed.

- *Basic Benefits*—In most plans, these benefits cover restorative work such as fillings, crowns, and inlays; endodontic procedures such as root canal fillings; and periodontic procedures to prevent or treat gum disease.

- *Prosthodontics Benefits*—These benefits cover the construction of bridges and dentures, called dental **prostheses,** and the repair of existing prosthetic appliances. Most dental contracts limit the number and timing of prosthesis replacements.

- *Orthodontic Benefits*—These benefits cover the use of braces and other devices to straighten teeth.

- *Oral and Maxillofacial Surgery*—**Oral surgery** and **maxillofacial surgery** (surgical procedures relating to the face and jaw) as well as the necessary general anesthesia are covered.

Carriers do not normally pay the same percentage for every type of procedure. For example, many plans cover the cost of prophylaxes and examinations in full, but they may pick up only 50 to 90 percent of other procedures.

Medicare offers no dental coverage. However, it does cover oral surgery procedures for conditions such as tumors or jaw disease under its medical benefits. Some dental procedures are covered under Medicaid; the fees are set by the individual states. Most Blue Cross and Blue Shield plans include dental coverage contracts.

Professional Focus

Dental Injury Claims and Workers' Compensation

The steps for processing dental injury claims are similar to medical workers' compensation procedures. The dentist must complete a first report of injury for the carrier's workers' compensation plan, usually within five days of the patient's visit. This report describes the condition of the patient's teeth and gums before the injury, the nature and extent of the injury, the repair and/or replacement of teeth required, and the cost. The report includes the employer's name and address, the employee's supervisor, the date and time of the accident, and the patient's description of the injury.

Authorization must be obtained from the carrier before treatment for anything other than emergency care. Payment will be made only for care required because of a job-related injury.

PROCESSING DENTAL CLAIMS

Dental patients complete patient information forms similar to those used in medical offices. The patient provides personal and employment information, dental insurance information, and account information. The dental patient information form usually has a signature line for authorization of release of information. The encounter form, too, is similar to that used in medical offices. An example is shown in Figure 14-4 (on page 262).

Dental Coding

In general, dental insurance claims require procedure codes, but not diagnosis codes. Surgical procedures submitted on a medical claim form are the exception. In these cases, diagnosis codes are also required. Dental procedure codes are five-digit codes that begin with the letter D to make them different from numbers in other coding systems. The second

Michael Davis, DDS

Provider: _____
_____
_____

ID #: _____   Tax ID: _____

Name: _____   Pat#: _____   Document: 8889
Address: _____   Code: _____   Date: 09-09-2010
_____   Phone: _____   Time: _____

Codes	— Services —	Codes	— X Rays —
D0120	PERIODIC ORAL EVALUATION	D0272	BITEWINGS 2 FILMS
D0140	LIMITED ORAL EVALUATION - PROBLEM FOCUSED	D0274	BITEWINGS 4 FILMS
D1203	FLUORIDE-TOPICAL CHILD (PROPHY NOT INCLUDED)		
D1351	SEALANT, PER TOOTH		
D2140	AMAL 1 SURF PRIMARY OR PERM	Codes	— Payments —
D2330	RESIN-BASED COMP 1 SURFACE ANTERIOR		
D2530	INLAY METALLIC - THREE SURF OR MORE	PMTDUE	PAYMENT DUE
D2750	PORC CRN FUSED TO HIGH NOBLE METAL	CASH	CASH PAYMENT—THANK YOU!
D2751	PORC CRN FUSED TO PREDOMINATELY BASE METAL	CHECK	CHECK—THANK YOU!
D2790	FULL CAST CROWN HIGH NOBLE METAL	MO	Money Order Paymnt—Thank You
D2920	RECMT CROWN		
D2930	PREFAB. SS CROWN - PRIMARY TOOTH		
D2932	PREFAB. RESIN CROWN		
D2940	SEDATIVE FILLING		
D2950	CORE BUILDUPS INCLUDING ANY PINS		
D2952	CAST POST & CORE/ADD. TO CR.		
D3110	PULP CAP DIRECT (EXCLUDING FINAL RESTORATION)		
D3320	ROOT CANAL, BICUSPID (EXCLUDING FINAL RESTORATION)		
D3330	ROOT CANAL, MOLARI (EXCLUDING FINAL RESTORATION)		
D5110	COMP DENTURE—MAXILLARY		
D5130	IMMEDIATE DENTURE—MAXILLARY		
D5213	PARTIAL DENTURE—MAXILLARY		
D5214	PARTIAL DENTURE—MANDIBULAR		
D5710	REBASE COMP MAXILLARY DENTURE		
D5750	RELINE COMP MAXILLARY DENTURE		
D5751	RELINE COMP MANDIBULAR DENTURE		
D6750	FIXED PARTIAL DENTURE (RETAINER) CROWN: PORCELAIN FUSED TO HIGH NOBLE METAL		
D6790	FIXED PARTIAL DENTURE (RETAINER) CROWN: FULL CAST HIGH NOBLE METAL		
D6950	PRECISION ATTACHMENT		
D7111	EXTRACTION: CORONAL REMNANTS		
D9940	OCCLUSAL GUARD, BY REPORT		

Description: _____

Family Aging Balances

Current	30	60	90
:____:	:____:	:____:	:____:

Remarks: _____

Next Appointment: _____

Previous Balance   :_____:
Today's Charges   :_____:
Amount Paid   :_____:
New Balance   :_____:

Figure 14-4 Dental Office Encounter Form

number of the code indicates the category of dental service. There are twelve categories:

Category of Service		Code Series
I.	Diagnostic	D0100–D0999
II.	Preventive	D1000–D1999
III.	Restorative	D2000–D2999
IV.	Endodontics	D3000–D3999
V.	Periodontics	D4000–D4999
VI.	Prosthodontics, Removable	D5000–D5899
VII.	Maxillofacial Prosthetics	D5900–D5999
VIII.	Implant Services	D6000–D6199
IX.	Prosthodontics, Fixed	D6200–D6999
X.	Oral and Maxillofacial Surgery	D7000–D7999
XI.	Orthodontics	D8000–D8999
XII.	Adjunctive General Services	D9000–D9999

The American Dental Association (ADA) develops and publishes the dental code set, **Current Dental Terminology (CDT).** The diagnosis codes for claims involving oral surgery or maxillofacial surgery are usually taken from the ICD-9-CM.

Case Study 14-1

Procedure: Performed root canal filling on Tooth 18.

Procedure code (refer to Figure 14-4):

_____

Case Study 14-2

Procedure: Established patient Toru Hayashi complained of pain in the upper or lower right area during his annual checkup. Two bitewings (X-rays designed to show the crowns of the upper and lower teeth at the same time) were taken of the area. Indicated requirement for filling; appointment made for March 22.

Procedure codes (refer to Figure 14-4):

_____

Dental Claim Forms

Compliance Tip

If blank 4 is answered yes, blanks 5 through 11 should be completed. The information in blanks 5 through 11 is used to determine which other carriers, if any, have primary liability for the provided treatment.

A dental claim form is used for two purposes: (1) to report the **Dentist's Pretreatment Estimate** to an insurance carrier before the service is performed, for an analysis of what will be reimbursed, and (2) to submit the **Dentist's Statement of Actual Services** for claim processing and payment.

A Dentist's Pretreatment Estimate may be submitted for a number of reasons. The primary reason is to find out whether the procedure is covered and how much of the cost will be reimbursed. In addition, this estimate helps to resolve the disagreements that at times arise between a dentist and a carrier about appropriate treatments. Also, dental patients often have choices regarding treatments. For example, one type of crown material may look better than another, but it may also be more expensive. If the dental insurance coverage has a set rate for a crown, a patient who desires the more expensive material may have to pay a higher cost.

Some dental office staff members process claims for patients or may help patients with completing claims. Many dental practitioners complete the universal claim form called the **ADA Dental Claim Form** for patients to attach to their own carriers' claim forms. The ADA Dental Claim Form is approved and updated by the American Dental Association (see Figures 14-5a and 14-5b). It has eleven sections. The top portion contains patient coverage information, the middle portion contains details about the examination and treatment plan, and the lower portion contains information on authorizations and billing details, such as the billing dentist.

When treatment involves a medical claim for oral or maxillofacial surgery, the claim must be submitted using the electronic HIPAA claim or the CMS-1500 paper claim form, depending on the carrier. The state Medicare carrier has specific guidelines for using the electronic HIPAA claim.

Filling Out the ADA Dental Claim Form

The instructions for completing the ADA Dental Claim Form are similar to those for other claims. Step-by-step instructions on how to fill in each blank on the form appear on the back of the form and are shown in Figure 14-5b on page 266.

Explore the Internet

Visit the website of the American Dental Association. Go to the A-Z topics section in the panel entitled Your Oral Health, and research the topic of insurance. What types of dental plans are available today?

ADA. Dental Claim Form

HEADER INFORMATION

1. Type of Transaction (Check all applicable boxes)

☐ Statement of Actual Services – OR – ☐ Request for Predetermination/Preauthorization

☐ EPSDT/Title XIX

2. Predetermination/Preauthorization Number

PRIMARY PAYER INFORMATION

3. Name, Address, City, State, Zip Code

OTHER COVERAGE

4. Other Dental or Medical Coverage? ☐ No (Skip 5-11)   ☐ Yes (Complete 5-11)

5. Subscriber Name (Last, First, Middle Initial, Suffix)

6. Date of Birth (MM/DD/CCYY) | **7. Gender** ☐ M ☐ F | **8. Subscriber Identifier (SSN or ID#)**

9. Plan/Group Number | **10. Relationship to Primary Subscriber (Check applicable box)** ☐ Self ☐ Spouse ☐ Dependent ☐ Other

11. Other Carrier Name, Address, City, State, Zip Code

PRIMARY SUBSCRIBER INFORMATION

12. Name (Last, First, Middle Initial, Suffix), Address, City, State, Zip Code

13. Date of Birth (MM/DD/CCYY) | **14. Gender** ☐ M ☐ F | **15. Subscriber Identifier (SSN or ID#)**

16. Plan/Group Number | **17. Employer Name**

PATIENT INFORMATION

18. Relationship to Primary Subscriber (Check applicable box) ☐ Self ☐ Spouse ☐ Dependent Child ☐ Other | **19. Student Status** ☐ FTS ☐ PTS

20. Name (Last, First, Middle Initial, Suffix), Address, City, State, Zip Code

21. Date of Birth (MM/DD/CCYY) | **22. Gender** ☐ M ☐ F | **23. Patient ID/Account # (Assigned by Dentist)**

RECORD OF SERVICES PROVIDED

	24. Procedure Date (MM/DD/CCYY)	25. Area of Oral Cavity	26. Tooth System	27. Tooth Number(s) or Letter(s)	28. Tooth Surface	29. Procedure Code	30. Description	31. Fee
1								
2								
3								
4								
5								
6								
7								
8								
9								
10								

MISSING TEETH INFORMATION

34. (Place an 'X' on each missing tooth)

Permanent: 1 2 3 4 5 6 7 8 9 10 11 12 13 14 15 16 / 32 31 30 29 28 27 26 25 24 23 22 21 20 19 18 17

Primary: A B C D E F G H I J / T S R Q P O N M L K

32. Other Fee(s)

33. Total Fee

35. Remarks

AUTHORIZATIONS

36. I have been informed of the treatment plan and associated fees. I agree to be responsible for all charges for dental services and materials not paid by my dental benefit plan, unless prohibited by law, or the treating dentist or dental practice has a contractual agreement with my plan prohibiting all or a portion of such charges. To the extent permitted by law, I consent to your use and disclosure of my protected health information to carry out payment activities in connection with this claim.

X_____

Patient/Guardian signature   Date

37. I hereby authorize and direct payment of the dental benefits otherwise payable to me, directly to the below named dentist or dental entity.

X_____

Subscriber signature   Date

BILLING DENTIST OR DENTAL ENTITY (Leave blank if dentist or dental entity is not submitting claim on behalf of the patient or insured/subscriber)

48. Name, Address, City, State, Zip Code

49. NPI | **50. License Number** | **51. SSN or TIN**

52. Phone Number (   )   –

ANCILLARY CLAIM/TREATMENT INFORMATION

38. Place of Treatment (Check applicable box) ☐ Provider's Office ☐ Hospital ☐ ECF ☐ Other

39. Number of Enclosures (00 to 99) Radiograph(s) Oral Image(s) Model(s)

40. Is Treatment for Orthodontics? ☐ No (Skip 41-42) ☐ Yes (Complete 41-42)

41. Date Appliance Placed (MM/DD/CCYY)

42. Months of Treatment Remaining | **43. Replacement of Prosthesis?** ☐ No ☐ Yes (Complete 44) | **44. Date Prior Placement (MM/DD/CCYY)**

45. Treatment Resulting from (Check applicable box) ☐ Occupational illness/injury ☐ Auto accident ☐ Other accident

46. Date of Accident (MM/DD/CCYY) | **47. Auto Accident State**

TREATING DENTIST AND TREATMENT LOCATION INFORMATION

53. I hereby certify that the procedures as indicated by date are in progress (for procedures that require multiple visits) or have been completed and that the fees submitted are the actual fees I have charged and intend to collect for those procedures.

X_____

Signed (Treating Dentist)   Date

54. NPI | **55. License Number**

56. Address, City, State, Zip Code

57. Phone Number (   )   – | **58. Treating Provider Specialty**

©American Dental Association, 2006
J515 (Same as ADA Dental Claim Form) – J516, J517, J518, J519

To Reorder call 1-800-947-4746
or go online at www.adacatalog.org

Figure 14-5a Front of ADA Dental Claim Form

General Instructions:

The form is designed so that the Primary Payer's name and address (Item 3) is visible in a standard #10 window envelope. Please fold the form using the 'tick-marks' printed in the left and right margins. The upper-right blank space is provided for insertion of the third-party payer's claim or control number.
a) All data elements are required unless noted to the contrary on the face of the form, or in the Data Element Specific Instructions that follow.
b) When a name and address field is required, the full entity or individual name, address and zip code must be entered (i.e., Items 3, 11, 12, 20 and 48).
c) All dates must include the four-digit year (i.e., Items 6, 13, 21, 24, 36, 37, 41, 44, and 53).
d) If the number of procedures being reported exceeds the number of lines available on one claim form the remaining procedures must be listed on a separate, fully completed claim form. Both claim forms are submitted to the third-party payer.

Data Element Specific Instructions

1. **EPSDT / Title XIX** -- Mark box if patient is covered by state Medicaid's **E**arly and **P**eriodic **S**creening, **D**iagnosis and **T**reatment program for persons under age 21.
2. Enter number provided by the payer when submitting a claim for services that have been predetermined or preauthorized.
4-11. Leave blank if no other coverage.
8. The subscriber's Social Security Number (SSN) or other identifier (ID#) assigned by the payer.
15. The subscriber's Social Security Number (SSN) or other identifier (ID#) assigned by the payer.
16. Subscriber's or employer group's Plan or Policy Number. May also be known as the Certificate Number. [Not the subscriber's identification number.]
19-23. Complete only if the patient is **not** the Primary Subscriber. (i.e., "Self" not checked in Item 18)
19. Check "FTS" if patient is a dependent and full-time student; "PTS" if a part-time student. Otherwise, leave blank.
23. Enter if dentist's office assigns a unique number to identify the patient that is **not** the same as the Subscriber Identifier number assigned by the payer (e.g., Chart #).
25. Designate tooth number or letter when procedure code directly involves a tooth. Use area of the oral cavity code set from ANSI/ADA/ISO Specification No. 3950 'Designation System for Teeth and Areas of the Oral Cavity'.
26. Enter applicable ANSI ASC X12 code list qualifier: Use "**JP**" when designating teeth using the ADA's Universal/National Tooth Designation System. Use "**JO**" when using the ANSI/ADA/ISO Specification No. 3950.
27. Designate tooth number when procedure code reported directly involves a tooth. If a range of teeth is being reported use a hyphen ('-') to separate the first and last tooth in the range. Commas are used to separate individual tooth numbers or ranges applicable to the procedure code reported.
28. Designate tooth surface(s) when procedure code reported directly involves one or more tooth surfaces. Enter up to five of the following codes, without spaces: **B** = Buccal; **D** = Distal; **F** = Facial; **L** = Lingual; **M** = Mesial; and **O** = Occlusal.
29. Use appropriate dental procedure code from current version of *Code on Dental Procedures and Nomenclature*.
31. Dentist's full fee for the dental procedure reported.
32. Used when other fees applicable to dental services provided must be recorded. Such fees include state taxes, where applicable, and other fees imposed by regulatory bodies.
33. Total of all fees listed on the claim form.
34. Report missing teeth on each claim submission.
35. Use "Remarks" space for additional information such as 'reports' for '999' codes or multiple supernumerary teeth.
36. Patient Signature: The patient is defined as an individual who has established a professional relationship with the dentist for the delivery of dental health care. For matters relating to communication of information and consent, this term includes the patient's parent, caretaker, guardian, or other individual as appropriate under state law and the circumstances of the case.
37. Subscriber Signature: Necessary when the patient/insured and dentist wish to have benefits paid directly to the provider. This is an authorization of payment. It does not create a contractual relationship between the dentist and the payer.
38. ECF is the acronym for **E**xtended **C**are **F**acility (e.g., nursing home).
48-52. Leave blank if dentist or dental entity is **not** submitting claim on behalf of the patient or insured/subscriber.
48. The individual dentist's name or the name of the group practice/corporation responsible for billing and other pertinent information. This may differ from the actual treating dentist's name. This is the information that should appear on any payments or correspondence that will be remitted to the billing dentist.
49. Identifier assigned to Billing Dentist of Dental Entity other than the SSN or TIN. Necessary when assigned by carrier receiving the claim
50. Refers to the license number of the billing dentist. This may differ from that of the treating (rendering) dentist that appears in the treating dentist's signature block.
52. The Internal Revenue Service requires that either the Social Security Number (SSN) or Tax Identification Number (TIN) of the billing dentist or dental entity be supplied **only** if the provider accepts payment directly from the third-party payer.
   When the payment is being accepted directly report the: 1) SSN if the billing dentist in unincorporated; 2) Corporation TIN if the billing dentist is incorporated; or 3) Entity TIN when the billing entity is a group practice or clinic.
53. The treating, or rendering, dentist's signature and date the claim form was signed. Dentists should be aware that they have ethical and legal obligations to refund fees for services that are paid in advance but not completed.
56. Full address, including city, state and zip code, where treatment performed by treating (rendering) dentist.
58. Enter the code that indicates the type of dental professional rendering the service from the 'Dental Service Providers' section of the *Healthcare Providers Taxonomy* code list. The current list is posted at: http://www.wpc-edi.com/codes/codes.asp. The available taxonomy codes, as of the first printing of this claim form, follow printed in **boldface**.

122300000X Dentist -- A dentist is a person qualified by a doctorate in dental surgery (D.D.S.) or dental medicine (D.M.D.) licensed by the state to practice dentistry, and practicing within the scope of that license.

Many dentists are general practitioners who handle a wide variety of dental needs.
1223G0001X General Practice

Other dentists practice in one of nine specialty areas recognized by the American Dental Association:
1223D0001X Dental Public Health
1223E0200X Endodontics
1223P0106X Oral & Maxillofacial Pathology
1223D0008X Oral and Maxillofacial Radiology
1223S0112X Oral & Maxillofacial Surgery
1223X0400X Orthodontics
1223P0221X Pediatric Dentistry (Pedodontics)
1223P0300X Periodontics
1223P0700X Prosthodontics

Figure 14-5b Back of ADA Dental Claim Form

Chapter Summary

1. The major parts of the mouth are the lips, cheeks, teeth, gums, tongue, palate, and throat. Each tooth has an outer coating, the enamel; a core, called the dentin; and pulp, containing the nerves and blood supply. The main sections of a tooth are the crown, the neck, and the root.

2. Many dental terms are based on anatomy. For example, the word *malocclusion* means a condition of poor alignment of the upper and lower teeth.

3. Six types of dental benefits offered by dental insurance plans are preventive, diagnostic, basic, prosthodontic, orthodontic, and those for oral and maxillofacial surgeries.

4. The procedures shown on dental insurance claims are coded with CDT-4 codes. Unless the claim is for oral or maxillofacial surgery, ICD-9-CM diagnosis codes are not required. The universal dental claim form approved by the American Dental Association is called the ADA Dental Claim Form. In dentistry, the electronic HIPAA claim or the CMS-1500 paper claim form is used only to report medical claims for oral and maxillofacial surgeries.

Check Your Understanding

Part 1. Choose the best answer.

_____ **1.** The maxilla is the:
    a. upper jawbone
    b. lower jawbone
    c. joint connecting the upper and lower jawbones

_____ **2.** The gingivae are the:
    a. contacts between upper and lower teeth
    b. gums
    c. incisors

_____ **3.** On a dental claim form, a treated tooth is indicated by:
    a. the name of the tooth
    b. the letter of the tooth
    c. the number of the tooth

_____ **4.** A regular cleaning of the teeth by a dentist to prevent disease is called:
    a. prosthesis
    b. prophylaxis
    c. impaction

_____ **5.** A set of dentures is a:
    a. prosthesis
    b. prophylaxis
    c. impaction

_____ **6.** In general, claims for dental treatments require:
    a. diagnosis codes
    b. procedure codes
    c. neither a nor b

_____ **7.** CDT codes begin with:
    a. a C
    b. an R
    c. a D

_____ **8.** Claims for oral surgery are reported on the:
    a. HIPAA or CMS-1500 form
    b. ADA form
    c. CMS-1450 form

_____ **9.** A dental claim form may be submitted for:
    a. a pretreatment estimate
    b. payment
    c. both a and b

_____ **10.** When completing a dental claim form for a dental treatment:
    a. indicate treatments due to illness, injury, or accidents
    b. complete the deductible and maximum allowable blanks
    c. be sure the office manager signs the form

Part 2. Using the most recent CDT-4 available, complete the following case studies. (If you do not have access to the CDT-4, ask your instructor for a list of dental procedure codes.)

1. Procedure: Patient Sarah Rabinowitz, age eight; first examination.

   Code: _____

2. Procedure: Patient Rory Wetsell, two-surface amalgam/filling on Tooth 15, permanent tooth; local anesthesia.

   Codes: _____

Part 3. Identify the numbers of the form locators on the ADA Dental Claim Form where the following data should be entered.

_____ **1.** Blue Cross and Blue Shield claim

_____ **2.** The fact that the patient has another dental plan

_____ **3.** The insured's date of birth when the insured is not the patient

_____ **4.** The name of the dental practice or dentist responsible for generating the charges shown on the claim

_____ **5.** Date of prior placement of a prosthesis

Part 4. Enter the correct CDT-4 code for each of the following procedures or services.

_____ **1.** Pulp vitality tests

_____ **2.** Prophylaxis—child

_____ **3.** Surgical incision to remove a foreign body from skin

_____ **4.** Extraction of coronal remnants

_____ **5.** Inlay—resin-based composite—three surfaces

_____ **6.** Nasal prosthesis

_____ **7.** Repair missing teeth in complete dentures

_____ **8.** Gingivectomy or gingivoplasty—four contiguous teeth per quadrant

_____ **9.** Endodontic therapy of molar (without final restoration)

_____ **10.** Recement crown

CHAPTER 15

Hospital Insurance

Learning Outcomes

After completing this chapter, you will be able to define the key terms and:

15-1 Compare inpatient and outpatient hospital services.

15-2 List the major steps relating to hospital claims processing.

15-3 Describe two differences in coding diagnoses for hospital inpatient cases and physician office services.

15-4 Describe the procedure codes used in hospital coding.

15-5 Discuss the important items that are reported on the HIPAA hospital claim, the 837I.

Key Terms

admitting diagnosis
ambulatory care
attending physician
charge master (charge ticket)
CMS-1450
diagnosis-related group
  (DRG)
837I claim

emergency care
health information
  management (HIM)
inpatient
master patient index
MS-DRGs
present on admission (POA)
  indicator

principal diagnosis
principal procedure
Prospective Payment
  System (PPS)
registration
UB-92
UB-04

Why This Chapter Is Important to You

The information in this chapter will enable you to:

- Become familiar with the coding systems used in hospitals.
- Learn the basic billing process that hospitals follow.
- Understand the format and use of the UB-04 claim form.

What Do You Think?

There are many working and financial agreements between physicians and hospitals; physicians in practices may have staff privileges at hospitals or may be associated with hospitals as medical specialists. Medical insurance specialists often prepare claims for surgery and other procedures performed by the physicians who employ them. Why do you think it is important to be aware of the coding systems and the billing process used in hospitals?

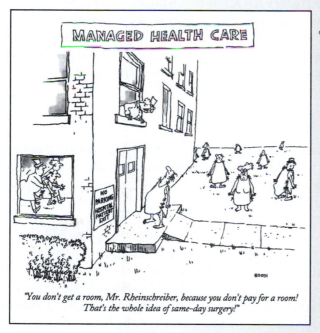

"You don't get a room, Mr. Rheinschreiber, because you don't pay for a room! That's the whole idea of same-day surgery!"

HEALTH CARE FACILITIES: INPATIENT VERSUS OUTPATIENT

General hospitals accept all types of patients. Specialized health care hospitals offer services such as acute care, psychiatric care, and rehabilitation. Private hospitals are either investor-owned for-profit institutions or nonprofit facilities. Public hospitals are those owned by the federal government (such as veterans' and military hospitals), by states (such as long-term psychiatric facilities and teaching hospitals), and by local governments such as counties and cities. The sizes of hospitals, measured by the number of beds, vary from small to very large.

Inpatient Care

Inpatient facilities are equipped for patients to stay overnight. In addition to hospital admission, inpatient care may be provided in:

- *Skilled Nursing Facilities* (SNF)—Facilities that provide skilled nursing or rehabilitation services to help with recovery after a hospital stay. Skilled nursing care includes care given by licensed nurses under the direction of a physician, such as intravenous injections, tube feeding, and changing sterile dressings on a wound.
- *Long-Term Care Facilities*—This term describes facilities such as nursing homes that provide care for patients with chronic disabilities and prolonged illnesses.
- *Hospital Emergency Rooms or Departments*—**Emergency care** involves a situation in which a delay in the treatment of the patient would lead to a significant increase in the threat to life or a body part. Emergency care differs from urgently needed care, in which the condition must be treated right away but is not life-threatening.

Outpatient or Ambulatory Care

Many hospitals have expanded beyond inpatient services to offer a variety of outpatient settings. Outpatient care, often called **ambulatory care,** covers all types of health services that do not require overnight hospital stays, such as same-day surgery. Most hospitals, for example, have outpatient departments that provide these services.

Different types of outpatient services are also provided in patients' home settings. Home health care services include care given at home, such as physical therapy or skilled nursing care. Home health care is provided by a home health agency (HHA), an organization that provides home care services, including skilled nursing care, physical therapy, occupational therapy, speech therapy, and care by home health aides. At-home recovery care is a different category that includes help with the activities of daily living (ADLs), such as bathing and eating. Hospice care is a special approach to caring for people with terminal illnesses in a familiar and comfortable place, either a special hospice facility or the patient's home.

HOSPITAL CLAIMS PROCESSING

Hospitals generally have large departments that are responsible for major business functions. The admissions department records the patient's personal and financial information. As in medical offices, hospital admissions staff must be sure patients give written consent for the work to be done and for the claim reporting that follows. The patient accounting department handles billing, and there is often a separate collections department. Organizing and maintaining patient medical records in hospitals are the duties of the **health information management (HIM)** department. Hospitals are also structured into departments for patient care. For example, there are professional services departments, such as laboratory, radiology, and surgery, as well as support services departments, such as food service and housekeeping.

From the insurance perspective, the three major steps in a patient's hospital stay are:

1. Admission, for creating or updating the patient's medical record, verifying patient insurance coverage, securing consent for release of information to payers, and collecting advance payments as appropriate.
2. Treatment, during which the various departments' services are provided and charges generated.
3. Discharge from the hospital or transfer to another facility, at which point the patient's record is compiled, claims or bills are created, and payment is followed up on.

Admission

HIPAA Tip

Under the HIPAA Privacy Rule, hospitals must give patients a copy of their privacy practices at registration and ask them to sign an acknowledgment that they have received this notice. Patients have many privacy rights, such as choosing whether they wish their names to appear in the hospital's registry.

Patients are admitted to hospitals in a process called **registration**. Like physician practices, hospitals must keep clear, accurate records of their patients' diagnoses and treatments. The record begins at a patient's first admission to the facility. More information is gathered for a hospital admission than is required for a visit to a physician practice. Special points about the patient's care, such as language requirements, religion, or disabilities, are also entered in the record.

CMS requires hospitals to give Medicare patients a copy of the two-page printout entitled "An Important Message from Medicare About Your Rights" on registration. The printout explains the beneficiary's rights as a hospital patient as well as his or her appeal rights regarding hospital discharge (see Figures 15-1(a) and (b) on pages 274 and 275).

The HIM department keeps a health record system that permits storage and retrieval of clinical information by patient name or number, by **attending physician** (the physician who is primarily responsible for the care of the patient during the hospital stay), and by diagnosis and procedure. At almost every facility, a part or all of the records are stored in a computer system. Each patient is listed in a patient register under a unique number. These numbers make up the **master patient index**—the main database that identifies patients.

Outpatient department and emergency room insurance claims are often delayed because it is difficult to verify insurance coverage in these settings.

Patient Name: _____

Patient ID Number: _____

Physician: _____

DEPARTMENT OF HEALTH AND HUMAN SERVICES
CENTERS FOR MEDICARE & MEDICAID SERVICES
OMB Approval No. 0938-0692

AN IMPORTANT MESSAGE FROM MEDICARE ABOUT YOUR RIGHTS

AS A HOSPITAL INPATIENT YOU HAVE THE RIGHT TO:

- Receive Medicare covered services. This includes medically necessary hospital services and services you may need after you are discharged, if ordered by your doctor. You have a right to know about these services, who will pay for them, and where you can get them.

- Be involved in any decisions about your hospital stay, and know who will pay for it.

- Report any concerns you have about the quality of care you receive to the Quality Improvement Organization (QIO) listed here:

_____

Name of QIO

_____

Telephone Number of QIO

_____

YOUR MEDICARE DISCHARGE RIGHTS

Planning For Your Discharge: During your hospital stay, the hospital staff will be working with you to prepare for your safe discharge and arrange for services you may need after you leave the hospital. When you no longer need inpatient hospital care, your doctor or the hospital staff will inform you of your planned discharge date.

If you think you are being discharged too soon:

- You can talk to the hospital staff, your doctor and your managed care plan (if you belong to one) about your concerns.

- You also have the right to an appeal, that is, a review of your case by a Quality Improvement Organization (QIO). The QIO is an outside reviewer hired by Medicare to look at your case to decide whether you are ready to leave the hospital.

    ◦ **If you want to appeal, you must contact the QIO no later than your planned discharge date and before you leave the hospital.**

    ◦ If you do this, you will not have to pay for the services you receive during the appeal (except for charges like copays and deductibles).

- If you do not appeal, but decide to stay in the hospital past your planned discharge date, you may have to pay for any services you receive after that date.

- **Step by step instructions for calling the QIO and filing an appeal are on page 2.**

To speak with someone at the hospital about this notice, call _____.

Please sign and date here to show you received this notice and understand your rights.

Signature of Patient or Representative	Date

Form CMS-R-193 (approved 05/07)

Figure 15-1a Printout Entitled "An Important Message from Medicare About Your Rights" (Page 1)

STEPS TO APPEAL YOUR DISCHARGE

- **STEP 1:** You must contact the QIO no later than your planned discharge date and before you leave the hospital. If you do this, you will not have to pay for the services you receive during the appeal (except for charges like copays and deductibles).

    - Here is the contact information for the QIO:

      _____
      Name of QIO *(in bold)*

      _____
      Telephone Number of QIO

      _____

    - You can file a request for an appeal any day of the week. **Once you speak to someone or leave a message, your appeal has begun.**

    - Ask the hospital if you need help contacting the QIO.

    - The name of this hospital is:

Hospital Name	Provider ID Number

- **STEP 2:** You will receive a detailed notice from the hospital or your Medicare Advantage or other Medicare managed care plan (if you belong to one) that explains the reasons they think you are ready to be discharged.

- **STEP 3:** The QIO will ask for your opinion. You or your representative need to be available to speak with the QIO, if requested. You or your representative may give the QIO a written statement, but you are not required to do so.

- **STEP 4:** The QIO will review your medical records and other important information about your case.

- **STEP 5:** The QIO will notify you of its decision within 1 day after it receives all necessary information.

    - If the QIO finds that you are not ready to be discharged, Medicare will continue to cover your hospital services.

    - If the QIO finds you are ready to be discharged, Medicare will continue to cover your services until noon of the day after the QIO notifies you of its decision.

IF YOU MISS THE DEADLINE TO APPEAL, YOU HAVE OTHER APPEAL RIGHTS:

- You can still ask the QIO or your plan (if you belong to one) for a review of your case:

    - If you have Original Medicare: Call the QIO listed above.

    - If you belong to a Medicare Advantage Plan or other Medicare managed care plan: Call your plan.

- If you stay in the hospital, the hospital may charge you for any services you receive after your planned discharge date.

For more information, call 1-800-MEDICARE (1-800-633-4227), or TTY: 1-877-486-2048.

ADDITIONAL INFORMATION:

Figure 15-1b Printout Entitled "An Important Message from Medicare About Your Rights" (Page 2)

The emergency department has its own registration system because people who come for emergency and urgent treatment must receive care immediately. Both outpatient and emergency room procedures must be established so as to collect the maximum amount of information available at that time. Many admissions departments as well as emergency departments join online insurance verification systems so that payers can be contacted during the registration process and verification can be received in seconds.

Records of Treatments and Charges During the Hospital Stay

The patient's hospital medical record contains (1) a face sheet (similar to a patient registration form that has been computer-generated); (2) notes of the attending physician and of other treating physicians; (3) ancillary documents like nurses' notes, medication administration records, and pathology, radiology, and laboratory reports; (4) patient data, including insurance information for patients who have been in the hospital before; and (5) a correspondence section that contains signed consent forms and other documents. In line with HIPAA security requirements, the confidentiality and security of patients' medical records are guarded by all hospital staff members. Both technical means, such as passwords and encryption, and legal protections, such as requiring staff members to sign confidentiality pledges, are used to ensure privacy.

Inpatients are usually charged by hospitals for the following services (the *technical component* of procedures):

- Room and board.
- Medications.
- Ancillary tests and procedures, such as laboratory workups.
- Equipment used during surgery or therapy.
- The amount of time spent in an operating room, recovery room, or intensive care unit.

Patients are charged according to the type of accommodations and services they receive. For example, the rate for a private room is higher than for a semiprivate room, and intensive care unit or recovery room charges are higher than charges for standard rooms. When patients are transferred to these various services, this activity is tracked. In an outpatient or an emergency department encounter, there is no room and board charge; instead, there is a visit charge.

Average service charges vary according to the type of care the hospital provides. For example, at a one-hundred-bed hospital that provides basic services, a large bill may be $15,000; but at a large five-hundred-bed hospital performing complicated surgeries such as open-heart procedures, a large bill is often more than $100,000.

Discharge and Billing

By the time patients are discharged from the hospital, their accounts have usually been totaled and insurance claims or bills created. The goal in most cases is to file a claim or bill within seven days after discharge. The items to be billed are recorded on the hospital's charge description master file, usually called the **charge master** or **charge ticket,** which is similar to a computerized medical office encounter form but with many more entries. This master list contains the following information for each billable item:

- The hospital's code for the service and a brief description of it.
- The charge for the service.
- The hospital department (such as laboratory).
- The hospital's cost to provide the service.
- A procedure code for the service.

The hospital's computer system tracks the patient's services. For example, if the patient is sent to the intensive care unit after surgery, the intensive care department's billing group reports the specific items performed for the patient, and these charges are entered on the patient's account.

INPATIENT (HOSPITAL) CODING

The HIM department is also responsible for diagnostic and procedural coding of the patients' medical records, based on the discharge summary signed by the attending physician. Coding is done by inpatient medical coders as soon as the patient is discharged. Some inpatient coders are generalists; others may have special skills in a certain area, like surgical coding or Medicare. Volumes 1 and 2 of the ICD-9-CM are used to code inpatient diagnoses, and Volume 3 is used to code procedures performed during hospitalization.

Hospital Diagnostic Coding

Different rules apply for assigning inpatient codes than for physician office diagnoses. The rules are extensive; three of them are described briefly below to illustrate some of the major differences in inpatient versus outpatient coding.

Rule 1   Principal Diagnosis

For ICD-9-CM diagnostic coding in medical practices, the first code listed is the primary diagnosis, defined as the main reason for the patient's encounter with the provider. Under hospital inpatient rules, the **principal diagnosis** is listed first. The principal diagnosis is the condition established *after study* to be chiefly responsible for the admission. This diagnosis is listed even if the patient has other, more severe diagnoses. In some cases, the **admitting diagnosis**—the condition identified by the physician at admission to the hospital—is also reported.

Rule 2   Suspected or Unconfirmed Diagnoses

When the patient is admitted for workups to uncover the cause of a problem, inpatient medical coders can also use a suspected or unconfirmed condition (rule out) if it is listed as the admitting diagnosis. The admitting diagnosis may not match the principal diagnosis once a final decision is made.

Rule 3 Comorbidities and Complications

The inpatient coder also lists all the other conditions that have an effect on the patient's hospital stay or course of treatment. Other conditions at admission that affect care during the hospitalizations are called comorbidities, meaning coexisting conditions. Conditions that develop as complications of surgery or other treatments are coded as complications.

Comorbidities and complications are shown in the patient medical record with the initials *CC*. Coding CCs is important because their presence may increase the hospital's reimbursement level for the care. The hospital insurance claim form discussed later in this chapter allows for up to eight additional conditions to be reported.

CMS has also put into place the requirement for a **present on admission (POA) indicator** for every reported diagnosis code for a patient upon discharge. *Present on admission* means that a condition existed at the time the order for inpatient admission occurs. This requirement is based on a federal mandate to Medicare to stop paying for conditions that hospitals cause or allow to develop during inpatient stays. Such conditions are now referred to as "never events," meaning that payers will not ever pay for them. Medicare will not assign an inpatient hospital discharge to a higher-paying MS-DRG if a selected hospital-acquired condition was not POA. The case will be paid as though the secondary diagnosis was not present.

Hospital Procedural Coding

In inpatient coding, ICD-9-CM, Volume 3, *Procedures,* is used to assign procedure codes. Reporting Volume 3 codes when appropriately documented may increase the hospital's reimbursement level for a patient's care because some procedures require more hospital time for recovery. For example, codes in range 93.31 to 93.39 are assigned when patients require physical therapy procedures such as whirlpool therapy.

Volume 3 of the ICD-9-CM has an Alphabetic Index and a Tabular List similar to those in Volumes 1 and 2. The Alphabetic Index is used to locate the procedure, and the Tabular List is used to confirm the code selection. Codes are either three or four digits. The fourth digit must be assigned if available.

The **principal procedure** assigned by the inpatient medical coder is the procedure that is most closely related to the treatment of the principal diagnosis. It is usually a surgical procedure. If no surgery is performed, the principal procedure may be a therapeutic procedure.

> ✔ **Compliance Tip**
>
> The inpatient coding rules apply only to inpatient services. Both hospital-based outpatient services and physician-office services are reported using Volumes 1 and 2 of the ICD-9-CM and using the outpatient rules and CPT codes for procedures.

PAYERS AND PAYMENT METHODS

Medicare and Medicaid both provide coverage for eligible patients' hospital services. Medicare Part A, known as hospital insurance, helps pay for inpatient hospital care, skilled nursing facilities (SNF), hospice care, and home health care. Private payers also offer hospitalization insurance. Most employees have coverage for hospital services through employers' programs.

Medicare Inpatient Payment System

Medicare's actions to control the cost of hospital services began with **diagnosis-related groups (DRGs).** Under the DRG classification system, the hospital stays of patients who had similar diagnoses were studied. Groupings were created based on the relative value of the resources that physicians and hospitals nationally used for patients with similar conditions. The calculations combine data about the patient's diagnosis and procedures with factors that affect the outcome of treatment, such as age, gender, comorbidities, and complications. At the same time the DRG system was created, Medicare changed the way hospitals were paid. Payment changed from a fee-for-service approach to the Medicare **Prospective Payment System (PPS).** In the PPS, the payment for each type of service is set ahead of time based on the DRG.

When DRGs were established, Medicare also set up Peer Review Organizations (PROs), which were later renamed Quality Improvement Organizations (QIOs). Made up of practicing physicians and other health care experts, these organizations are contracted by CMS in each state to review Medicare and Medicaid claims for the appropriateness of hospitalization and clinical care. QIOs aim to ensure that payment is made only for medically necessary services. QIOs are also resources for investigating patients' complaints regarding the quality of care at a given facility or through a managed care plan.

In 2008 Medicare adopted a new type of DRG called **MS-DRGs** (Medicare-Severity DRGs) to better reflect the different severity of illness among patients who have the same basic diagnosis. The system recognizes the higher cost of treating patients with more complex conditions. There are 258 sets of MS-DRGs that are split into two or three subgroups based on the presence or absence of a complication or comorbidity (CC) or a major CC (MCC).

Medicare Outpatient Payment Systems

The use of DRGs under a PPS system proved to be very effective in controlling costs. In 2000, this approach was implemented for outpatient hospital services, which previously were paid on a fee-for-service basis. For example, the Hospital Outpatient Prospective Payment System (PPS) is used to pay for hospital outpatient services. In place of DRGs, patients are grouped under an ambulatory patient classification (APC) system. Reimbursement is made according to preset amounts based on the value of each APC.

Private Insurance Companies

Because of the expense involved with hospitalization, private payers encourage providers to minimize the number of days patients stay in the hospital. Most private payers establish the standard number of days allowed for various conditions and compare this number to the patient's actual stay. Many private payers have also adopted the DRG method of setting prospective payments for hospital services. Hospitals and the payers, which may include Blue Cross and Blue Shield or other managed care plans, negotiate the rates for each DRG.

CLAIMS AND FOLLOW UP

Hospitals must submit claims for Medicare Part A reimbursement to Medicare fiscal intermediaries using the HIPAA health care claim called **837I.** Similar to the 837 claim (Chapter 6), this format is called I for "institutional"; the physicians' claim is 837P for "professional."

In some situations, a paper claim form called the **UB-92** (uniform billing 1992), also known as the **CMS-1450,** is also accepted by most other payers. As of May 2007, the new version of this form, the **UB-04,** must be used.

837I Health Care Claim Completion

The 837I, like the 837P, has sections requiring data elements for the billing and the pay-to provider, the subscriber and patient, and the payer, plus claim and service level details. Most of the data elements report the same information as summarized below for the paper claim.

UB-04 Claim Form Completion

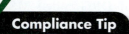

✓ Compliance Tip

Like physician practice coding, the correct level of service must be reported to avoid fraud. For example, a patient has pulmonary edema (fluid in the lungs) that is due to the principal diagnosis of congestive heart failure (CHF). The correct ICD-9-CM code order leads to a DRG 127 classification. If the coder incorrectly reports pulmonary edema and respiratory failure, the patient is assigned DRG 87, which has a higher relative value, resulting in an improperly high payment.

The UB-04 claim form is complex and requires multiple entries. The form is shown in Figure 15-2. It is used to report patient data, information on the insured, facility/patient type, the source of the admission, various conditions that affect payment, whether Medicare is the primary payer (for Medicare claims), the principal and other diagnosis codes, the admitting diagnosis, the principal procedure code, the attending physician, other key physician, and charges. The information for the form locators often requires choosing from a list of codes. All dates should show the year as four digits.

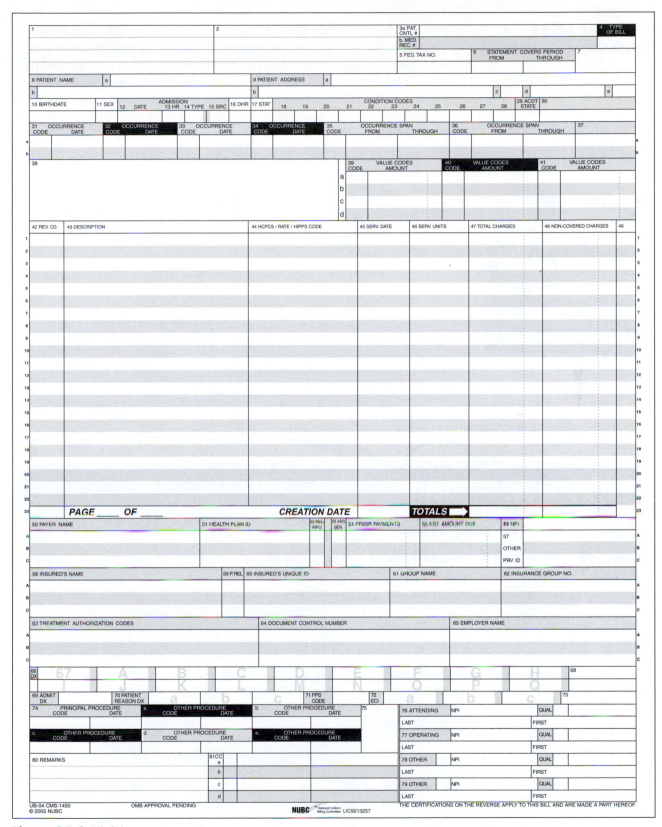

Figure 15-2 UB-04

Remittance Advice Processing

Hospitals receive a remittance advice when payments are transmitted to their accounts. The patient accounting department and then the health information management (HIM) department check that appropriate payment has been received. Unless the software used for billing automatically reports that the billed code is not the same as the paid code, procedures to find and follow up these exceptions must be set up between the two departments.

Explore the Internet

Using your favorite search engine, locate information about the hospital insurance program, Medicare Part A, on the CMS website. What are the eligibility requirements for this program?

Professional Focus

Career Opportunities in Hospitals

Provider Relations Representative

Provider relations representatives speak for an institution to its network of physicians. Because they establish networks of providers, many hospitals employ provider relations representatives to enroll physicians in their networks and to monitor their status. These employees process the documents needed for providers to become participants in the network, maintain the current list of providers, and answer questions from providers about policies and procedures.

Medical Coder—Hospital

Medical coding specialists who work in the hospital setting are called hospital or facility coders. They may work in an inpatient setting, an outpatient clinic, or another institution such as a skilled nursing facility. Hospital coders review patients' medical records and assign diagnosis and procedure codes. They are knowledgeable about the coding rules and procedures for hospital coding, and they may be certified by either the American Academy of Professional Coders (AAPC) or the American Health Information Management Association (AHIMA). Hospital coders need to become experienced in working with lengthy, complicated records of patients' stays, including operative, laboratory, pathology, and radiology reports. Accurate coding is a critical part of ensuring that claims follow the legal and ethical requirements of Medicare and other third-party payers.

Chapter Summary

1. Inpatient (involving an overnight stay) services are provided by general and specialized hospitals, skilled nursing facilities, and long-term care facilities. Outpatient services are provided by ambulatory surgical centers or units, by home health agencies, and by hospice staff.

2. The first major step in the hospital claim processing sequence is admission, when the patient is registered. Personal and financial information is entered in the hospital's health record system; insurance coverage is verified; and consent forms are signed by the patient. In the second step, the patient's treatments and transfer among the various departments in the hospital are tracked and recorded. The third step, discharge and billing, follows the discharge of the patient from the facility and completion of the patient's record. Payments are based on the appropriate diagnosis-related group (DRG) and are set in advance (prospective in nature).

3. Two ways in which inpatient coding differs from physician and outpatient diagnostic coding are that (a) the main diagnosis, called the principal diagnosis, is established after study in the hospital setting, and (b) unconfirmed conditions (rule outs) may be coded as the admitting diagnosis.

4. Volume 3 of the ICD-9-CM, *Procedures,* is used to report the procedures for inpatient services. The three- or four-digit codes are assigned based on the principal diagnosis.

5. In hospital billing, the HIPAA claim for institutions, known as the 837I—or in some situations, the paper UB-04 claim form (CMS-1450)—is used to report patient data, information on the insured, facility/patient type, the source of the admission, various conditions that affect payment, whether Medicare is the primary payer (for Medicare claims), the principal and other diagnosis codes, the admitting diagnosis, the principal procedure code, the attending physician, other key physician, and charges.

Check Your Understanding

Part 1. Write "T" or "F" in the blank to indicate whether you think the statement is true or false.

_____ **1.** Skilled nursing facilities (SNF) are classified as outpatient facilities.

_____ **2.** Emergency care involves a life-threatening situation.

_____ **3.** An inpatient's insurance coverage is usually verified in the discharge process.

_____ **4.** The master patient index contains the name of each patient's attending physician.

_____ **5.** Hospital services are covered by Medicare Part A.

_____ **6.** At-home care is considered outpatient care.

_____ **7.** The hospital's charge master serves the same purpose as a medical office's encounter form.

_____ **8.** The principal diagnosis is based on the admitting diagnosis.

_____ **9.** Inpatient coding rules do not permit the reporting of suspected or unconfirmed diagnoses.

_____ **10.** ICD-9-CM, Volume 3, is used to report inpatient procedures.

Part 2. Choose the best answer.

_____ **1.** When the hospital staff collects data on a patient who is being admitted for services, the process is called:
   a. health information management
   b. registration
   c. MSP

_____ **2.** Which of the following hospital departments has different procedures for collecting patients' personal and insurance information?
   a. accounting department
   b. surgery department
   c. emergency department

_____ **3.** Patient charges in hospitals vary according to:
   a. their accommodations
   b. their services
   c. their accommodations and services

_____ **4.** Conditions that arise during the patient's hospital stay as a result of treatments are called:
   a. comorbidities
   b. admitting diagnoses
   c. complications

_____ **5.** In inpatient coding, the initials CC mean:
   a. chief complaint
   b. comorbidities and complications
   c. cubic centimeters

_____ **6.** The code 76.23 is an example of which type of code?
   a. CPT-4
   b. ICD-9-CM, Volume 1
   c. ICD-9-CM, Volume 3

_____ **7.** Under a prospective payment system, payments for services are:
   a. set in advance
   b. calculated based on the provider's fees
   c. based on a discount to the provider's usual fees

_____ **8.** When preparing claims for Medicare Part A reimbursement, hospitals must use the:
   a. CMS-1500
   b. 837P
   C. 837I

CHAPTER 16

Medisoft Claim Simulations

Chapter 16 first provides Part I, an introduction to the Medisoft Advanced Patient Accounting program. Then, in Parts II and III, you will use the program to complete seven claims. In Part II you are given step-by-step instructions on completing Case Study 16-1 and optional Case Study 16-2. In Part III you will complete five claims on your own.

PART I: INTRODUCTION TO MEDISOFT

The Medisoft introduction is in two parts:

- An overview describes the program's database structure, how claims are created in Medisoft, and the major dialog boxes that are used for data entry in creating claims.
- Getting Started with Medisoft contains instructions on downloading the Medisoft Student Data files that are used in the simulations in Parts II and III and practice in using Medisoft menus.

Overview of Medisoft

Medisoft Advanced Patient Accounting, a computerized patient billing system that is widely used in medical offices, is used in this textbook as an example of the type of program with which medical insurance specialists often work. Processing information to complete insurance claim forms is one of the main functions of the Medisoft program.

How Medisoft Is Organized

The Medisoft program is designed to collect information and store it in databases. A database is a collection of related facts. For example, a provider database contains information about a practice's physicians while a patient database contains each patient's unique chart number and personal information, including address, phone, employer, assigned provider, and so on. The major databases in the Medisoft program are:

- Provider
- Patient/Guarantor
- Insurance Carriers
- Diagnosis Codes
- Procedure Codes
- Transactions

When a command is given, such as the command to create a patient statement, the program pulls together the required data by drawing on information from the various databases.

How Insurance Claims Are Created in Medisoft

Three major steps are followed to create insurance claims using Medisoft: (1) setting up the practice, (2) entering patient and transaction information, and (3) creating insurance claims.

Setting Up the Practice

Before Medisoft can be used to store information about patients and their visits, basic facts about the practice itself must be entered in several of the databases listed above. Information about the practice's providers is recorded in the provider database, including each provider's National Provider Identifier (NPI) and other secondary provider identification numbers for different carriers. In addition, frequently used diagnosis and procedure codes are entered in their own databases with code descriptions. Finally, insurance carrier data is entered. The insurance carrier database contains information about the carriers that most patients use, as well as options for electronic claim submission and paper claim printing. These databases are created once during the setup of the practice. However, they may be updated as often as necessary.

Entering Patient and Transaction Information

Entering patient and transaction information in the database is an ongoing process. After a patient visits a physician in the practice, the medical insurance specialist organizes the information gathered on the patient information form and encounter form. After analyzing and checking the data, each element is entered in Medisoft. A new record must be created for a new patient, and information on established patients may need to be updated. Next, the appropriate insurance carrier for the visit is selected. Usually, this is the patient's primary insurance carrier, but in workers' compensation cases, for example, the carrier will be different. Then, the purposes of the visit, the diagnosis codes, and the procedure codes are identified, with the appropriate charges.

Creating Insurance Claims

When all patient and transaction information has been entered and checked, the medical insurance specialist issues the command to Medisoft to create an insurance claim form. Medisoft then organizes the necessary databases. Within Medisoft, each database is linked, or related, to each of the others by having at least one fact in common. For example, the patient's chart number appears both in the patient/guarantor database and the transaction database, thereby linking the two. Medisoft selects data from each database as needed. The program then follows the instructions for printing or transmitting the form electronically to the designated receiver, which is often a clearinghouse.

Data Entry in Medisoft

The following section provides an overview of the main areas in Medisoft where data are entered for creating insurance claims.

Patient/Guarantor Information

The Patient/Guarantor dialog box is where basic information about patients is entered. The dialog box has three tabs that are used to enter information about patients. Tabs are so named because they resemble the tabs on file folders. When a tab name is clicked, the entire contents of that tab are displayed. Each tab contains fields where data are keyed. The first tab in the Patient/Guarantor dialog box is called the Name, Address tab. In addition to the patient's name and address, the patient's unique chart number is entered in this tab. If the user does not enter a chart number, Medisoft assigns a number automatically.

Many Medisoft dialog boxes include default entries to save time when various types of data are entered. For example, in the Country field in the Name, Address tab, the entry "USA" automatically appears. If this entry is correct, the user moves on to the next entry, accepting the default. This information is stored when the user clicks the Save button. If the default entry is not correct, other data may be entered and stored in its place.

The second tab in the Patient/Guarantor dialog box, called the Other Information tab, contains information about the patient's employment and other miscellaneous data. The third tab, Payment Plan, is used to enter the terms for the patient's payment plan, provided the practice offers payment plans and the patient requests one.

Figure 16-1 shows the Name, Address tab in Medisoft's Patient/Guarantor dialog box for a sample patient.

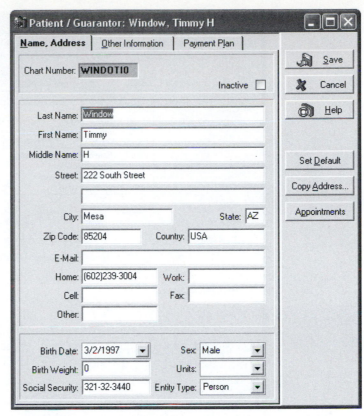

Figure 16-1 Sample Patient/Guarantor Dialog Box with Name, Address Tab Active

Case Information

Most information about a patient's account, insurance coverage, and medical condition is stored in the Case dialog box in Medisoft. Once a patient's personal information has been entered in the Patient/Guarantor dialog box, a new case can be created in the Case dialog box each time the patient visits the medical office with a different complaint. A new case is also set up if the insurance carrier differs from the patient's primary carrier, such as in workers' compensation, in order to keep the information separate from other office visits.

The Case dialog box contains eleven tabs for entering a patient's case information: Personal, Account, Diagnosis, Policy 1, Policy 2, Policy 3, Condition, Miscellaneous, Medicaid and Tricare, Comment, and EDI. These tabs contain information about the patient's billing account, insurance coverage, medical condition, and other information that may be required to create insurance claims. Figure 16-2 on page 290 shows a sample Policy 1 tab with the Insurance Carrier drop-down list displayed. Figure 16-3 on page 291 shows a sample Diagnosis tab with the Diagnosis drop-down list displayed.

Transaction Entry

Transactions—patients' visits and charges, as well as payments or adjustments—are entered in the Transaction Entry dialog box (see Figure 16-4 on page 291). When the patient's chart number and case are selected, Medisoft displays information previously entered in other dialog boxes, such as the patient's name and birth date, case name, and insurance

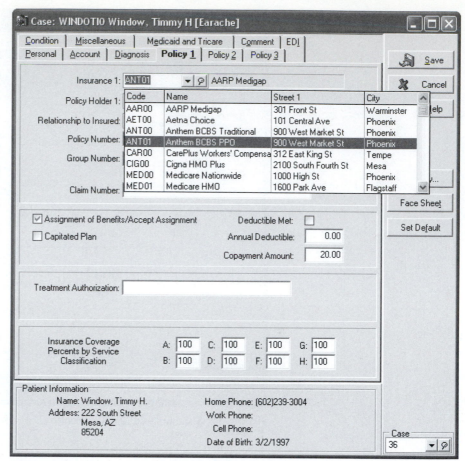

Figure 16-2 Sample Policy 1 Tab in Case Dialog Box

carrier information, in the upper portion of the Transaction Entry dialog box for easy reference.

The middle and lower portions of the dialog box are used to record transactions. Procedure codes and their corresponding charges are recorded in the middle portion, called the Charges tab. Payments received from patients and insurance carriers are recorded in the Payments, Adjustments, And Comments tab in the lower portion of the dialog box.

In the Charges tab, procedures are selected from a drop-down list of Procedure Codes (see Figure 16-5 on page 292). To display the drop-down list, the inside of the Procedure box is clicked and then the triangle button that appears is clicked. The list shows the CPT codes and descriptions that are frequently used by the practice. If the correct procedure is not included in the list, a dialog box can be accessed for the purpose of adding it.

Similarly, in the Payments, Adjustments, And Comments tab in the lower portion of the Transaction Entry dialog box, a payment type is selected in the Pay/Adj Code field using a drop-down list of codes already set up in the database.

Transaction entries must be saved by clicking the Save Transactions button in the bottom right corner of the dialog box. Any transaction can be edited by clicking in the field to be edited and making the change.

When transaction entry is complete, a walkout receipt can be printed for the patient by clicking the Print Receipt button at the bottom of the

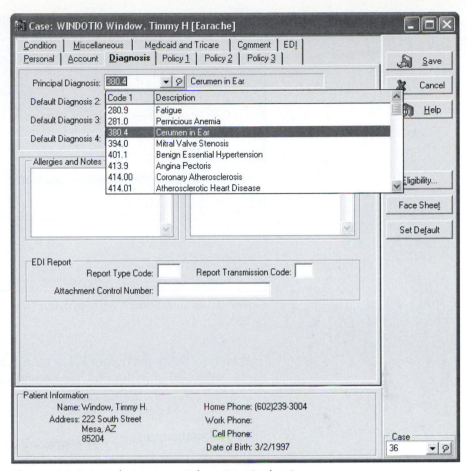

Figure 16-3 Sample Diagnosis Tab in Case Dialog Box

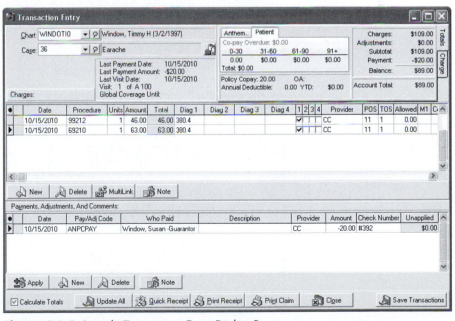

Figure 16-4 Sample Transaction Entry Dialog Box

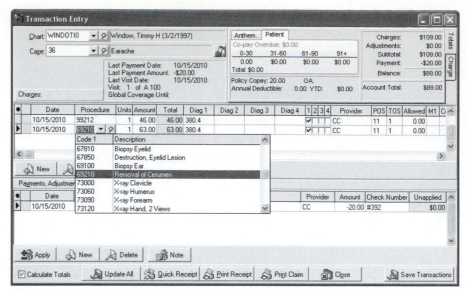

Figure 16-5 Transaction Entry Dialog Box with Procedure Code Drop-Down List

Transaction Entry dialog box. This receipt lists the charges and payments for the visit. Patients who file their own insurance claims use this information to complete the claim form.

Claim Management

Once a patient's transaction entries have been completed for a visit, a claim can be created. Claims are created in Medisoft using the Create Claims button in the Claim Management dialog box (see Figure 16-6). The Claim Management dialog box is used to (1) create batches of claims for transmission, (2) transmit claims electronically or print them on paper forms, and (3), if necessary, make corrections to existing claims. Medisoft lists the claims that have been sent by either mode (print or electronic) so that each claim can be marked with its status when RA reports arrive from carriers.

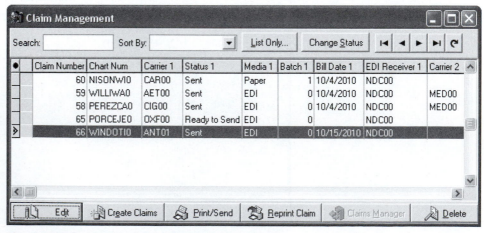

Figure 16-6 Sample Claim Management Dialog Box

When a claim is created in Medisoft, the program selects data from each database as needed and creates a claim file in the CMS-1500 format. The program then follows the instructions for transmitting the claim electronically to the designated receiver, which is usually a clearinghouse. As most insurance carriers now require claims in the HIPAA format, the clearinghouse converts the Medisoft CMS-1500 claim file into HIPAA format and then transmits the file to the carrier. CMS-1500 claim forms can also be printed if required by a carrier, although most carriers now prefer to work with the electronic format.

Reports

Once patient and transaction data have been recorded, and claims have been generated, a number of standard and custom reports, such as day sheets and aging reports, can be produced by selecting an option on Medisoft's Reports menu.

Day sheets list the daily financial activity in the practice. Insurance aging reports detail how long a payer has taken to respond to each claim. Patient aging reports show how long a patient has taken to pay the amount owed on the patient statement. These reports are reviewed by the practice manager to determine areas for improvement in the cash flow of the practice.

Figure 16-7 displays a sample patient day sheet for October 1, 2010. The report data is grouped alphabetically by patient and includes procedures performed for each patient on that day, as well as charges, payments received, and each patient's current balance.

Getting Started with Medisoft

As mentioned in the Overview, before a medical practice begins to use Medisoft, basic information about the practice and its patients must be entered in the computer. This preliminary work has been done for you. The medical practice with which you will work is called Central Practice

---

Central Practice Center
Patient Day Sheet

October 01, 2010
10/1/2010

Entry	Date	Document	POS	Description	Provider	Code	Modifiers	Amount
NISONWI0	**Nisonson, William**							
38	10/1/2010	0810060000	11	NP Expanded Problem Focused	SJ	99202		75.00
39	10/1/2010	0810060000	11	Tibia & Fibula Fracture, Shaft	SJ	27750		681.00

Patient's Charges	Patient's Receipts	Insurance Receipts	Adjustments	Patient Balance
$756.00	$0.00	$0.00	$0.00	$0.00

Entry	Date	Document	POS	Description	Provider	Code	Modifiers	Amount
PEREZCA0	**Perez, Carmen**							
65	10/1/2010	0810010000	11	EP Expanded Problem Focused	CC	99213		62.00
67	10/1/2010	0810010000	11	Cigna HMO Plus Copayment	CC	CIGCPAY		-20.00

Patient's Charges	Patient's Receipts	Insurance Receipts	Adjustments	Patient Balance
$62.00	-$20.00	$0.00	$0.00	$42.00

Entry	Date	Document	POS	Description	Provider	Code	Modifiers	Amount
WILLIWA0	**Williams, Walter**							
61	10/1/2010	0810010000	11	EP Problem Focused	CC	99212		46.00
62	10/1/2010	0810010000	11	ECG Complete	CC	93000		70.00
64	10/1/2010	0810010000	11	Aetna Copayment	CC	AETCPAY		-15.00

Patient's Charges	Patient's Receipts	Insurance Receipts	Adjustments	Patient Balance
$116.00	-$15.00	$0.00	$0.00	$101.00

Figure 16-7 Sample Patient Day Sheet Report

Center (CPC). Check with your instructor to determine whether the Medisoft Student Data, which contains the CPC database, has already been loaded on our computer.

If your instructor has not already loaded the data, go to the Online Learning Center at www.mhhe.com/fp2p6e to download it. You will need to load the student data before you resume with the practice session and claim simulations that follow in the remainder of the chapter.

Practice Selecting Menu Options

The first step in becoming acquainted with Medisoft is to use the program's menu system. Medisoft offers program choices through a group of nine menus. The Medisoft menu bar lists the name of each Medisoft menu: File, Edit, Activities, Lists, Reports, Tools, Window, Services, and Help.

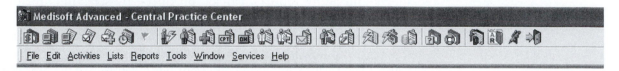

The two menus used the most in the Medisoft exercises in this text are the Lists menu and the Activities menu.

The Lists Menu

Some of the data already entered for Central Practice Center is accessed through the Lists menu. Use the following steps to practice selecting some of the options on the Lists menu.

1. Click the menu name, Lists, to display the Lists menu.

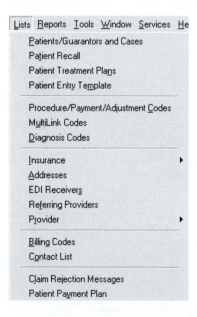

2. Click the first option, Patients/Guarantors and Cases. The Patient List dialog box is displayed. This dialog box contains the names and chart numbers of all the established patients for the medical office.

3. Click the Close button to return to the main Medisoft window.

4. Again, click the menu name, Lists.

5. When the Lists menu is displayed, click Procedure/Payment/Adjustment Codes. The list that appears contains the CPT codes and descriptions for the procedures that are most frequently used by this medical office. Scroll to the bottom of the list. Notice the list also contains a number of codes for accounting purposes, such as take back, withhold, adjustment, copayment, deductible, and payment codes.

6. Click the Close button to return to the main Medisoft window.

7. To learn more about the program, access two more options from the Lists menu, Diagnosis Codes and Insurance Carriers. The Diagnosis List dialog box lists the ICD codes and descriptions of the diagnoses that are most frequently used by this medical office. The Insurance Carrier List dialog box displays a list of the carriers where most of this office's claims are filed.

8. When you are finished viewing the lists, return to the main Medisoft window.

The Activities Menu

Other than the patients' personal and case information, much of the data necessary to create claims is entered through options on the Activities menu. Follow the steps below to view two major dialog boxes that are accessed through the Activities menu:

1. Click Activities on the menu bar to display the Activities menu.

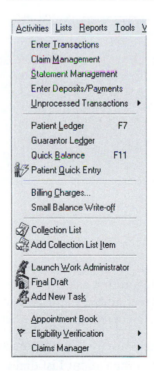

2. Click the first option, Enter Transactions. The Transaction Entry dialog box is displayed. This dialog box is used to enter data about patient transactions and to record charges and payments.

3. Click the Close button.

4. Again, open the Activities menu.

5. Click Claim Management. The dialog box that appears is used to create and transmit (or print) electronic and paper claims.

6. Click the Close button.

The menu options in Medisoft provide insight into the type of data that is stored in the program. In Parts II and III, you will use the dialog boxes connected with these menus to create claims.

PART II: GUIDED CLAIM SIMULATIONS

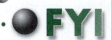

NOTE: Before completing the claim simulations in Part II, be sure you have followed the instructions in Part I, "Getting Started with Medisoft," to download the Medisoft Student Data files for Central Practice Center, the sample medical practice used in these simulations.

In Case Study 16-1 you will use Medisoft to:

- Edit an established patient's record.
- Enter the patient's diagnosis code.
- Enter the transactions for an office visit.
- Print a walkout receipt.
- Create an electronic claim with a claim verification report.

Case Study 16-1

Robin Caruthers, an established patient at Central Practice Center, comes to the office for a routine visit. As the medical insurance specialist, you enter the transactions for the office visit. After entering the transactions, you create an electronic claim and view the claim verification report for the claim.

Follow the steps on pages 296–306 to complete Case Study 16-1.

Edit an Established Patient's Record

When Robin Caruthers arrives at the medical office for her routine appointment, you first ask her to verify her current address. You determine that her street address and phone number need to be updated. Follow these steps to correct Mrs. Caruthers' address:

1. Select Patients/Guarantors and Cases from the Lists menu.

2. When the Patient List dialog box appears, key *C* in the Search For box to highlight the entry for Caruthers, Robin.

3. Click the Edit Patient button in the bottom-left corner of the Patient List dialog box. The Patient/Guarantor dialog box for Robin Caruthers is displayed.

4. Press the Tab key three times to move to the Street field, or click in the Street box.

5. Key the correct street address, *22 Bayside Drive.*

6. Click in the Home (phone) box.

7. Edit the home phone to display *(602) 629-0222.* The Patient/ Guarantor dialog box should look like the one below.

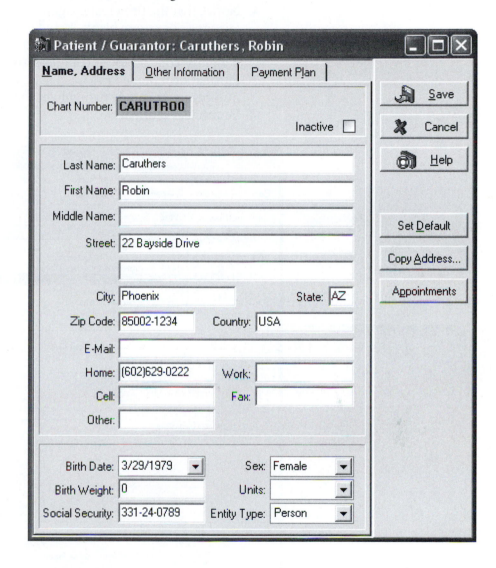

8. Click the Save button to save the changes and return to the Patient List dialog box.

Enter Diagnosis Information

After Mrs. Caruthers finishes her appointment with the doctor, she hands you the encounter form from the visit. Before you can enter the transactions on the encounter form, you need to enter the diagnosis code on the encounter form in Mrs. Caruthers' Case dialog box. In Medisoft, transactions must be linked to at least one diagnosis code. If they are not, the claim created for the transactions will be rejected by the insurance company.

1. With Robin Caruthers' Chart Number and Case information still displayed in the Patient List dialog box, click the line that reads Ventricular Fibrillation on the right side of the dialog box to select this case.
2. Click the Edit Case button at the bottom of the dialog box.
3. The eleven tabs for this case appear. Click the Diagnosis tab.
4. Notice that the Principal Diagnosis box and the three Default Diagnosis boxes are blank. As today's appointment was a routine visit in connection with her ventricular fibrillation case, the diagnosis code on the encounter form is 427.41 (Ventricular Fibrillation). In the Principal Diagnosis box, key the first two numbers of this code to highlight the diagnosis code for Ventricular Fibrillation.

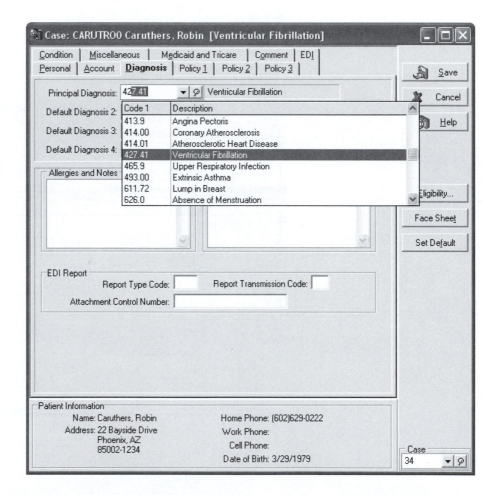

5. Press Tab to select the diagnosis, and then click the Save button to save your work.
6. The entry is saved and you are returned to the Patient List dialog box. Click the Close button to exit the Patient List dialog box.

. . . .

Enter New Transactions

Now that Robin Caruthers' diagnosis code has been recorded, follow the steps below to enter the transactions for the visit. In addition to the encounter form, Mrs. Caruthers hands you a check for $20 because her PPO requires a $20 copay per visit. Therefore, there are two transactions to be recorded for Mrs. Caruthers' visit today—a procedural charge for the office visit and a check copayment.

1. Select Enter Transactions from the Activities menu to display the Transaction Entry dialog box.

2. Key *C* in the Chart box to locate the entry for Robin Caruthers, and then press Enter twice to display her information.

3. Notice that Robin Caruthers' current case (Ventricular Fibrillation) and insurance information, including her policy copayment requirement, are displayed in the top section of the Transaction Entry dialog box.

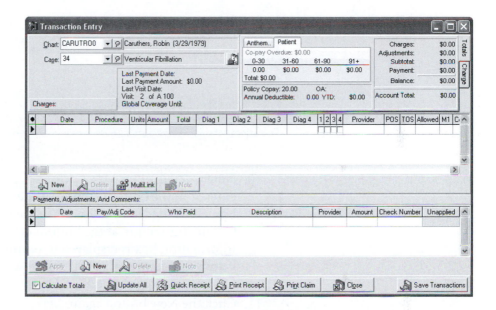

4. To enter a charge transaction, click the New button in the middle of the Transaction Entry dialog box, in the section labeled Charges.

5. Today's date is displayed as the default date in the Date field. For the purposes of this simulation, change the date in the Date box to 10/15/2010 by clicking inside the Date box and then keying *10/15/2010* over the current entry.

6. Press the Tab key to save the date entry and move to the Procedure field.

7. Click the Triangle button in the Procedure field. A drop-down list of procedure codes and descriptions is displayed.

8. From Mrs. Caruthers' encounter form, you see that the procedure code for today's visit is 99212 (EP Problem focused). First key *9* in the Procedure box. Notice that the first code beginning with 9 is highlighted.

9. Key another *9*, and then key the rest of the procedure code— *212*—and press the Tab key. Medisoft inserts the code in the Procedure box and displays the default unit of 1 in the Units box

and the default amount of $46.00 in the Amount box. Notice that the Diagnosis code entered earlier in the Case dialog box, 427.41, is also displayed.

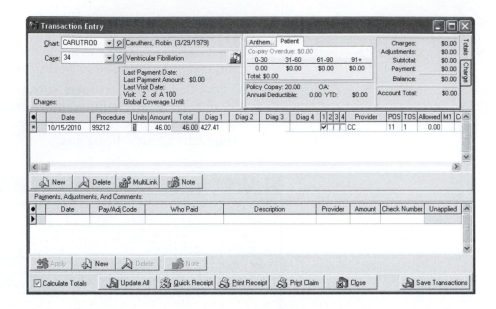

10. Now you will enter Mrs. Caruthers' payment. Payments are entered in the bottom section of the Transaction Entry dialog box. Click the New button in the Payments, Adjustments, and Comments section at the bottom of the dialog box. (An Information box is displayed to remind you that Robin Caruthers' insurance requires a $20.00 copayment for each visit. Click the OK button to continue.)

11. Click the New button again. Make sure the date in the Date box is still 10/15/2010. Press the Tab key twice to save the date entry and move to the Pay/Adj Code box.

12. Click the Triangle button to display the list of payment codes and descriptions.

13. Scroll through the list to locate the code for Mrs. Caruthers' copayment. (Notice, at the top of the Transaction Entry dialog box, that her insurance carrier is Anthem BCBS PPO. Therefore, you are looking for the copayment code for this carrier.) Click the code ANPCPAY for "Anthem BCBS PPO Copayment" to insert it in the Pay/Adj Code box, and then press the Tab key.

14. Medisoft inserts the code in the Pay/Adj Code box and displays the name of the guarantor in the Who Paid box, and the default amount of "-20.00" in the Amount box for this transaction. The minus sign indicates a payment rather than a charge. Notice the Unapplied box at the end of the transaction line also displays the amount of the payment.

15. Click inside the Check Number box, and then key *339* to record the number on Mrs. Caruthers' check. The dialog box should now look like this:

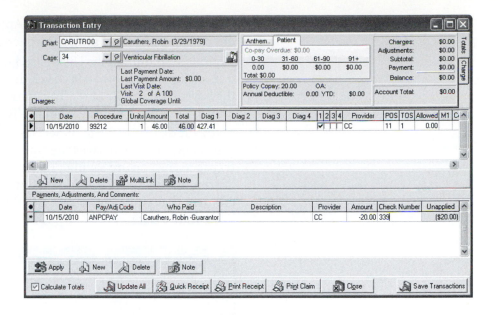

16. The last step in recording the payment is to apply the payment just entered to its corresponding charge. To do this, click the Apply button at the bottom of the Payments, Adjustments, and Comments section of the dialog box.

17. The Apply Payment to Charges dialog box appears. Click the white background of the This Payment box on the line with the office visit procedure charge (the only procedure charge in this case).

18. Key *20* and press Tab. The payment appears in the This Payment column and the Unapplied box in the upper right corner displays a zero amount. (If the box does not yet display zero, click anywhere in the white space underneath the This Payment column to update it.) The copayment has now been applied to the corresponding office visit charge. (*Note:* It is the usual procedure at Central Practice Center to apply a patient's copayment to the office visit charge before any other charges.)

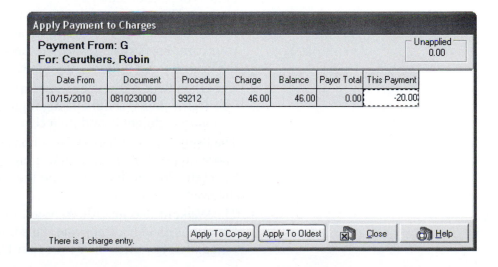

19. Click the Close button to close the Apply Payment to Charges dialog box and return to the Transaction Entry dialog box.

20. Notice the amount in the Unapplied box at the end of the transaction line is now $0.00. Click the Save Transactions button in the lower right corner of the Transaction Entry dialog box to save the information you have entered in the Transaction Entry dialog box.

21. Medisoft displays a Date of Service Validation box for each new transaction before it saves the transaction if the date of the transactions you are saving (10/15/2010) is later than the current date on your computer system. This box asks you to confirm that you want to save the transaction, even though it has a future date.

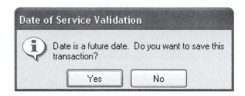

22. For the purposes of the simulations in this book, click Yes each time this box appears. In the present Transaction Entry screen, you will need to click Yes two times, as there are two new transactions.

You have successfully recorded one charge and one payment in the Transaction Entry dialog box. Keep the Transaction Entry dialog box open for now, as you will use it in the next section.

Create a Walkout Receipt

If a patient makes a payment during an office visit, the patient is usually given a walkout receipt at the time of the visit. After the transactions for the visit have been entered in the Transaction Entry dialog box, the Print Receipt button at the bottom of the Transaction Entry dialog box is used to print a walkout receipt. Follow these steps to create a walkout receipt for Robin Caruthers' visit.

1. With Robin Caruthers' transactions for 10/15/2010 still displayed in the Transaction Entry dialog box, click the Print Receipt button. (*Note:* Although the Quick Receipt button can also be used to print a walkout receipt, because of the likely difference in your computer's system date and the date used in the simulations, the Print Receipt button is used in these simulations.)

2. The Open Report dialog box appears. The option Walkout Receipt (All Transactions) should be highlighted. If it is not, click this option to highlight it, and then click the OK button.

3. The Print Report Where? Dialog box appears, giving you the option to print the report, view it on screen, or export it to a file. Select the Preview the Report on the Screen option, and then click the Start button.

4. The Walkout Receipt (All Transactions): Data Selection Questions dialog box appears. This box is to used to specify a range of dates. Click inside the first Date From Range box in this

dialog box, and key *10/15/2010* to change the date to 10/15/2010. Press Tab and key the same date in the second Date From Range box, as you are printing a walkout receipt for today's transactions only.

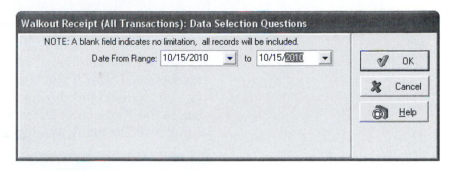

5. With the date range specified, click the OK button.
6. The Preview Report window appears with Robin Caruthers' walkout receipt displayed. Use the scroll bar to view the full length of the page.
7. If you are connected to a printer, click the printer icon located at the top of the screen.
8. When the Print dialog box appears, click the OK button to begin printing. After a few seconds, the receipt will be printed.
9. Click the Close button at the top of the screen to exit the Preview Report window.
10. You are back at the Transaction Entry dialog box. Click the Close button to close the Transaction Entry dialog box.

Create an Electronic Claim and Print a Claim Verification Report

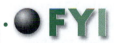

Note: Because you are in an instructional setting and your system is not set up to send claims, you will not actually be able to transmit the claim electronically. This is the case for all the electronic claims in the simulations in this chapter. However, you will go through the steps leading up to the point of transmission, including verifying the details of the claim in a claim verification report.

In most medical offices, claims are created and transmitted in batches, often at the end of the day. The batch method is more efficient, given the number of claims that are created daily. For instructional purposes, in this book claims are created and viewed as soon as the transactions for the claim have been recorded. The method of creating and sending claims is the same in both cases. When individual claims are created, the filtering option is set to a single chart number. When more than one claim is created, a range of chart numbers is specified. Follow the steps below to create an electronic claim for Robin Caruthers' transactions on 10/15/2010.

1. To create a claim, click Claim Management on the Activities menu. The Claim Management dialog box is displayed. Claims that have already been created are listed in the dialog box.
2. To create a new claim, click the Create Claims button. The Create Claims dialog box appears. This dialog box is used to set the range of claims you want to create. In this instance, enter the date *10/15/2010* in both of the Transaction Dates range boxes, and then press Tab.
3. Depending on your computer's system date, when you enter the 10/15/2010 date, the program will display a Confirm box, asking if you want to change the future date you have entered. In both instances, click No and continue.

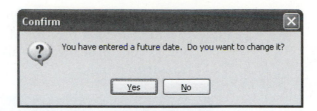

Confirm

? You have entered a future date. Do you want to change it?

Yes   No

4. In both of the Chart Numbers range boxes, to select the claim for Robin Caruthers, key *C* and then press Tab. Leave the other boxes blank. (*Note:* If you were creating claims for all the patients' transactions during the day, you would enter today's date in the Transaction Dates boxes and leave the Chart Numbers boxes blank to select all chart numbers.)

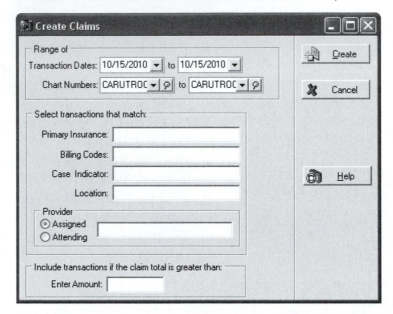

5. To create the claim for the transactions indicated, click the Create button.

6. The Create Claim dialog box closes, and you are returned to the Claim Management dialog box. Notice that the claim for Robin Caruthers is added to the list of created claims in the Claim Management dialog box. The Status 1 column in the Claim Management dialog box indicates the claim is "Ready to Send," and the Media 1 column indicates that the claim will be sent as an electronic file (EDI, "electronic data interchange"). This is because the default claim type for Mrs. Caruthers' insurance carrier is set to electronic.

7. To send the claim for Robin Caruthers to the clearinghouse, first click on the claim for Robin Caruthers in the Claim Management dialog box to highlight it, and then click the Print/Send button.

8. The Print/Send Claims dialog box appears. Because Robin Caruthers' claim is an electronic claim, click the Electronic radio button in the billing method portion of the dialog box. In the Electronic Claim Receiver box, select NDC, which stands for National Data Corporation, the name of the clearinghouse, if it is not already selected.

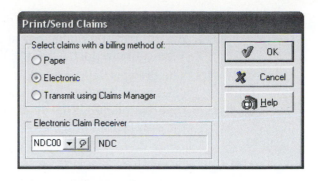

9. Click the OK button.

10. The Send Electronic Claims dialog box is displayed, with NDC displayed as the receiver.

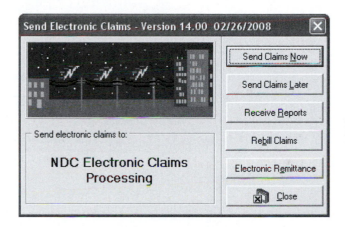

11. Click the Send Claims Now button. The Data Selection Questions dialog box appears. The various range boxes provide options for filtering the claims. In the first Chart Number Range box, key *C* to select Robin Caruthers, and then press Tab. Follow the same steps to fill in the second Chart Number Range box.

12. For the purposes of this simulation, delete the date displayed in the second Date Created Range box.

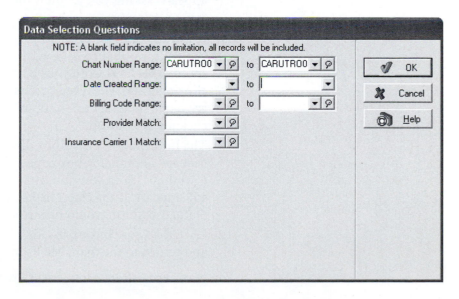

13. Click the OK button.

14. An Information dialog box appears, asking if you want to view a Verification report. Click the Yes button.

15. The Preview Report window appears with a copy of an EMC (Electronic Media Claim) Verification report displayed. The report contains all the details of Robin Caruthers' claim, which is the only claim in the batch.

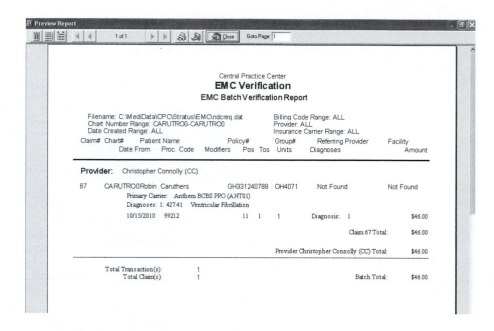

16. Click the Close button when finished viewing the report. The Preview Report window closes, and an Information dialog box appears, asking you if you want to continue with the transmission.

17. If you were in a medical office, you would click the Yes button and the claim would be sent electronically (for example, over a high-speed cable line) from your computer to a computer at the clearinghouse. However, because you are in a school setting and are not actually set up to submit electronic claims at this time, click the No button.

18. The Information dialog box disappears and the Claim Management dialog box appears as before. Because Robin Caruthers' claim was not actually sent, the "Ready to Send" status still appears. If the claim had actually been sent electronically, the Status 1 column would now read "Sent."

19. Click the Close button to close the Claim Management dialog box and return to the main Medisoft window.

You have successfully completed Case Study 16-1.

Additional guided practice in using Medisoft to create claims is available by printing out Case Study 16-2 from the text's Online Learning Center (OLC). Similar to Case Study 16-1, Case Study 16-2 provides step-by-step instructions, with emphasis on printing a claim on paper rather than sending it electronically.

In Case Study 16-2 you will use Medisoft to:

- Enter insurance information for a new patient.
- Enter the patient's diagnosis code.
- Enter the transactions for an office visit.
- Create and print a paper claim.

To access the PDF file for Case Study 16-2:

1. Go to the text's OLC at www.mhhe.com/fp2p6e.
2. In the Student Edition section. select the link for Case Study 16-2. Follow the instructions for printing out the file.
3. Follow the steps in the Case Study 16-2 printout to create a workers' compensation claim for Shih-Chi Yang.

Backing Up Data While Exiting Medisoft

When entering data in Medisoft, it is important to back up your work regularly for safekeeping. A backup copy of the database files prevents you from losing your work if the hard drive fails, or if you accidentally delete data while working. If you are working in an instructional environment where you share computers, it is essential that you back up your work on exiting the program, so that you can restore it at the beginning of the next session.

In the next section, you will back up the data entered during the last two simulations.

1. You can back up your data at any time using the Backup option on the File menu. However, by default, Medisoft also gives you the opportunity to back up your data each time you exit the program. Click the Exit option on the File menu to exit Medisoft.
2. The Backup Reminder dialog box appears. You will back up your data to the folder on your hard drive where you stored the original Student Data file, CPC.mbk, only you will back it up under a new name, using your initials. Click the Back Up Data Now button.
3. The Backup dialog box appears. The Destination File Path and Name box at the top should already show the name of the folder on your hard drive where CPC.mbk is stored (whichever file was last used is displayed by default). If it does not show this path, use the Find button to locate this folder on your hard drive.
4. To back up the data under a new name, change the file name CPC. mbk at the end of the path name to **CPCxxx.mbk** (where xxx stands for your initials) as follows. Press the right arrow key on your keyboard to move the cursor to the end of the file name.

Then use the left arrow key to position the cursor in the file name and make the changes. The dialog box should now look like this:

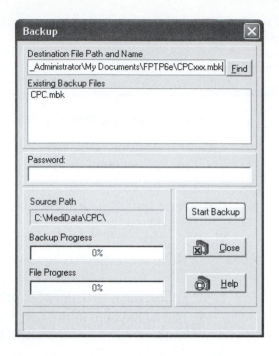

5. Click the Start Backup button.

6. Medisoft backs up the data under the new name and displays an Information box indicating that the backup is complete.

7. Click the OK button to close the Information dialog box and exit the Medisoft program.

8. For safekeeping, copy your new backup file from your hard drive to an external storage device, such as a flash drive or a CD-ROM. A separate backup copy prevents you from losing your work if the hard drive fails or if you or someone else accidentally deletes data on the computer.

Restoring a Backup File

If you are sharing a computer with other students in an instructional environment, you will need to perform a restore before a new Medisoft session to be certain you are working with your own data. If necessary, follow these steps to restore your latest backup file.

To restore the file *CPCxxx.mbk* to *C:\Medidata\CPC:*

1. Copy your backup file from your external storage device to the assigned location on your hard drive. (Ask your instructor if you are not sure which folder this is.)

2. Start Medisoft.

3. Check the title bar at the top of the screen to make sure the Central Practice Center data set is the active data set. (If it is not, use the Open Practice option on the File menu to select it.)

4. Open the File menu, and click Restore Data.

5. When the Warning box appears, click OK. The Restore dialog box appears.

6. Use the Find button if necessary to locate your assigned storage folder on the hard drive (the folder used in step 1 above). Locate CPCxxx.mbk in the list of existing backup files displayed for that folder, and click on it to attach it to the Backup File Path and Name at the top of the dialog box. The end of the path name should read \ . . . \CPCxxx.mbk.

7. The Destination Path at the bottom of the box should already be C:\MediData\CPC. The dialog box should now look like this:

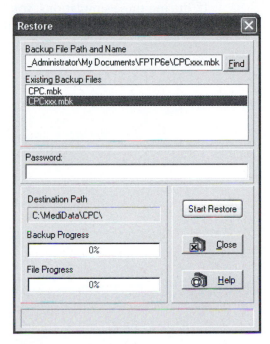

8. Click the Start Restore button.

9. When the Confirm box appears, click OK.

10. An Information box appears indicating that the restore is complete. Click OK to continue.

11. The Restore dialog box disappears. You are ready to begin the next session.

PART III: CLAIM SIMULATIONS

In Part III, you will complete five claim simulations on your own, using what you learned in the guided simulations in Part II. Each simulation will test your knowledge of a different type of medical insurance:

- Case Study 16-3 Blue Cross and Blue Shield (PPO)
- Case Study 16-4 Medicare
- Case Study 16-5 Medicaid (HMO)
- Case Study 16-6 TRICARE
- Case Study 16-7 Workers' Compensation

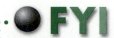

REMINDER: If you are in an instructional environment where you share computers, you may need to restore your work from the previous session before you begin the simulations in Part III of this chapter. See the instructions on Restoring a Backup File above (pp. 308–309).

For each of the five case studies, the following information has already been entered in the database from the patient information form: provider information, patient information, and insurance coverage. You will use the encounter form provided in each case study to carry out the remaining tasks:

1. Enter a diagnosis code.
2. Enter office visit transactions. (Remember to apply all patient copayments to the corresponding office visit charge.)
3. Print a walkout receipt (if a payment is received from the patient).
4. Create an electronic claim with a claim verification report.

If, during these simulations, you have questions about any procedures, notify your instructor or lab facilitator.

CENTRAL PRACTICE CENTER

Vijay Singh, M.D.–Cardiovascular Disease
1122 E. University Drive
Mesa, AZ 85204
602–969–4237

PATIENT NAME	APPT. DATE/TIME
John O'Rourke	10/20/2010 11:00am

PATIENT NO.	DX
OROURJO0	1. 414.00 coronary artherosclerosis

PAYMENT RECEIVED	
$20 copay, check #1922	2. 3. 4.

DESCRIPTION	✓	CPT	FEE	DESCRIPTION	✓	CPT	FEE
EXAMINATION				**PROCEDURES**			
New Patient				Diagnostic Anoscopy		46600	
Problem Focused		99201		ECG Complete	✓	93000	70
Expanded Problem Focused		99202		I&D, Abscess		10060	
Detailed	✓	99203	103	Pap Smear		88150	
Comprehensive		99204		Removal of Cerumen		69210	
Comprehensive/Complex		99205		Removal 1 Lesion		17000	
Established Patient				Removal 2-14 Lesions		17003	
Minimum		99211		Removal 15+ Lesions		17004	
Problem Focused		99212		Rhythm ECG w/Report		93040	
Expanded Problem Focused		99213		Rhythm ECG w/Tracing		93041	
Detailed		99214		Sigmoidoscopy, diag.		45330	
Comprehensive/Complex		99215					
				LABORATORY			
PREVENTIVE VISIT				Bacteria Culture		87081	
New Patient				Fungal Culture		87101	
Age 12-17		99384		Glucose Finger Stick		82948	
Age 18-39		99385		Lipid Panel	✓	80061	64
Age 40-64		99386		Specimen Handling		99000	
Age 65+		99387		Stool/Occult Blood		82270	
Established Patient				Tine Test		85008	
Age 12-17		99394		Tuberculin PPD		86580	
Age 18-39		99395		Urinalysis		81000	
Age 40-64		99396		Venipuncture	✓	36415	16
Age 65+		99397					
				INJECTION/IMMUN.			
CONSULTATION: OFFICE/ER				DT Immun		90702	
Requested By:				Hepatitis A Immun		90632	
Problem Focused		99241		Hepatitis B Immun		90746	
Expanded Problem Focused		99242		Influenza Immun		90660	
Detailed		99243		Pneumovax		90732	
Comprehensive		99244					
Comprehensive/Complex		99245		**TOTAL FEES**			

CENTRAL PRACTICE CENTER
Christopher Connolly, M.D.–General Practice
1122 E. University Drive
Mesa, AZ 85204
602–969–4237

PATIENT NAME	APPT. DATE/TIME
Donna Gaeta	10/07/2010 3:30pm

PATIENT NO.	DX
GAETADO0	1. v70.0 routine medical exam
PAYMENT RECEIVED	2.
	3.
	4.

DESCRIPTION	✓	CPT	FEE	DESCRIPTION	✓	CPT	FEE
EXAMINATION				**PROCEDURES**			
New Patient				Diagnostic Anoscopy		46600	
Problem Focused		99201		ECG Complete	✓	93000	29
Expanded Problem Focused		99202		I&D, Abscess		10060	
Detailed		99203		Pap Smear	✓	88150	29
Comprehensive		99204		Removal of Cerumen		69210	
Comprehensive/Complex		99205		Removal 1 Lesion		17000	
Established Patient				Removal 2-14 Lesions		17003	
Minimum		99211		Removal 15+ Lesions		17004	
Problem Focused		99212		Rhythm ECG w/Report		93040	
Expanded Problem Focused		99213		Rhythm ECG w/Tracing		93041	
Detailed		99214		Sigmoidoscopy, diag.		45330	
Comprehensive/Complex		99215					
				LABORATORY			
PREVENTIVE VISIT				Bacteria Culture		87081	
New Patient				Fungal Culture		87101	
Age 12-17		99384		Glucose Finger Stick		82948	
Age 18-39		99385		Lipid Panel		80061	
Age 40-64		99386		Specimen Handling		99000	
Age 65+	✓	99387	142	Stool/Occult Blood		82270	
Established Patient				Tine Test		85008	
Age 12-17		99394		Tuberculin PPD		86580	
Age 18-39		99395		Urinalysis	✓	81000	16
Age 40-64		99396		Venipuncture	✓	36415	16
Age 65+		99397					
				INJECTION/IMMUN.			
CONSULTATION: OFFICE/ER				DT Immun		90702	
Requested By:				Hepatitis A Immun		90632	
Problem Focused		99241		Hepatitis B Immun		90746	
Expanded Problem Focused		99242		Influenza Immun		90660	
Detailed		99243		Pneumovax		90732	
Comprehensive		99244					
Comprehensive/Complex		99245					
				TOTAL FEES			

CENTRAL PRACTICE CENTER
David Rosenberg, M.D.–Dermatology
1122 E. University Drive
Mesa, AZ 85204
602–969–4237

PATIENT NAME	APPT. DATE/TIME
Otto Kaar	10/14/2010 1:30pm

PATIENT NO.	DX
KAAROTT0	**1.** 682.1 abscess on neck
	2.
PAYMENT RECEIVED	**3.**
$15 copay, check #331	**4.**

DESCRIPTION	✓	CPT	FEE	DESCRIPTION	✓	CPT	FEE
EXAMINATION				**PROCEDURES**			
New Patient				Diagnostic Anoscopy		46600	
Problem Focused		99201		ECG Complete		93000	
Expanded Problem Focused		99202		I&D, Abscess	✓	10060	57
Detailed		99203		Pap Smear		88150	
Comprehensive		99204		Removal of Cerumen		69210	
Comprehensive/Complex		99205		Removal 1 Lesion		17000	
Established Patient				Removal 2-14 Lesions		17003	
Minimum		99211		Removal 15+ Lesions		17004	
Problem Focused		99212		Rhythm ECG w/Report		93040	
Expanded Problem Focused	✓	99213	39	Rhythm ECG w/Tracing		93041	
Detailed		99214		Sigmoidoscopy, diag.		45330	
Comprehensive/Complex		99215					
				LABORATORY			
PREVENTIVE VISIT				Bacteria Culture		87081	
New Patient				Fungal Culture		87101	
Age 12-17		99384		Glucose Finger Stick		82948	
Age 18-39		99385		Lipid Panel		80061	
Age 40-64		99386		Specimen Handling		99000	
Age 65+		99387		Stool/Occult Blood		82270	
Established Patient				Tine Test		85008	
Age 12-17		99394		Tuberculin PPD		86580	
Age 18-39		99395		Urinalysis		81000	
Age 40-64		99396		Venipuncture		36415	
Age 65+		99397					
				INJECTION/IMMUN.			
CONSULTATION: OFFICE/ER				DT Immun		90702	
Requested By:				Hepatitis A Immun		90632	
Problem Focused		99241		Hepatitis B Immun		90746	
Expanded Problem Focused		99242		Influenza Immun		90660	
Detailed		99243		Pneumovax		90732	
Comprehensive		99244					
Comprehensive/Complex		99245					
				TOTAL FEES			

CENTRAL PRACTICE CENTER

Nancy Ronkowski, M.D.–Obstetrics & Gynecology
1122 E. University Drive
Mesa, AZ 85204
602–969–4237

PATIENT NAME				APPT. DATE/TIME			
Robyn Janssen				10/13/2010 10:00am			

PATIENT NO.				DX			
JANSSRO0				1. 626.0 absence of menstruation			

PAYMENT RECEIVED				2.			
$10 copay, check #2088				3.			
				4.			

DESCRIPTION	✓	CPT	FEE	DESCRIPTION	✓	CPT	FEE
EXAMINATION				**PROCEDURES**			
New Patient				Diagnostic Anoscopy		46600	
Problem Focused		99201		ECG Complete		93000	
Expanded Problem Focused		99202		I&D, Abscess		10060	
Detailed		99203		Pap Smear		88150	
Comprehensive		99204		Removal of Cerumen		69210	
Comprehensive/Complex		99205		Removal 1 Lesion		17000	
Established Patient				Removal 2-14 Lesions		17003	
Minimum		99211		Removal 15+ Lesions		17004	
Problem Focused		99212		Rhythm ECG w/Report		93040	
Expanded Problem Focused	✓	99213	62	Rhythm ECG w/Tracing		93041	
Detailed		99214		Sigmoidoscopy, diag.		45330	
Comprehensive/Complex		99215					
				LABORATORY			
PREVENTIVE VISIT				Bacteria Culture		87081	
New Patient				Fungal Culture		87101	
Age 12-17		99384		Glucose Finger Stick		82948	
Age 18-39		99385		Lipid Panel		80061	
Age 40-64		99386		Specimen Handling		99000	
Age 65+		99387		Stool/Occult Blood		82270	
Established Patient				Tine Test		85008	
Age 12-17		99394		Tuberculin PPD		86580	
Age 18-39		99395		Urinalysis		81000	
Age 40-64		99396		Venipuncture		36415	
Age 65+		99397					
				INJECTION/IMMUN.			
CONSULTATION: OFFICE/ER				DT Immun		90702	
Requested By:				Hepatitis A Immun		90632	
Problem Focused		99241		Hepatitis B Immun		90746	
Expanded Problem Focused		99242		Influenza Immun		90660	
Detailed		99243		Pneumovax		90732	
Comprehensive		99244					
Comprehensive/Complex		99245					
				TOTAL FEES			

Case Study 16-7

CENTRAL PRACTICE CENTER
Christopher Connolly, M.D.–General Practice
1122 E. University Drive
Mesa, AZ 85204
602–969–4237

PATIENT NAME	APPT. DATE/TIME
Marilyn Grogan	10/16/2010 10:30am

PATIENT NO.	DX
GROGAMA0	**1.** 465.9 upper respiratory infection
PAYMENT RECEIVED	**2.**
	3.
	4.

DESCRIPTION	✓	CPT	FEE	DESCRIPTION	✓	CPT	FEE
EXAMINATION				**PROCEDURES**			
New Patient				Diagnostic Anoscopy		46600	
Problem Focused	✓	99201	56	ECG Complete		93000	
Expanded Problem Focused		99202		I&D, Abscess		10060	
Detailed		99203		Pap Smear		88150	
Comprehensive		99204		Removal of Cerumen		69210	
Comprehensive/Complex		99205		Removal 1 Lesion		17000	
Established Patient				Removal 2-14 Lesions		17003	
Minimum		99211		Removal 15+ Lesions		17004	
Problem Focused		99212		Rhythm ECG w/Report		93040	
Expanded Problem Focused		99213		Rhythm ECG w/Tracing		93041	
Detailed		99214		Sigmoidoscopy, diag.		45330	
Comprehensive/Complex		99215					
				LABORATORY			
PREVENTIVE VISIT				Bacteria Culture		87081	
New Patient				Fungal Culture	✓	87101	35
Age 12-17		99384		Glucose Finger Stick		82948	
Age 18-39		99385		Lipid Panel		80061	
Age 40-64		99386		Specimen Handling		99000	
Age 65+		99387		Stool/Occult Blood		82270	
Established Patient				Tine Test		85008	
Age 12-17		99394		Tuberculin PPD		86580	
Age 18-39		99395		Urinalysis		81000	
Age 40-64		99396		Venipuncture		36415	
Age 65+		99397					
				INJECTION/IMMUN.			
CONSULTATION: OFFICE/ER				DT Immun		90702	
Requested By:				Hepatitis A Immun		90632	
Problem Focused		99241		Hepatitis B Immun		90746	
Expanded Problem Focused		99242		Influenza Immun		90660	
Detailed		99243		Pneumovax		90732	
Comprehensive		99244					
Comprehensive/Complex		99245		**TOTAL FEES**			

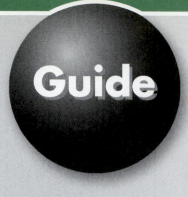

Guide to the Interactive Simulated CMS-1500 Form

This Guide introduces you to the interactive simulated CMS-1500 form that was created for use with this text. The simulated form is a PDF file that can be used with Adobe Reader to create and print CMS-1500 insurance claims. The form provides an easy-to-use alternative to filling in claim forms by hand, and may be used to complete the various claim case studies contained in the end-of-chapter exercises. The Guide shows you how to download the form, enter data, print a claim, and save the data in the form as a text file.

COMPUTER SUPPLIES AND EQUIPMENT

To use the interactive simulated CMS-1500 form with this text, the following items are required:

- Windows Vista, XP, or 2000 operating system
- 128 MB of RAM minimum, 256 MB or greater recommended
- Up to 100 MB of available hard-disk space
- Microsoft Internet Explorer 5.5 or higher
- Adobe Reader version 7 or 8 (version 8 is recommended)
- Printer
- Active Internet connection to access the Online Learning Center

> **Tip**
>
> Adobe Reader software is available for download, free of charge, from the Adobe website at www.adobe.com.

DOWNLOADING THE CMS-1500 FORM FROM THE ONLINE LEARNING CENTER

A copy of the simulated form (CMS-1500.pdf) is available for download at the text's Online Learning Center (OLC). To download the file:

1. Create a folder on your computer under My Documents for storing the file.
2. Go to the text's OLC at www.mhhe.com/fp2p6e, and click *Student Edition.*
3. Under Course-wide Content, select Simulated CMS-1500 Form and the corresponding link to download the file.
4. A blank CMS-1500 form appears on your screen in Adobe Reader. To save a copy of the blank form to your computer, open the File menu and click the Save a Copy option.
5. In the Save a Blank Copy of this Form dialog box that appears, click the Save a Blank Copy button.

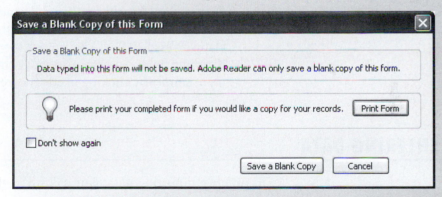

6. The Save a Copy dialog box appears. In the Save In field at the top of the dialog box, select the folder where you want to copy the blank form (see step 1 above), and then click the Save button.
7. A copy is saved to your computer. Click the Exit option on the File menu to exit the Adobe Reader program.
8. Exit the OLC.

NAVIGATING THROUGH THE FORM

1. From the desktop, locate the folder where you stored the simulated form and double click the file name (CMS-1500.pdf) to open it.

2. Use the scroll bar or the up and down arrows in the right margin of the screen to scroll through the file. Notice that the first page contains the front of the CMS-1500 form, and the second page contains the back. Return to the first page.

3. Open the Zoom option on the View menu to display the available zoom options. If it is not already selected, select the Fit Width option to show the full width of the form on the screen. Because the type on the form is small, the Fit Width option is the recommended viewing option.

4. Rollover text describing the contents is supplied for each field (also known as Form Locators, or FLs) on the form. Without clicking inside the field, let the cursor hover over FL 11a (Insured's Date of Birth) in the YY section until the following rollover text appears.

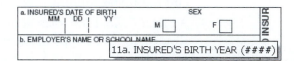

5. To practice navigating through the form, click the Self box in FL 6 (Patient Relationship to Insured) and press TAB five times. The TAB key moves the cursor forward through each field on the claim. Press SHIFT TAB to move the cursor backwards through the same fields. You can also move the cursor to any field on the form simply by clicking inside the field.

ENTERING DATA

To practice inputting data, you will fill in the first five FLs for Medicare patient Sharon Diaz. In the claim form examples in this text, upper case characters are used to make the claim easier to read. However, mixed case characters may also be used when entering data.

1. In FL 1, click the Medicare box and then key an X.

2. According to the formatting rules, data in FL1a (Insured's I.D. Number) is entered without spaces or hyphens. Since Sharon's I.D. number is 499-68-3301A, key 499683301A.

3. The patient's name is reported in FL 2, in the order of last name, first name, and middle initial, using commas to separate each part. For Sharon Diaz, key DIAZ, SHARON.

4. In FL 3 (Patient's Birthdate), enter the date 01/25/1940. As indicated by the rollover text, use two digits for the month and

day, and four digits for the year. Then key an X in the box marked F to indicate that the patient's gender is female.

5. Because the insured's name and the patient's name in this case are the same, FL 4 (Insured's name) is left blank.

6. Click inside FL 5 and enter the following address, using the Tab key to move from one section to the next: 123 SNOW DRIVE, ALLIANCE, OH, 44601.

7. According to the formatting rules, no spaces or dashes are used when entering phone numbers. Therefore, for telephone number (555) 492-6606, key 555 for the area code, press Tab, and then key 4926606.

PRINTING A CLAIM

Now that you are familiar with entering data, you are ready to practice printing. When using Adobe Reader to fill in a form, you cannot save the data you enter in the form when you exit. Therefore, you must print the claim before you exit to have a record of your work. Follow the steps below to practice printing a claim form.

1. Assume you have finished filling in the claim for Sharon Diaz. To save a copy of your work, click the Print option on the File menu.

2. The Print dialog box appears, as shown here.

Tip

Adobe Reader Versus Adobe Acrobat

In Adobe Reader, a filled-in form can be printed, but it cannot be saved to a PDF file. To save a filled-in form to a PDF file, the form must be completed in Adobe Acrobat, version 8—a full scale software program that is purchased separately. Although the claim exercises in this text can be completed with either program, because of the high cost of the Adobe Acrobat software, the text assumes the use of Adobe Reader.

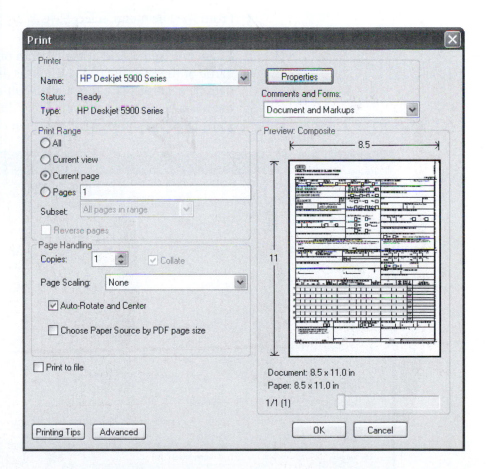

3. In the Printer section, verify the correct printer is selected in the Name box.

4. In the Print Range section, if you do not want a copy of page 2 (the back of the claim form), change the print range to print page 1 only, or click the Current Page option. To print both pages, leave the print range setting as it is.

5. In the Page Handling section, set the Page Scaling option to None. (Note: If text in the margins is cut off when you print the form, change this option to Shrink to Printable Area or Fit to Printable Area.)

6. Click the OK button at the bottom of the dialog box to print the claim.

USING THE SAVE AS TEXT OPTION

Although you cannot save the data and the form together, Adobe Reader provides a Save as Text option that enables you to save the data that is on-screen into a separate text file. You lose the layout of the form, but the data itself is saved. The text file, a Windows Notepad file, lists the names of the thirty-three FLs together with the data currently displayed in each. Follow the steps below to practice using the Save as Text option.

1. From the File menu, select Save as Text. The Save As dialog box appears.

2. In the File Name field at the bottom of the dialog box, the original name of the PDF file (CMS-1500) is displayed. The Save as Type field below it displays the new default extension (.txt) to indicate the file is being saved as a text file. Edit the file name to CMS-1500-DIAZ, as shown here, and then click the Save button.

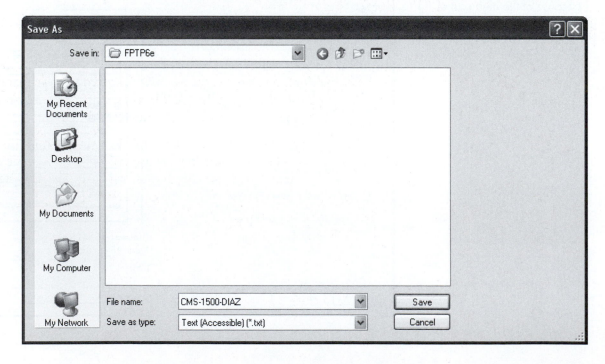

3. The new text file is saved, and the Save As dialog box closes. To view the text file, you must open it in Windows Notepad. First, exit Adobe Reader by clicking the X in the top right corner of the screen.

4. Open Windows Explorer, and locate the folder where you are storing your work for this text. The new text file (CMS-1500-DIAZ) will be displayed in the same folder. Double click on the file name to open it.

5. The file opens in Windows Notepad, as shown here.

```
CMS-1500-DIAZ - Notepad
File  Edit  Format  View  Help
(PAYER NAME AND ADDRESS:
1st Line - Name)
(text)
(text)
(text)
(text)
(text)
(text)
(PAYER NAME AND ADDRESS:
3rd Line - Second line of address (leave blank if none))
(PAYER NAME AND ADDRESS:
4th Line - City, State (2 digits), and Zip Code)
(1. MEDICARE #) X
(1. MEDICAID #)
(1. TRICARE CHAMPUS (Sponsor's SSN))
(1. CHAMPVA (Member ID#))
(1. GROUP HEALTH PLAN (SSN or ID))
(1. FECA BLK LUNG (SSN))
(1. OTHER (ID))
(1a. INSURED'S I.D. NUMBER) 499683301A
(2. PATIENT'S NAME (Last Name, First Name, Middle Initial)) DIAZ, SHARON
(3. PATIENT'S BIRTH MONTH (##)) 01
(3. PATIENT'S BIRTH DAY (##)) 25
(3. PATIENT'S BIRTH YEAR (####)) 1940
(3. PATIENT'S SEX (M))
(3. PATIENT'S SEX (F)) X
(4. INSURED'S NAME (Last Name, First Name, Middle Initial))
(5. PATIENT'S ADDRESS (No., Street)) 123 SNOW DRIVE
(5. PATIENT'S ADDRESS (City)) ALLIANCE
(5. PATIENT'S ADDRESS (State)) OH
(5. PATIENT'S ADDRESS (Zip Code)) 44601
(5. PATIENT'S TELEPHONE (Area code)) 555
(5. PATIENT'S TELEPHONE) 4926606
```

6. Notice that each FL is listed in parentheses. Any data that was in the fields at the time the file was saved is listed after the parentheses. When finished viewing the text file, click the X in the upper right corner of the window to close the Notepad screen.

This completes the introduction to the interactive simulated CMS-1500 form. If you choose, you can now use the form to practice creating claims with the data in the end-of-chapter case studies (Chapter 6 and Chapters 8-12).

Glossary

837I claim The HIPAA (ASC X12N) institutional claim transaction.

837P claim (HIPAA 837 claim) The HIPAA (ASC X12N) professional claim transaction, used to file physicians' claims.

A

acceptance of assignment (V. accept assignment) A participating physician's agreement to accept the allowed charge as payment in full.

accounts receivable (A/R) Monies owed to a medical practice by its patients and third-party payers.

Acknowledgment of Receipt of Notice of Privacy Practices Form accompanying a covered entity's Notice of Privacy Practices; covered entities must make a good-faith effort to have patients sign the acknowledgment.

acute Describes an illness or condition having severe symptoms and a short duration; can also refer to a sudden exacerbation of a chronic condition.

ADA Dental Claim Form Authorized form for submitting dental insurance claims.

add-on code Procedures that are performed and reported only in addition to a primary procedure; indicated in CPT by a plus sign (+) next to the code.

adjudication The process followed by health plans to examine claims and determine benefits.

adjustment An amount (positive or negative) entered in a patient billing program to change a patient's account balance.

admitting diagnosis The patient's condition determined by a physician at admission to an inpatient facility.

administrative code set Under HIPAA, required codes for various data elements, such as taxonomy codes and place of service (POS) codes.

advance beneficiary notice of noncoverage (ABN) Medicare form used to inform a patient that a service to be provided is not likely to be reimbursed by the program.

aging report A report that shows the time span between issuing an invoice and receiving payment; used in medical offices to determine late payments and collect them.

allowed charge The maximum charge that a health plan pays for a specific service or procedure; also called allowable charge, maximum fee, and other terms.

Alphabetic Index The section of the ICD-9-CM in which diseases and injuries with corresponding diagnosis codes are presented in alphabetical order.

ambulatory care Outpatient care.

ambulatory patient classification (APC) A Medicare payment classification for outpatient services.

American Academy of Professional Coders (AAPC) National association that fosters the establishment and maintenance of professional, ethical, educational, and certification standards for medical coding.

American Association of Medical Assistants National association that fosters the profession of medical assisting.

American Association for Medical Transcription National association fostering the profession of medical transcription.

American Health Information Management Association (AHIMA) National association of health information management professionals; promotes valid, accessible, yet confidential health information and advocates quality health care.

American Medical Association (AMA) Member organization for physicians; goals are to promote the art and science of medicine, improve public health, and promote ethical, educational, and clinical standards for the medical profession.

American National Standards Institute (ANSI) Organization that sets standards for electronic data interchange on a national level.

Accredited Standards Committee X12, Insurance Subcommittee (ASC X12N) The ANSI-accredited standards development organization that maintains the administrative and financial electronic transactions standards adopted under HIPAA.

appeal A request sent to a payer for reconsideration of a claim adjudication.

assignment of benefits Authorization by policyholder that allows a health plan to pay benefits directly to a provider.

at-home recovery care Assistance with the activities of daily living provided for a patient in the home.

attending physician The clinician primarily responsible for the care of the patient from the beginning of a hospitalization.

audit Methodical review; in medical insurance, a formal examination of a physician's accounting or patient medical records.

audit-edit claim response Report from a receiver of an electronic claim transmitted to its sender regarding the status and completeness of the claim.

authorization Document signed by a patient that permits release of particular medical information under the specific stated conditions.

B

balance billing Collecting the difference between a provider's usual fee and a payer's lower allowed charge from the insured.

benefits The amount of money a health plan pays for services covered in an insurance policy.

billing provider The person or organization (often a clearinghouse or billing service) sending a HIPAA claim, as distinct from the pay-to provider that receives payment.

billing service Company that provides billing and claims processing services.

birthday rule The guideline that determines which of two parents with medical coverage has the primary insurance for a child; the parent whose day of birth is earlier in the calendar year is considered primary.

BlueCard Program A Blue Cross and Blue Shield program that provides benefits for plan subscribers who are away from their local areas.

BlueCard Worldwide The international component of the BlueCard Program that allows BCBS plan members traveling or living abroad to receive the benefits they would receive at home.

Blue Cross A primarily non-profit corporation that offers prepaid medical benefits for hospital services, and some outpatient, home care, and other institutional services.

Blue Cross and Blue Shield Association (BCBS) The national licensing agency of Blue Cross and Blue Shield Plans.

Blue Shield A primarily non-profit corporation which offers prepaid medical benefits for physician, dental, and vision services, and other outpatient care.

bundled code Single procedure code used to report a group of related procedures.

C

CHAMPUS Now the TRICARE program; formerly the Civilian Health and Medical Program of the Uniformed Services (Army, Navy, Air Force, Marine Corps, Coast Guard, Public Health Service, and the National Oceanic and Atmospheric Administration) that serves spouses and children of active-duty service members, military retirees and their families, some former spouses, and survivors of deceased military members.

CHAMPVA The Civilian Health and Medical Program of the Veterans Administration (now known as the Department of Veterans Affairs) which shares health care costs for families of veterans with 100 percent service-connected disability and the surviving spouses and children of veterans who die from service-connected disabilities.

CHAMPVA for Life Program for beneficiaries who are both Medicare and CHAMPVA eligible; extends benefits to spouses or dependents who are age sixty-five and over.

CMS See Centers for Medicare and Medicaid Services.

CMS-1450 Paper claim for hospital services; also known as the UB-92.

CMS-1500 Paper claim for physician services.

CPT The abbreviation that refers to the American Medical Association's publication *Current Procedural Terminology*.

canines Two of the 32 permanent adult teeth.

capitation Payment method in which a prepayment covers the provider's services to a plan member for a specified period of time.

capitation rate (cap rate) The contractually set periodic prepayment to a provider for specified services to each enrolled plan member.

carrier Health plan; also known as insurance company, payer, or third-party payer.

carrier block Date entry area located in the upper right of the CMS-1500 that allows for a four-line address for the payer.

case Group of related data about a patient's personal/insurance account information and a particular medical condition.

cash flow The inflow of payments from patients and payers to a medical practice and the outflow from the practice of payments to suppliers and staff; based on the actual movement of money rather than amounts that are receivable or payable.

catastrophic cap The maximum annual amount a TRICARE beneficiary must pay for deductible and cost share.

category In the ICD-9-CM, a three-digit code used to classify a particular disease or injury.

Category I code Procedure codes in the six major sections of the CPT: evaluation and management, anesthesia, surgery, pathology/laboratory, radiology, and medicine.

Category II code Optional CPT codes that track performance measures for a medical goal such as reducing tobacco use.

Category III code Temporary codes for emerging technology, services, and procedures; to be used, rather than an unlisted code, when available.

categorically needy A person who receives assistance from government programs such as Temporary Assistance for Needy Families (TANF).

Centers for Medicare and Medicaid Services (CMS) Federal agency within the Department of Health and Human Services (HHS) that runs Medicare, Medicaid, Clinical Laboratories (under the CLIA program), and other governmental health programs. Formerly Health Care Financing Administration (HCFA.)

certificate Term for Blue Cross and Blue Shield medical insurance policy.

charge master (or charge ticket) A hospital's list of the codes and charges for its services.

chief complaint (CC) A patient's description of the symptoms or other reasons for seeking medical care for a provider encounter.

chronic An illness or condition with a long duration.

Civilian Health and Medical Program of the Veterans Administration See CHAMPVA.

Civil Service Retirement System (CSRS) A disability program for employees of the federal government.

claim adjustment reason code Code used by a health plan on a remittance advice to describe payment information.

claim attachment Documentation that a provider sends to a payer in support of a health care claim.

claim control number Unique number assigned by the sender to a health care claim.

claim filing indicator code Administrative code used to identify the type of health plan.

claim frequency code (claim submission reason code) Administrative code that identifies the claim as original, replacement, or void/cancel action.

claim scrubber Software that checks claims to permit error correction for "clean" claims.

clean claim A claim that is accepted by a health plan for adjudication.

clearinghouse A company that converts, for a fee, nonstandard data formats into HIPAA standard transactions and transmits the data to health plans; or also handles the reverse process, changing HIPAA formatted transactions from health plans into nonstandard formats for providers.

code linkage The connection between a service and a patient's condition or illness; establishes the medical necessity of the procedure.

code set Alphabetic and/or numeric representations for data. Medical code sets are systems of medical terms that are required for HIPAA transactions. Administrative (non-medical) code sets, such as taxonomy codes and Zip codes, are also used in HIPAA transactions.

coding The process of assigning numerical codes to diagnoses and procedures/services.

coexisting condition Additional illness that either has an effect on the patient's primary illness or is also treated during the encounter.

coinsurance The portion of charges that an insured person must pay for health care services after payment of the deductible amount; usually stated as a percentage.

compliance plan A medical practice's written plan for (a) the appointment of a compliance officer and committee, (b) a code of conduct for physicians' business arrangements and employees' compliance, (c) training plans, (d) properly prepared and updated coding tools such as job reference aids, encounter forms, and documentation templates, (e) rules for prompt identification and refunding of overpayments, and (f) ongoing monitoring and auditing of claim preparation.

condition code Two-digit numeric or alphanumeric code used to report a special condition or unique circumstance about a claim; reported in Item Number 10d on the CMS-1500 claim form.

consultation Service performed by a physician to advise a requesting physician about a patient's condition and care; the consultant does not assume responsibility for the patient's care and must send a written report back to the requestor.

consumer-driven health plan (CDHP) Type of medical insurance that combines a high-deductible health plan with a medical savings plan which covers some out-of-pocket expenses.

conventions Typographic techniques or standard practices that provide visual guidelines for understanding printed material.

coordination of benefits (COB) A clause in an insurance policy that explains how the policy will pay if more than one insurance policy applies to the claim.

copayment An amount that a health plan requires a beneficiary to pay at the time of service for each health care encounter.

Correct Coding Initiative (CCI) Computerized Medicare system of CPT code edits to prevent overpayment for procedures.

cost-share The term meaning coinsurance for a TRICARE or CHAMPVA beneficiary.

covered entity (CE) Under HIPAA, a health plan, clearinghouse, or provider that transmits any health information in electronic form in connection with a HIPAA transaction. In the law, "health plan" does not specifically include workers' compensation programs, property and casualty programs, or disability insurance programs.

crossover claim Claim for services to a Medicare/Medicaid beneficiary; Medicare is the primary payer and automatically transmits claim information to Medicaid as the secondary payer.

cross-reference Directions in printed material that tell a reader where to look for additional information.

Current Dental Terminology (CDT-4) Publication of the American Dental Association containing a standardized classification system for reporting dental procedures and services.

Current Procedural Terminology (CPT) Publication of the American Medical Association containing the HIPAA-mandated standardized classification system for reporting medical procedures and services performed by physicians.

D

database An organized collection of related data items having a specific structure.

data element The smallest unit of information in a HIPAA transaction.

data format An arrangement of electronic data for transmission.

day sheet In a medical office, a report that summarizes the business day's charges and payments, drawn from all the patient ledgers for the day.

deductible An amount that an insured person must pay, usually on an annual basis, for health care services before a health plan's payment begins.

Defense Enrollment Eligibility Reporting System (DEERS) The worldwide database of TRICARE and CHAMPVA beneficiaries.

de-identified health information Medical data from which individual identifiers have been removed; also known as a redacted or blinded record.

dentin The hard material that fills 80 to 90 percent of the tooth.

Dentist's Pretreatment Estimate A dentist's estimate of dental work required for a patient that is submitted to an insurance carrier before the service is performed.

Dentist's Statement of Actual Services A dental claim form that reports the services a dentist has performed for a patient.

dependent A person other than the insured, such as a spouse or child, who is covered under a health plan.

destination payer In HIPAA claims, the health plan receiving the claim.

determination A payer's decision regarding the benefits due for a claim.

diagnoses A physician's opinion of the nature of patients' illnesses or injuries.

diagnosis code The number assigned to a diagnosis in the International Classification of Diseases.

diagnosis-related groups (DRGs) A system of analyzing conditions and treatments for similar groups of patients used to establish Medicare fees for hospital inpatient services.

direct payment Payment for procedures that is made by an insurance company or a patient to a provider.

disability compensation program A plan that reimburses the insured for lost income when the insured cannot work because of an illness or injury, whether or not it is work-related.

disallowed charge An item on a remittance advice that identifies the difference between the allowable charge and the amount the physician charged for a service.

discounted fee-for-service A negotiated payment schedule for health care services based on a reduced percentage of a provider's usual charges.

documentation The systematic, logical, and consistent recording of a patient's health status—history, examinations, tests, results of treatments, and observations—in chronological order in a patient's medical record.

downcoding A payer's review and reduction of a procedure code (often an E/M code) to a lower level than reported by the provider.

durable medical equipment (DME) Medicare term for reusable physical supplies such as wheelchairs and hospital beds that are ordered by the provider for use in the home; reported with HPCPS Level II codes.

Dx Abbreviation for diagnosis.

E

E code An alphanumeric ICD code for an external cause of injury or poisoning.

E/M code See evaluation and management codes.

Early and Periodic Screening, Diagnosis, and Treatment (EPSDT) Medicaid's prevention, early detection, and treatment program for eligible children under the age of 21.

edit In an electronic claim, a computer check for missing data or other mistakes, such as outdated codes.

electronic claim A health care claim that is transmitted electronically; also known as an electronic media claim (EMC).

electronic data interchange (EDI) The exchange (system to system) of data in a standardized format.

electronic funds transfer (EFT) Electronic routing of funds between banks.

electronic media Electronic storage media, such as hard drives and removable media, and transmission media used to exchange information already in electronic storage media, such as the Internet. Paper transmission via fax and voice transmission via telephone are not electronic transmission.

electronic health records (EHR) A running collection of health information that provides immediate electronic access by authorized users.

electronic remittance Payment made through electronic funds transfer.

electronic remittance advice See remittance advice.

emergency care Care received in a situation in which a delay in the treatment of the patient would lead to a significant increase in the threat to life or body part.

enamel The outer coating of the tooth.

encounter An office visit between a patient and a medical professional.

encounter form A listing of the diagnoses, procedures, and charges for a patient's visit; also called the superbill.

encryption A method of scrambling transmitted data so it cannot be deciphered without the use of a confidential process or key.

eponym A name or phrase that is formed from or based on a person's name; usually describes a condition or procedure associated with that person.

established patient A patient who has received professional services from a provider (or another provider with the same specialty in the same practice) within the past three years.

ethics Standards of conduct based on moral principles.

etiology The cause or origin of a disease.

etiquette Standards of professional behavior.

evaluation and management (E/M) codes Procedure codes that cover physicians' services performed to determine the optimum course for patient care; listed in the Evaluation and Management section of CPT.

excluded service A service specified in a medical insurance contract as not covered.

explanation of benefits (EOB) A document from a payer sent to a patient that shows how the amount of a benefit was determined.

explanation of Medicare benefits (EOMB) See Medicare Summary Notice.

F

family deductible A fixed, periodic amount that must be met by the combination of payments for covered services to each individual of an insured/dependent group before benefits from a payer begin.

Federal Employees' Compensation Act (FECA) A federal law that provides workers' compensation insurance for civilian employees of the federal government.

Federal Employee Health Benefits (FEHB) plan The health insurance plan that covers employees of the federal government.

Federal Employees Retirement System (FERS) - Disability program for employees of the federal government.

Federal Insurance Contribution Act (FICA) The federal law that authorizes payroll deductions for the Social Security Disability Program.

Federal Medicaid Assistance Percentage (FMAP) Basis for federal government Medicaid allocations to individual states.

fee-for-service Method of charging under which a provider's payment is based on each service performed.

fee schedule List of charges for services performed.

final report A report filed by the physician in a state workers' compensation case when the patient is discharged.

first report of injury or illness A report filed in state workers' compensation cases that contains the employer's name and address, employee's supervisor, date and time of accident, geographic location of injury, and the patient's description of what happened.

fiscal agent An organization that processes claims for a government program.

fiscal intermediary A government contractor that processes claims for government programs; for Medicare, the fiscal intermediary (FI) processes Part A claims.

Flexible Blue The Blue Cross and Blue Shield consumer-driven health plan.

formulary A list of a health plan's selected drugs and their proper dosages; often a plan pays only for the drugs it lists.

fraud Intentional deceptive act to obtain a benefit.

G

gatekeeper See primary care physician.

gingivae (gingiva) The gums.

global period The number of days surrounding a surgical procedure during which all services relating to the procedure—preoperative, during the surgery, and postoperative—are considered part of the surgical package and are not additionally reimbursed.

group health plan Under HIPAA, an employee health plan that either has 50 or more participants or is administered by another business entity.

guardian An adult legally responsible for care and custody of a minor.

H

HCFA See Centers for Medicare and Medicaid Services.

HCFA-1450 See CMS-1450.

HCFA-1500 See CMS-1500.

health care claim An electronic transaction or a paper document filed with a health plan to receive benefits.

Health Care Financing Administration See Centers for Medicare and Medicaid Services.

Health Care Common Procedure Coding System (HCPCS) Procedure codes for Medicare claims, made up of CPT codes (Level I) and national codes (Level II).

health information management (HIM) Hospital department that organizes and maintains patient medical records; also profession devoted to managing, analyzing, and utilizing data vital for patient care, making it accessible to healthcare providers.

Health Insurance Portability and Accountability Act (HIPAA) Federal act that set forth guidelines for standardizing the electronic data interchange of administrative and financial transactions, exposing fraud and abuse in government programs, and protecting the security and privacy of health information.

health maintenance organization (HMO)   A managed health care system in which providers agree to offer health care to the organization's members for fixed periodic payments from the plan; usually members must receive medical services only from the plan's providers.

health plan   Under HIPAA, an individual or group plan that either provides or pays for the cost of medical care, including group health plan, health insurance issuer, health maintenance organization, Medicare Part A or B, Medicaid, TRICARE, and other governmental and nongovernmental plans.

HIPAA claim   Generic term for the HIPAA ASC X12N 837 professional health care claim transaction.

HIPAA Electronic Health Care Transactions and Code Sets (TCS)   The HIPAA rule governing the electronic exchange of health information.

HIPAA National Identifier   HIPAA-mandated identification systems for employers, health care providers, health plans, and patients; the NPI, National Provider System, and employer system are in place, health plan and patient systems are to be created.

HIPAA Privacy Rule   Law that regulates the use and disclosure of patients' protected health information (PHI).

HIPAA Security Rule   Law that requires covered entities to establish administrative, physical, and technical safeguards to protect the confidentiality, integrity and availability of health information.

HIPAA transaction   General term for the electronic transactions, such as claim status inquiries, health care claim transmittal, and coordination of benefits regulated under the HIPAA Health Care Transactions and Code Sets standards.

home plan   A Blue Cross and Blue Shield plan in the community where the subscriber has contracted for coverage.

hospice   A public or private organization that provides services for terminally ill people and their families.

host plan   A participating provider's local Blue Cross and Blue Shield plan.

I

ICD-9-CM   Abbreviated title of International Classification of Diseases, 9th Revision, Clinical Modification.

ICD code   A system of diagnostic codes based on the International Classification of Diseases.

incisors   Four of the 32 permanent adult teeth; the cutting teeth.

indemnity plan   An insurance company's agreement to reimburse a policy holder a predetermined amount for covered losses.

indirect payment   Payment made to a provider by an insurance company on behalf of a patient.

individual deductible   A fixed, periodic amount that must be met by each individual of an insured/dependent group before benefits from a payer begin.

individual relationship code   Administrative code that specifies the patient's relationship to the subscriber (insured).

informed consent   The process by which a patient authorizes medical treatment after discussion regarding the nature, indications, benefits, and risks of a treatment a physician recommends.

inpatient   A person admitted to a medical facility for services that require an overnight stay.

insurance aging report   A report grouping unpaid claims transmitted to payers by the length of time that they remain due, such as 30, 60, 90, or 120 days.

insurance carrier   Health plan; also known as insurance company, payer, or third-party payer.

insured   The policyholder or subscriber to a health plan or medical insurance policy; also known as guarantor.

International Classification of Diseases, 9th Revision, Clinical Modification (ICD-9-CM)   A publication containing the HIPAA-mandated standardized classification system for diseases and injuries; developed by the World Health Organization and modified for use in the United States.

L

legacy number   A provider's identification number issued by a payer before implementation of the National Provider Identification system.

liable   Legally responsible.

limiting charge   In Medicare, the highest fee (115 percent of the Medicare Fee Schedule) that nonparticipating physicians can charge for a particular service.

line item control number   On a HIPAA claim, the unique number assigned by the sender to each service line item reported.

local coverage determinations (LCDs)   Formerly called Local Medicare Review Policies (LMRPs), these are issued by Medicare to help clarify medical necessity issues.

M

main number   The five-digit procedure code listed in the CPT.

main term   The word in bold-faced type that identifies a disease or condition in the Alphabetic index in ICD-9-CM.

managed care   A system that combines the financing and the delivery of appropriate, cost-effective health care services to its members.

managed care organization (MCO)   Organization offering some type of managed health care plan.

mandible   The lower jaw bone.

master patient index   A hospital's main patient database.

maxilla   The upper jaw bone.

maxillofacial surgery   Surgical procedure related to the face and jaw.

Medicaid   A federal and state assistance program that pays for health care services for people who cannot afford them.

MediCal   California's state Medicaid program name.

medical coders   Medical office staff with specialized training who handle the diagnostic and procedural coding of medical records.

medical insurance   A financial plan that covers the cost of hospital and medical care due to illness or injury.

medical insurance specialist   The person in a medical office who handles patients' health care claims.

medical malpractice   Failure to use an acceptable level of professional skill when giving medical services that results in injury or harm to a patient.

medical necessity denial   Refusal by a health plan to pay for a reported procedure that does not meet its medical necessity criteria.

medical records   Files that contain the documentation of patients' medical history, record of care, progress notes, correspondence, and related billing/financial information.

Medical Savings Account (MSA)   The Medicare health savings account program.

medically indigent   Medically needy.

medically necessary   Payment criterion of payers that requires medical treatments to be appropriate and provided in accordance with generally accepted standards of medical practice. The reported procedure or service (1) matches the diagnosis, (2) is not elective, (3) is not experimental, (4) has not been performed for the convenience of the patient or the patient's family, and (5) has been provided at the appropriate level.

medically needy   Medicaid classification for people with high medical expenses and low financial resources, although not sufficiently low to receive cash assistance.

medically unlikely edits (MUEs)   CMS unit-of-service edits that check for clerical or software-based coding or billing errors, such as anatomically related mistakes.

Medicare   The federal health insurance program for people 65 or older and some people with disabilities.

Medicare Advantage   Medicare plans other than the Original Medicare Plan.

Medicare administrative contractor (MAC)   New entities assigned by CMS to replace the Part A fiscal intermediaries and the Part B carriers; also known as A/B MACs, they handle claims and related functions for both Parts A and B within specific multistate jurisdictions. DME MACs handle claims for durable medical equipment, supplies, and drugs billed by physicians.

Medicare beneficiary   A person covered by Medicare.

Medicare carrier   A private organization under contract with CMS to administer Medicare Part B claims in an assigned region.

Medicare Fee Schedule (MFS)   The RBRVS-based allowed fees that are reimbursable to Medicare participating physicians.

Medicare Modernization Act (MMA)   Short name for the Medicare Prescription Drug, Improvement, and Modernization Act of 2003.

Medicare Part A   The part of the Medicare program that pays for hospitalization, care in a skilled nursing facility, home health care, and hospice care.

Medicare Part B   The part of the Medicare program that pays for physician services, outpatient hospital services, durable medical equipment, and other services and supplies.

Medicare Part C   Managed care health plans offered to Medicare beneficiaries under the Medicare Advantage program.

Medicare Part D   Prescription drug reimbursement plans offered to Medicare beneficiaries.

Medicare-participating agreement   A phrase that describes physicians and other providers of medical services who have signed agreements with Medicare to accept assignment on all Medicare claims.

Medicare Remittance Notice (MRN)   Remittance advice from Medicare to providers that explains how payments for a batch of Medicare claims were determined.

Medicare Summary Notice (MSN)   Type of remittance advice from Medicare to plan beneficiaries to explain how their benefits were determined.

Medigap   Insurance plan offered by a private insurance carrier to supplement Medicare Original Plan coverage.

Medi-Medi beneficiary   Person who is eligible for both Medicare and Medicaid benefits.

member plan   Independent insurance company licensed to offer Blue Cross and Blue Shield health plans.

military treatment facility (MTF)   Government facility providing medical services for members and dependents of the Uniformed Services.

minimum necessary standard   Principle that individually identifiable health information should be disclosed only to the extent needed to support the purpose of the disclosure.

modifier   A number that is appended to a code to report particular facts. CPT modifiers report special circumstances involved with a procedure or service. HCPCS modifiers are often used to designate a body part, such as left side or right side.

molars   Six of the 32 permanent adult teeth.

MS-DRGs (Medicare-Severity DRGs)   Medicare Inpatient Prospective Payment System revision that takes into account whether certain conditions were present on admission.

N

National coverage determinations (NCDs)   Issued by Medicare to help clarify medical necessity issues.

National Patient ID (Individual Identifier)   Unique individual identification system to be created under HIPAA National Identifiers.

National Payer ID (Health Plan ID)   Unique health plan identification system to be created under HIPAA National Identifiers.

National Plan and Provider Enumeration System (NPPES)   A system set up by HHS which processes applications for NPIs, assigns them, and then stores the data and identifying numbers for both health plans and providers.

National Provider Identifier (NPI)   Under HIPAA, unique 10-digit identifier assigned to each provider by the National Provider System; replaces both the UPIN and Medicare PIN.

National Uniform Claim Committee (NUCC)   Organization responsible for the content of health care claims.

nationwide plan   A Blue Cross and Blue Shield national account health plan.

network   Providers and suppliers who participate in a particular managed care organization or health plan.

network model HMO   A type of health maintenance organization where physicians remain self-employed and provide services to both HMO-members and nonmembers.

new patient   A patient who has not received professional services from a provider (or another provider with the same specialty in the same practice) within the past three years.

nonavailability statement (NAS)   A form required for preauthorization when a TRICARE member seeks medical services in other than military treatment facilities.

noncovered (excluded) services   A service specified in a medical insurance contract as not eligible for benefits.

nonparticipating (nonPAR) physician   A physician or other health care provider who chooses not to join a particular government or other program or plan.

nontraumatic injury   A condition caused by the work environment over a period longer than one work day or shift. Also known as occupational disease or illness.

not elsewhere classified (NEC)   An ICD-9-CM abbreviation indicating the code to be used when an illness or condition cannot be placed in any other category.

Notice of Claim Filed   Notification from Social Security that a patient of a medical office has filed for disability compensation.

Notice of Exclusions from Medicare Benefits (NEMB)   Former form for notifying Medicare beneficiaries that a service is not covered by the program; now included in the Advance Beneficiary Notice of Noncoverage (ABN)

Notice of Privacy Practices (NPP)   A HIPAA-mandated description of a covered entity's principles and procedures related to the protection of patients' health information.

not otherwise specified (NOS)   An ICD-9-CM abbreviation indicating the code to be used when no information is available for assigning the illness or condition a more specific code.

O

occlusion   The contact between the upper and lower teeth.

occupational disease/illness   A condition caused by the work environment over a period longer than one work day or shift; also known as nontraumatic injury.

Occupational Safety and Health Administration (OSHA)   Federal agency that regulates workers' health and safety risks in the workplace.

Office of Civil Rights (OCR)   Government agency that enforces the HIPAA Privacy Act.

Office of the Inspector General (OIG)   Government agency that investigates and prosecutes fraud against government health care programs such as Medicare.

Office of Workers' Compensation Programs (OWCP)   The office of the U.S. Department of Labor that administers the Federal Employees' Compensation Act.

OIG Compliance Program Guidance for Individual and Small Group Physician Practices   OIG publication that explains the recommended features of compliance plans for small providers.

oral cavity   The inner section of the mouth.

oral surgery   Surgical procedure related to the face and jaw.

Original Medicare Plan   The Medicare fee-for-service plan.

out-of-area program   A Blue Cross and Blue Shield Association program that provides benefits for subscribers who are away from their local areas.

out-of-network   Providers or suppliers who do not participate in a managed care organization or health plan.

out-of-pocket   Expenses the insured must pay for a particular encounter before benefits begin.

outpatient   A patient who receives health care in a hospital setting without admission; the length of stay is generally less than 23 hours.

outside laboratory   Work performed by an independent laboratory rather than by a physician-operated in-office laboratory.

overpayment   An improper or excessive payment to a provider as a result of billing or claims processing errors for which a refund is owed by the provider.

P

palate   The roof of the mouth.

panel   In CPT, a single code grouping laboratory tests that are frequently done together.

participating (PAR) physician   A physician who agrees to provide medical services to a payer's policyholders according to the terms of the plan or program's contract.

password   Confidential authentication information composed of a string of characters.

patient aging report   A report grouping unpaid patients' bills by the length of time that they remain due, such as 30, 60, 90, or 120 days.

patient information form   A form that includes a patient's personal, employment, and insurance company data needed to complete a health care claim; also known as a registration form.

patient ledger   A record of all charges and payments made on a particular patient's account.

patient statement   A report that shows the services provided to a patient, the total payments made, total charges, adjustments, and the balance due.

payer   Insurance carrier; also known as insurance company, health plan, or third-party payer.

payer of last resort   Regulation that Medicaid pays last on a claim when a patient has other insurance coverage.

pay-to provider   The person or organization that is to receive payment for services reported on a HIPAA claim; may be the same as or different from the billing provider.

permanent disability   A condition that prevents a person with a disability compensation program from doing any job.

Physician Quality Reporting Initiative (PQRI)   A CMS program that provides a potential bonus for performance by physicians on selected measures addressing quality of care.

place of service (POS) code   A HIPAA administrative code that indicates where medical services have been provided, such as an office or hospital.

point-of-service (POS) plan   In HMOs, a plan that permits patients to receive medical services from non-network providers; this choice requires a larger patient payment than visits with network providers.

policyholder   A person who buys an insurance plan; the insured, subscriber, or guarantor.

preauthorization   Prior authorization from a payer for services to be provided; if not received, the charge is not usually covered.

preexisting condition   An illness or disorder of a beneficiary that existed before the effective date of insurance coverage.

preferred provider organization (PPO)   A managed care organization structured as a network of health care providers who agree to perform services for plan members at discounted fees; usually, plan members can receive services from non-network providers for a higher charge.

premium   The periodic amount of money the insured pays to a health plan for a health care policy.

premolars   Four of the 32 permanent adult teeth.

present on admission (POA) indicator   Indicator required by Medicare that identifies whether a coded condition was present at the time of hospital admission.

preventive medical services   Care that is provided to keep patients healthy or to prevent illness, such as routine checkups and screening tests.

Primary Care Manager (PCM)   Provider who coordinates and manages the care of TRICARE beneficiaries.

primary care physician (PCP)   A physician in a health maintenance organization who directs all aspects of a patient's care, including routine services, referrals to specialists within the system, and supervision of hospital admissions; also known as a gatekeeper.

primary diagnosis   A diagnosis that represents the patient's major illness or condition for an encounter.

primary insurance (payer)   The health plan that pays benefits first when a patient is covered by more than one plan.

primary procedure   The most resource-intensive (highest paid) CPT procedure done during a patient's encounter.

principal diagnosis   The condition that after study is established as chiefly responsible for a patient's admission to a hospital.

principal procedure   The main service performed for the condition listed as the principal diagnosis for a hospital inpatient.

prior authorization number   An identifying code assigned by a government program or health insurance plan when preauthorization is required; also called the certification number.

private disability insurance   An insurance plan that can be purchased to provide the insured benefits when illness or injury prevents employment.

procedure code   A code that identifies medical treatment or diagnostic services.

procedures   Medical treatments and services provided by physicians and other licensed medical professionals.

professional courtesy   Discounting fees or not charging a physician's family members or other physicians for work performed.

prognosis   The physician's prediction of outcome of disease and likelihood of recovery.

progress report   A report filed by the physician in state workers' compensation cases when a patient's medical condition or disability changes; also known as a supplemental report.

prophylaxes   Dental procedure to clean the teeth.

Prospective Payment System (PPS)   Medicare system for payment for institutional services.

prostheses (dental)   Dental bridges and dentures.

protected health information (PHI)   Individually identifiable health information that is transmitted or maintained by electronic media.

provider   A person or entity that supplies medical or health services and bills for or is paid for the services in the normal course of business. A provider may be a professional member of the health care team, such as a physician, or a facility, such as a hospital or skilled nursing home.

pulp   The soft core of the tooth containing the nerves and blood vessels.

Q

qualifier   A code indicating what a particular number represents.

R

real-time claims adjudication (RTCA)   Electronic health insurance claim processed at patient check-out; allows practice to know what the patient will owe for the visit.

reasonable fee   The lower of either the fee the physician bills or the usual fee, unless special circumstances apply.

referral   Transfer of patient care from one physician to another.

referral number   Authorization number given by a referring physician to the referred physician.

referring provider   The physician who refers the patient to another physician for treatment.

registration   The process of gathering personal and insurance information about a patient during admission to a hospital.

relative value scale (RVS)   System of assigning unit values to medical services based on an analysis of the skill and time required of the physician to perform them.

relative value unit (RVU)   A factor assigned to a medical service based on the relative skill and time required to perform it.

remittance   The statement of the results of the health plan's adjudication of a claim.

remittance advice (RA)   Health plan document describing a payment resulting from a claim adjudication; also called an explanation of benefits (EOB).

rendering provider   Term used to identify the physician or other medical professional who provides the procedure reported on a health care claim if other than the pay-to provider.

Resource-Based Relative Value Scale (RBRVS)   - Federally mandated relative value scale for establishing Medicare charges.

responsible party   Person or entity other than the insured or the patient who will pay a patient's charges.

retention schedule   A practice policy that governs which information from patients' medical records is to be stored, for how long it is to be retained, and the storage medium to be used.

rider   Document that modifies an insurance contract.

S

schedule of benefits   A list of the medical expenses that a health plan covers.

secondary insurance (payer)   The health plan that pays benefits after the primary plan when a patient is covered by more than one plan.

secondary procedure   A procedure performed in addition to the primary procedure.

secondary provider identifier   On HIPAA claims, identifiers that may be required by various plans in addition to the NPI, such as a plan identification number.

self-insured employer   A company that creates its own insurance plan for its employees, rather than using a carrier; the employer assumes all payment risk, contracts with physicians, and pays for claims from a company fund.

self-pay patient   A patient who does not have insurance coverage.

service line information   On a HIPAA claim, information about the services being reported.

small health plan   Under HIPAA, a health plan with under $5 million in annual receivables.

Social Security Disability Insurance (SSDI)   The federal disability compensation program for salaried and hourly wage earners, self-employed people who pay a special tax, and widows, widowers, and minor children with disabilities whose deceased spouse/parent would qualify for Social Security benefits if alive.

sponsor   The uniformed service member in a family qualified for TRICARE or CHAMPVA.

staff model HMO   A type of HMO in which member providers are employees of the organization and provide services for only HMO-member patients.

State Children's Health Insurance Program (SCHIP)   - Program offering health insurance coverage for uninsured children under Medicaid.

state compensation board/commission   The state agency that administers state workers' compensation laws.

State Disability Insurance (SDI)   State-based disability insurance program that covers all the employees in a state.

subcategory   In ICD-9-CM, a four-digit code number.

subclassification   In ICD-9-CM, a five-digit code number.

subpoena   A order of a court for a party to appear and testify in a court of law.

subpoena *duces tecum* An order of a court directing a party to appear, to testify, and to bring specified documents or items.

subscriber The insured.

subterm A word or phrase that describes a main term in the Alphabetic Index of the ICD-9-CM.

superbill A listing of the diagnoses, procedures, and charges for a patient's visit; also called the encounter form.

supplemental insurance An insurance plan, such as Medigap, that provides benefits for services which are not normally covered by a primary plan.

supplemental report A report filed by the physician in state workers' compensation cases when a patient's medical condition or disability changes; also known as progress report.

Supplemental Security Income (SSI) A government program that helps pay living expenses for low-income older people and those who are blind or have disabilities.

supplementary term A nonessential word or phrase that helps to define a code in the ICD-9-CM; usually enclosed in parentheses or brackets.

surgical package A combination of services included in a single procedure code for some surgical procedures in CPT.

T

Tabular List The section of the ICD-9-CM in which diagnosis codes are presented in numerical order.

taxonomy code Administrative code set under HIPAA that is used to report a physician's specialty when it affects payment.

Temporary Assistance for Needy Families (TANF) A government program that provides cash assistance for low-income families.

temporary disability A condition that keeps a person with a private disability compensation program from working at the usual job for a short time, but from which the worker is expected to recover completely and return to work.

third-party liability An obligation of an insurance plan or government program to pay all or part of medical costs.

third-party payer A private or governmental organization that insures or pays for health care on the behalf of beneficiaries: The insured person is the first party, the provider the second party, and the payer the third party.

timely filing The payer's guidelines for the deadline (in days from date of service) for sending claims; claims submitted after the deadline may be denied or reduced.

transactions Under HIPAA, a structured set of data transmitted between two parties to carry out financial or administrative activities related to health care; in a medical billing program, a financial exchange that is recorded, such as a patient's copayment or deposit of funds into the provider's bank account.

traumatic injury An injury caused by a specific event or series of events within a single work day or shift.

treatment, payment, and operations (TPO) Health care treatment, payment, and operations; under HIPAA, patients' protected health information may be shared for TPO.

TRICARE A government health program that serves dependents of active-duty service members, military retirees and their families, some former spouses, and survivors of deceased military members; formerly called CHAMPUS.

TRICARE Extra TRICARE'S managed care health plan that offers a network of civilian providers.

TRICARE for Life Program for beneficiaries who are both Medicare and TRICARE eligible.

TRICARE Prime The basic managed care health plan offered by TRICARE.

TRICARE Prime Remote A TRICARE plan that provides no-cost health care through civilian providers for eligible service members and their families who are on remote assignment.

TRICARE Standard The fee-for-service health plan offered by TRICARE.

TRICARE Reserve Select TRICARE health plan offered to certain members of the National Guard and Reserve activated on or after September 11, 2001.

U

UB-04 (formerly UB-92) Paper hospital claim, formerly a Medicare-required Part A (hospital) form; also known as the CMS-1450.

UB-92 See UB-04.

unbundle The incorrect billing practice of breaking a panel or package of services/ procedures into component parts and reporting them separately.

uncollectible account Monies that cannot be collected from the practice's payers or patients and must be written off.

unlisted procedures A service that is not listed in CPT; reported with an unlisted procedure code and requires a special report when used.

upcode Use of a procedure code that provides a higher payment than the code for the service actually provided.

urgently needed care In Medicare, a beneficiary's unexpected illness or injury requiring immediate treatment; Medicare plans pay for this service even if it is provided out of a plan's service area.

usual, customary, and reasonable (UCR) Setting fees by comparing the usual fee the provider charges for the service, the customary fee charged by most providers in the community, and what is reasonable considering the circumstances.

usual fee   Fee for a service or procedure that is charged by a provider for most patients under typical circumstances.

uvula   The cone-shaped structure at the end of the soft palate.

V

V code   An alphanumeric code in the ICD-9-CM that identifies factors that influence health status and encounters that are not due to illness or injury.

Veteran's Compensation Program   A federal disability program covering veterans of the uniformed services.

Veteran's Pension Program   A federal disability program covering veterans of the uniformed services.

W

walkout receipt   A medical billing program report given to a patient that lists the diagnoses, services provided, fees, and payments received and due after an encounter.

Welfare Reform Act   1996 law that established the Temporary Assistance for Needy Families program in place of the Aid to Families with Dependent Children program and tightened Medicaid eligibility requirements.

workers' compensation insurance   A state or federal plan that covers medical care and other benefits for employees who suffer accidental injury or become ill as a result of employment.

write off   (N. write-off) To deduct an amount from a patient's account because of a contractual agreement to accept a payer's allowed charge or other reason.

Index

1500

HEALTH INSURANCE CLAIM FORM

APPROVED BY NATIONAL UNIFORM CLAIM COMMITTEE 08/05

| | PICA | | | | | | | | PICA | |

1. MEDICARE ☐ (Medicare #) **MEDICAID** ☐ (Medicaid #) **TRICARE CHAMPUS** ☐ (Sponsor's SSN) **CHAMPVA** ☐ (Member ID#) **GROUP HEALTH PLAN** ☐ (SSN or ID) **FECA BLK LUNG** ☐ (SSN) **OTHER** ☐ (ID)

1a. INSURED'S I.D. NUMBER (For Program in Item 1)

2. PATIENT'S NAME (Last Name, First Name, Middle Initial)

3. PATIENT'S BIRTH DATE MM | DD | YY   **SEX** M ☐ F ☐

4. INSURED'S NAME (Last Name, First Name, Middle Initial)

5. PATIENT'S ADDRESS (No., Street)

6. PATIENT RELATIONSHIP TO INSURED Self ☐ Spouse ☐ Child ☐ Other ☐

7. INSURED'S ADDRESS (No., Street)

CITY   **STATE**

8. PATIENT STATUS Single ☐ Married ☐ Other ☐   Employed ☐ Full-Time Student ☐ Part-Time Student ☐

CITY   **STATE**

ZIP CODE   **TELEPHONE** (Include Area Code) ( )

ZIP CODE   **TELEPHONE** (INCLUDE AREA CODE) ( )

9. OTHER INSURED'S NAME (Last Name, First Name, Middle Initial)

10. IS PATIENT'S CONDITION RELATED TO:

11. INSURED'S POLICY GROUP OR FECA NUMBER

a. OTHER INSURED'S POLICY OR GROUP NUMBER

a. EMPLOYMENT? (CURRENT OR PREVIOUS) ☐ YES ☐ NO

a. INSURED'S DATE OF BIRTH MM | DD | YY   **SEX** M ☐ F ☐

b. OTHER INSURED'S DATE OF BIRTH MM | DD | YY   **SEX** M ☐ F ☐

b. AUTO ACCIDENT? ☐ YES ☐ NO   **PLACE** (State)

b. EMPLOYER'S NAME OR SCHOOL NAME

c. EMPLOYER'S NAME OR SCHOOL NAME

c. OTHER ACCIDENT? ☐ YES ☐ NO

c. INSURANCE PLAN NAME OR PROGRAM NAME

d. INSURANCE PLAN NAME OR PROGRAM NAME

10d. RESERVED FOR LOCAL USE

d. IS THERE ANOTHER HEALTH BENEFIT PLAN? ☐ YES ☐ NO   *If yes*, return to and complete item 9 a-d.

READ BACK OF FORM BEFORE COMPLETING & SIGNING THIS FORM.

12. PATIENT'S OR AUTHORIZED PERSON'S SIGNATURE I authorize the release of any medical or other information necessary to process this claim. I also request payment of government benefits either to myself or to the party who accepts assignment below.

SIGNED _____   DATE _____

13. INSURED'S OR AUTHORIZED PERSON'S SIGNATURE I authorize payment of medical benefits to the undersigned physician or supplier for services described below.

SIGNED _____

14. DATE OF CURRENT: MM | DD | YY ◄ ILLNESS (First symptom) OR INJURY (Accident) OR PREGNANCY(LMP)

15. IF PATIENT HAS HAD SAME OR SIMILAR ILLNESS. GIVE FIRST DATE MM | DD | YY

16. DATES PATIENT UNABLE TO WORK IN CURRENT OCCUPATION FROM MM | DD | YY TO MM | DD | YY

17. NAME OF REFERRING PHYSICIAN OR OTHER SOURCE

17a.
17b. NPI

18. HOSPITALIZATION DATES RELATED TO CURRENT SERVICES FROM MM | DD | YY TO MM | DD | YY

19. RESERVED FOR LOCAL USE

20. OUTSIDE LAB? ☐ YES ☐ NO   **$ CHARGES**

21. DIAGNOSIS OR NATURE OF ILLNESS OR INJURY. (Relate Items 1,2,3 or 4 to Item 24e by Line)

1. ____ . ____   3. ____ . ____
2. ____ . ____   4. ____ . ____

22. MEDICAID RESUBMISSION CODE   **ORIGINAL REF. NO.**

23. PRIOR AUTHORIZATION NUMBER

24. A. DATE(S) OF SERVICE From MM DD YY To MM DD YY	B. PLACE OF SERVICE	C. EMG	D. PROCEDURES, SERVICES, OR SUPPLIES (Explain Unusual Circumstances) CPT/HCPCS	MODIFIER	E. DIAGNOSIS POINTER	F. $ CHARGES	G. DAYS OR UNITS	H. EPSDT Family Plan	I. ID. QUAL.	J. RENDERING PROVIDER ID.#
1									NPI	
2									NPI	
3									NPI	
4									NPI	
5									NPI	
6									NPI	

25. FEDERAL TAX I.D. NUMBER   SSN ☐ EIN ☐

26. PATIENT'S ACCOUNT NO.

27. ACCEPT ASSIGNMENT? (For govt. claims, see back) ☐ YES ☐ NO

28. TOTAL CHARGE $

29. AMOUNT PAID $

30. BALANCE DUE $

31. SIGNATURE OF PHYSICIAN OR SUPPLIER INCLUDING DEGREES OR CREDENTIALS (I certify that the statements on the reverse apply to this bill and are made a part thereof.)

SIGNED _____   DATE _____

32. SERVICE FACILITY LOCATION INFORMATION

a. NPI   b.

33. BILLING PROVIDER INFO & PHONE # ( )

a. NPI   b.

NUCC Instruction Manual available at: www.nucc.org

BECAUSE THIS FORM IS USED BY VARIOUS GOVERNMENT AND PRIVATE HEALTH PROGRAMS, SEE SEPARATE INSTRUCTIONS ISSUED BY APPLICABLE PROGRAMS.

NOTICE: Any person who knowingly files a statement of claim containing any misrepresentation or any false, incomplete or misleading information may be guilty of a criminal act punishable under law and may be subject to civil penalties.

REFERS TO GOVERNMENT PROGRAMS ONLY

MEDICARE AND CHAMPUS PAYMENTS: A patient's signature requests that payment be made and authorizes release of any information necessary to process the claim and certifies that the information provided in Blocks 1 through 12 is true, accurate and complete. In the case of a Medicare claim, the patient's signature authorizes any entity to release to Medicare medical and nonmedical information, including employment status, and whether the person has employer group health insurance, liability, no-fault, worker's compensation or other insurance which is responsible to pay for the services for which the Medicare claim is made. See 42 CFR 411.24(a). If item 9 is completed, the patient's signature authorizes release of the information to the health plan or agency shown. In Medicare assigned or CHAMPUS participation cases, the physician agrees to accept the charge determination of the Medicare carrier or CHAMPUS fiscal intermediary as the full charge, and the patient is responsible only for the deductible, coinsurance and noncovered services. Coinsurance and the deductible are based upon the charge determination of the Medicare carrier or CHAMPUS fiscal intermediary if this is less than the charge submitted. CHAMPUS is not a health insurance program but makes payment for health benefits provided through certain affiliations with the Uniformed Services. Information on the patient's sponsor should be provided in those items captioned in "Insured"; i.e., items 1a, 4, 6, 7, 9, and 11.

BLACK LUNG AND FECA CLAIMS

The provider agrees to accept the amount paid by the Government as payment in full. See Black Lung and FECA instructions regarding required procedure and diagnosis coding systems.

SIGNATURE OF PHYSICIAN OR SUPPLIER (MEDICARE, CHAMPUS, FECA AND BLACK LUNG)

I certify that the services shown on this form were medically indicated and necessary for the health of the patient and were personally furnished by me or were furnished incident to my professional service by my employee under my immediate personal supervision, except as otherwise expressly permitted by Medicare or CHAMPUS regulations.

For services to be considered as "incident" to a physician's professional service, 1) they must be rendered under the physician's immediate personal supervision by his/her employee, 2) they must be an integral, although incidental part of a covered physician's service, 3) they must be of kinds commonly furnished in physician's offices, and 4) the services of nonphysicians must be included on the physician's bills.

For CHAMPUS claims, I further certify that I (or any employee) who rendered services am not an active duty member of the Uniformed Services or a civilian employee of the United States Government or a contract employee of the United States Government, either civilian or military (refer to 5 USC 5536). For Black-Lung claims, I further certify that the services performed were for a Black Lung-related disorder.

No Part B Medicare benefits may be paid unless this form is received as required by existing law and regulations (42 CFR 424.32).

NOTICE: Any one who misrepresents or falsifies essential information to receive payment from Federal funds requested by this form may upon conviction be subject to fine and imprisonment under applicable Federal laws.

NOTICE TO PATIENT ABOUT THE COLLECTION AND USE OF MEDICARE, CHAMPUS, FECA, AND BLACK LUNG INFORMATION
(PRIVACY ACT STATEMENT)

We are authorized by CMS, CHAMPUS and OWCP to ask you for information needed in the administration of the Medicare, CHAMPUS, FECA, and Black Lung programs. Authority to collect information is in section 205(a), 1862, 1872 and 1874 of the Social Security Act as amended, 42 CFR 411.24(a) and 424.5(a) (6), and 44 USC 3101;41 CFR 101 et seq and 10 USC 1079 and 1086; 5 USC 8101 et seq; and 30 USC 901 et seq; 38 USC 613; E.O. 9397.

The information we obtain to complete claims under these programs is used to identify you and to determine your eligibility. It is also used to decide if the services and supplies you received are covered by these programs and to insure that proper payment is made.

The information may also be given to other providers of services, carriers, intermediaries, medical review boards, health plans, and other organizations or Federal agencies, for the effective administration of Federal provisions that require other third parties payers to pay primary to Federal program, and as otherwise necessary to administer these programs. For example, it may be necessary to disclose information about the benefits you have used to a hospital or doctor. Additional disclosures are made through routine uses for information contained in systems of records.

FOR MEDICARE CLAIMS: See the notice modifying system No. 09-70-0501, titled, 'Carrier Medicare Claims Record,' published in the <u>Federal Register</u>, Vol. 55 No. 177, page 37549, Wed. Sept. 12, 1990, or as updated and republished.

FOR OWCP CLAIMS: Department of Labor, Privacy Act of 1974, "Republication of Notice of Systems of Records," <u>Federal Register</u> Vol. 55 No. 40, Wed Feb. 28, 1990, See ESA-5, ESA-6, ESA-12, ESA-13, ESA-30, or as updated and republished.

FOR CHAMPUS CLAIMS: <u>PRINCIPLE PURPOSE(S):</u> To evaluate eligibility for medical care provided by civilian sources and to issue payment upon establishment of eligibility and determination that the services/supplies received are authorized by law.

<u>ROUTINE USE(S):</u> Information from claims and related documents may be given to the Dept. of Veterans Affairs, the Dept. of Health and Human Services and/or the Dept. of Transportation consistent with their statutory administrative responsibilities under CHAMPUS/CHAMPVA; to the Dept. of Justice for representation of the Secretary of Defense in civil actions; to the Internal Revenue Service, private collection agencies, and consumer reporting agencies in connection with recoupment claims; and to Congressional Offices in response to inquiries made at the request of the person to whom a record pertains. Appropriate disclosures may be made to other federal, state, local, foreign government agencies, private business entities, and individual providers of care, on matters relating to entitlement, claims adjudication, fraud, program abuse, utilization review, quality assurance, peer review, program integrity, third-party liability, coordination of benefits, and civil and criminal litigation related to the operation of CHAMPUS.

<u>DISCLOSURES:</u> Voluntary; however, failure to provide information will result in delay in payment or may result in denial of claim. With the one exception discussed below, there are no penalties under these programs for refusing to supply information. However, failure to furnish information regarding the medical services rendered or the amount charged would prevent payment of claims under these programs. Failure to furnish any other information, such as name or claim number, would delay payment of the claim. Failure to provide medical information under FECA could be deemed an obstruction.

It is mandatory that you tell us if you know that another party is responsible for paying for your treatment. Section 1128B of the Social Security Act and 31 USC 3801-3812 provide penalties for withholding this information.

You should be aware that P.L. 100-503, the "Computer Matching and Privacy Protection Act of 1988", permits the government to verify information by way of computer matches.

MEDICAID PAYMENTS (PROVIDER CERTIFICATION)

I hereby agree to keep such records as are necessary to disclose fully the extent of services provided to individuals under the State's Title XIX plan and to furnish information regarding any payments claimed for providing such services as the State Agency or Dept. of Health and Human Services may request.

I further agree to accept, as payment in full, the amount paid by the Medicaid program for those claims submitted for payment under that program, with the exception of authorized deductible, coinsurance, co-payment or similar cost-sharing charge.

SIGNATURE OF PHYSICIAN (OR SUPPLIER): I certify that the services listed above were medically indicated and necessary to the health of this patient and were personally furnished by me or my employee under my personal direction.

NOTICE: This is to certify that the foregoing information is true, accurate and complete. I understand that payment and satisfaction of this claim will be from Federal and State funds, and that any false claims, statements, or documents, or concealment of a material fact, may be prosecuted under applicable Federal or State laws.

According to the Paperwork Reduction Act of 1995, no persons are required to respond to a collection of information unless it displays a valid OMB control number. The valid OMB control number for this information collection is 0938-0008. The time required to complete this information collection is estimated to average 10 minutes per response, including the time to review instructions, search existing data resources, gather the data needed, and complete and review the information collection. If you have any comments concerning the accuracy of the time estimate(s) or suggestions for improving this form, please write to: CMS, Attn: PRA Reports Clearance Officer, 7500 Security Boulevard, Baltimore, Maryland 21244-1850.

HEALTH INSURANCE CLAIM FORM

APPROVED BY NATIONAL UNIFORM CLAIM COMMITTEE 08/05

☐ PICA ☐ ☐ | PICA ☐☐☐

CARRIER →

1. MEDICARE ☐ (Medicare #)	MEDICAID ☐ (Medicaid #)	TRICARE CHAMPUS ☐ (Sponsor's SSN)	CHAMPVA ☐ (Member ID#)	GROUP HEALTH PLAN ☐ (SSN or ID)	FECA BLK LUNG ☐ (SSN)	OTHER ☐ (ID)	1a. INSURED'S I.D. NUMBER (For Program in Item 1)

2. PATIENT'S NAME (Last Name, First Name, Middle Initial)	3. PATIENT'S BIRTH DATE MM ¦ DD ¦ YY SEX M ☐ F ☐	4. INSURED'S NAME (Last Name, First Name, Middle Initial)

5. PATIENT'S ADDRESS (No., Street)	6. PATIENT RELATIONSHIP TO INSURED Self ☐ Spouse ☐ Child ☐ Other ☐	7. INSURED'S ADDRESS (No., Street)

CITY	STATE	8. PATIENT STATUS Single ☐ Married ☐ Other ☐	CITY	STATE

ZIP CODE	TELEPHONE (Include Area Code) ( )	Employed ☐ Full-Time Student ☐ Part-Time Student ☐	ZIP CODE	TELEPHONE (INCLUDE AREA CODE) ( )

9. OTHER INSURED'S NAME (Last Name, First Name, Middle Initial)	10. IS PATIENT'S CONDITION RELATED TO:	11. INSURED'S POLICY GROUP OR FECA NUMBER

a. OTHER INSURED'S POLICY OR GROUP NUMBER	a. EMPLOYMENT? (CURRENT OR PREVIOUS) YES ☐ NO ☐	a. INSURED'S DATE OF BIRTH MM ¦ DD ¦ YY SEX M ☐ F ☐

b. OTHER INSURED'S DATE OF BIRTH MM ¦ DD ¦ YY SEX M ☐ F ☐	b. AUTO ACCIDENT? YES ☐ NO ☐ PLACE (State)	b. EMPLOYER'S NAME OR SCHOOL NAME

c. EMPLOYER'S NAME OR SCHOOL NAME	c. OTHER ACCIDENT? YES ☐ NO ☐	c. INSURANCE PLAN NAME OR PROGRAM NAME

d. INSURANCE PLAN NAME OR PROGRAM NAME	10d. RESERVED FOR LOCAL USE	d. IS THERE ANOTHER HEALTH BENEFIT PLAN? YES ☐ NO ☐ If yes, return to and complete item 9 a-d.

PATIENT AND INSURED INFORMATION →

READ BACK OF FORM BEFORE COMPLETING & SIGNING THIS FORM.

12. PATIENT'S OR AUTHORIZED PERSON'S SIGNATURE I authorize the release of any medical or other information necessary to process this claim. I also request payment of government benefits either to myself or to the party who accepts assignment below.

SIGNED _____ DATE _____

13. INSURED'S OR AUTHORIZED PERSON'S SIGNATURE I authorize payment of medical benefits to the undersigned physician or supplier for services described below.

SIGNED _____

14. DATE OF CURRENT: MM ¦ DD ¦ YY ◄ ILLNESS (First symptom) OR INJURY (Accident) OR PREGNANCY(LMP)	15. IF PATIENT HAS HAD SAME OR SIMILAR ILLNESS. GIVE FIRST DATE MM ¦ DD ¦ YY	16. DATES PATIENT UNABLE TO WORK IN CURRENT OCCUPATION FROM MM ¦ DD ¦ YY TO MM ¦ DD ¦ YY

17. NAME OF REFERRING PHYSICIAN OR OTHER SOURCE	17a. 17b. NPI	18. HOSPITALIZATION DATES RELATED TO CURRENT SERVICES FROM MM ¦ DD ¦ YY TO MM ¦ DD ¦ YY

19. RESERVED FOR LOCAL USE		20. OUTSIDE LAB? YES ☐ NO ☐ $ CHARGES

21. DIAGNOSIS OR NATURE OF ILLNESS OR INJURY. (Relate Items 1,2,3 or 4 to Item 24e by Line) 1. └── . ── 3. └── . ── 2. └── . ── 4. └── . ──	22. MEDICAID RESUBMISSION CODE ORIGINAL REF. NO.
	23. PRIOR AUTHORIZATION NUMBER

24. A. DATE(S) OF SERVICE From MM DD YY To MM DD YY	B. PLACE OF SERVICE	C. EMG	D. PROCEDURES, SERVICES, OR SUPPLIES (Explain Unusual Circumstances) CPT/HCPCS ¦ MODIFIER	E. DIAGNOSIS POINTER	F. $ CHARGES	G. DAYS OR UNITS	H. EPSDT Family Plan	I. ID. QUAL.	J. RENDERING PROVIDER ID.#
1								NPI	
2								NPI	
3								NPI	
4								NPI	
5								NPI	
6								NPI	

25. FEDERAL TAX I.D. NUMBER SSN ☐ EIN ☐	26. PATIENT'S ACCOUNT NO.	27. ACCEPT ASSIGNMENT? (For govt. claims, see back) YES ☐ NO ☐	28. TOTAL CHARGE $	29. AMOUNT PAID $	30. BALANCE DUE $

31. SIGNATURE OF PHYSICIAN OR SUPPLIER INCLUDING DEGREES OR CREDENTIALS (I certify that the statements on the reverse apply to this bill and are made a part thereof.) SIGNED _____ DATE _____	32. SERVICE FACILITY LOCATION INFORMATION a. NPI b.	33. BILLING PROVIDER INFO & PHONE # ( ) a. NPI b.

PHYSICIAN OR SUPPLIER INFORMATION →

NUCC Instruction Manual available at: www.nucc.org

BECAUSE THIS FORM IS USED BY VARIOUS GOVERNMENT AND PRIVATE HEALTH PROGRAMS, SEE SEPARATE INSTRUCTIONS ISSUED BY APPLICABLE PROGRAMS.

NOTICE: Any person who knowingly files a statement of claim containing any misrepresentation or any false, incomplete or misleading information may be guilty of a criminal act punishable under law and may be subject to civil penalties.

REFERS TO GOVERNMENT PROGRAMS ONLY

MEDICARE AND CHAMPUS PAYMENTS: A patient's signature requests that payment be made and authorizes release of any information necessary to process the claim and certifies that the information provided in Blocks 1 through 12 is true, accurate and complete. In the case of a Medicare claim, the patient's signature authorizes any entity to release to Medicare medical and nonmedical information, including employment status, and whether the person has employer group health insurance, liability, no-fault, worker's compensation or other insurance which is responsible to pay for the services for which the Medicare claim is made. See 42 CFR 411.24(a). If item 9 is completed, the patient's signature authorizes release of the information to the health plan or agency shown. In Medicare assigned or CHAMPUS participation cases, the physician agrees to accept the charge determination of the Medicare carrier or CHAMPUS fiscal intermediary as the full charge, and the patient is responsible only for the deductible, coinsurance and noncovered services. Coinsurance and the deductible are based upon the charge determination of the Medicare carrier or CHAMPUS fiscal intermediary if this is less than the charge submitted. CHAMPUS is not a health insurance program but makes payment for health benefits provided through certain affiliations with the Uniformed Services. Information on the patient's sponsor should be provided in those items captioned in "Insured"; i.e., items 1a, 4, 6, 7, 9, and 11.

BLACK LUNG AND FECA CLAIMS

The provider agrees to accept the amount paid by the Government as payment in full. See Black Lung and FECA instructions regarding required procedure and diagnosis coding systems.

SIGNATURE OF PHYSICIAN OR SUPPLIER (MEDICARE, CHAMPUS, FECA AND BLACK LUNG)

I certify that the services shown on this form were medically indicated and necessary for the health of the patient and were personally furnished by me or were furnished incident to my professional service by my employee under my immediate personal supervision, except as otherwise expressly permitted by Medicare or CHAMPUS regulations.

For services to be considered as "incident" to a physician's professional service, 1) they must be rendered under the physician's immediate personal supervision by his/her employee, 2) they must be an integral, although incidental part of a covered physician's service, 3) they must be of kinds commonly furnished in physician's offices, and 4) the services of nonphysicians must be included on the physician's bills.

For CHAMPUS claims, I further certify that I (or any employee) who rendered services am not an active duty member of the Uniformed Services or a civilian employee of the United States Government or a contract employee of the United States Government, either civilian or military (refer to 5 USC 5536). For Black-Lung claims, I further certify that the services performed were for a Black Lung-related disorder.

No Part B Medicare benefits may be paid unless this form is received as required by existing law and regulations (42 CFR 424.32).

NOTICE: Any one who misrepresents or falsifies essential information to receive payment from Federal funds requested by this form may upon conviction be subject to fine and imprisonment under applicable Federal laws.

NOTICE TO PATIENT ABOUT THE COLLECTION AND USE OF MEDICARE, CHAMPUS, FECA, AND BLACK LUNG INFORMATION
(PRIVACY ACT STATEMENT)

We are authorized by CMS, CHAMPUS and OWCP to ask you for information needed in the administration of the Medicare, CHAMPUS, FECA, and Black Lung programs. Authority to collect information is in section 205(a), 1862, 1872 and 1874 of the Social Security Act as amended, 42 CFR 411.24(a) and 424.5(a) (6), and 44 USC 3101;41 CFR 101 et seq and 10 USC 1079 and 1086; 5 USC 8101 et seq; and 30 USC 901 et seq; 38 USC 613; E.O. 9397.

The information we obtain to complete claims under these programs is used to identify you and to determine your eligibility. It is also used to decide if the services and supplies you received are covered by these programs and to insure that proper payment is made.

The information may also be given to other providers of services, carriers, intermediaries, medical review boards, health plans, and other organizations or Federal agencies, for the effective administration of Federal provisions that require other third parties payers to pay primary to Federal program, and as otherwise necessary to administer these programs. For example, it may be necessary to disclose information about the benefits you have used to a hospital or doctor. Additional disclosures are made through routine uses for information contained in systems of records.

FOR MEDICARE CLAIMS: See the notice modifying system No. 09-70-0501, titled, 'Carrier Medicare Claims Record,' published in the Federal Register, Vol. 55 No. 177, page 37549, Wed. Sept. 12, 1990, or as updated and republished.

FOR OWCP CLAIMS: Department of Labor, Privacy Act of 1974, "Republication of Notice of Systems of Records," Federal Register Vol. 55 No. 40, Wed Feb. 28, 1990, See ESA-5, ESA-6, ESA-12, ESA-13, ESA-30, or as updated and republished.

FOR CHAMPUS CLAIMS: PRINCIPLE PURPOSE(S): To evaluate eligibility for medical care provided by civilian sources and to issue payment upon establishment of eligibility and determination that the services/supplies received are authorized by law.

ROUTINE USE(S): Information from claims and related documents may be given to the Dept. of Veterans Affairs, the Dept. of Health and Human Services and/or the Dept. of Transportation consistent with their statutory administrative responsibilities under CHAMPUS/CHAMPVA; to the Dept. of Justice for representation of the Secretary of Defense in civil actions; to the Internal Revenue Service, private collection agencies, and consumer reporting agencies in connection with recoupment claims; and to Congressional Offices in response to inquiries made at the request of the person to whom a record pertains. Appropriate disclosures may be made to other federal, state, local, foreign government agencies, private business entities, and individual providers of care, on matters relating to entitlement, claims adjudication, fraud, program abuse, utilization review, quality assurance, peer review, program integrity, third-party liability, coordination of benefits, and civil and criminal litigation related to the operation of CHAMPUS.

DISCLOSURES: Voluntary; however, failure to provide information will result in delay in payment or may result in denial of claim. With the one exception discussed below, there are no penalties under these programs for refusing to supply information. However, failure to furnish information regarding the medical services rendered or the amount charged would prevent payment of claims under these programs. Failure to furnish any other information, such as name or claim number, would delay payment of the claim. Failure to provide medical information under FECA could be deemed an obstruction.

It is mandatory that you tell us if you know that another party is responsible for paying for your treatment. Section 1128B of the Social Security Act and 31 USC 3801-3812 provide penalties for withholding this information.

You should be aware that P.L. 100-503, the "Computer Matching and Privacy Protection Act of 1988", permits the government to verify information by way of computer matches.

MEDICAID PAYMENTS (PROVIDER CERTIFICATION)

I hereby agree to keep such records as are necessary to disclose fully the extent of services provided to individuals under the State's Title XIX plan and to furnish information regarding any payments claimed for providing such services as the State Agency or Dept. of Health and Human Services may request.

I further agree to accept, as payment in full, the amount paid by the Medicaid program for those claims submitted for payment under that program, with the exception of authorized deductible, coinsurance, co-payment or similar cost-sharing charge.

SIGNATURE OF PHYSICIAN (OR SUPPLIER): I certify that the services listed above were medically indicated and necessary to the health of this patient and were personally furnished by me or my employee under my personal direction.

NOTICE: This is to certify that the foregoing information is true, accurate and complete. I understand that payment and satisfaction of this claim will be from Federal and State funds, and that any false claims, statements, or documents, or concealment of a material fact, may be prosecuted under applicable Federal or State laws.

1500

HEALTH INSURANCE CLAIM FORM

APPROVED BY NATIONAL UNIFORM CLAIM COMMITTEE 08/05

☐☐ PICA

PICA ☐☐

1. MEDICARE ☐ (Medicare #)   **MEDICAID** ☐ (Medicaid #)   **TRICARE CHAMPUS** ☐ (Sponsor's SSN)   **CHAMPVA** ☐ (Member ID#)   **GROUP HEALTH PLAN** ☐ (SSN or ID)   **FECA BLK LUNG** ☐ (SSN)   **OTHER** ☐ (ID)

1a. INSURED'S I.D. NUMBER (For Program in Item 1)

2. PATIENT'S NAME (Last Name, First Name, Middle Initial)

3. PATIENT'S BIRTH DATE MM | DD | YY   **SEX** M ☐ F ☐

4. INSURED'S NAME (Last Name, First Name, Middle Initial)

5. PATIENT'S ADDRESS (No., Street)

6. PATIENT RELATIONSHIP TO INSURED Self ☐ Spouse ☐ Child ☐ Other ☐

7. INSURED'S ADDRESS (No., Street)

CITY   STATE

8. PATIENT STATUS Single ☐ Married ☐ Other ☐   Employed ☐ Full-Time Student ☐ Part-Time Student ☐

CITY   STATE

ZIP CODE   TELEPHONE (Include Area Code) ( )

ZIP CODE   TELEPHONE (INCLUDE AREA CODE) ( )

9. OTHER INSURED'S NAME (Last Name, First Name, Middle Initial)

10. IS PATIENT'S CONDITION RELATED TO:

11. INSURED'S POLICY GROUP OR FECA NUMBER

a. OTHER INSURED'S POLICY OR GROUP NUMBER

a. EMPLOYMENT? (CURRENT OR PREVIOUS) YES ☐ NO ☐

a. INSURED'S DATE OF BIRTH MM | DD | YY   **SEX** M ☐ F ☐

b. OTHER INSURED'S DATE OF BIRTH MM | DD | YY   SEX M ☐ F ☐

b. AUTO ACCIDENT? YES ☐ NO ☐ PLACE (State)

b. EMPLOYER'S NAME OR SCHOOL NAME

c. EMPLOYER'S NAME OR SCHOOL NAME

c. OTHER ACCIDENT? YES ☐ NO ☐

c. INSURANCE PLAN NAME OR PROGRAM NAME

d. INSURANCE PLAN NAME OR PROGRAM NAME

10d. RESERVED FOR LOCAL USE

d. IS THERE ANOTHER HEALTH BENEFIT PLAN? YES ☐ NO ☐ *If yes*, return to and complete item 9 a-d.

READ BACK OF FORM BEFORE COMPLETING & SIGNING THIS FORM.
12. PATIENT'S OR AUTHORIZED PERSON'S SIGNATURE I authorize the release of any medical or other information necessary to process this claim. I also request payment of government benefits either to myself or to the party who accepts assignment below.

SIGNED _____ DATE _____

13. INSURED'S OR AUTHORIZED PERSON'S SIGNATURE I authorize payment of medical benefits to the undersigned physician or supplier for services described below.

SIGNED _____

14. DATE OF CURRENT: MM | DD | YY ◄ ILLNESS (First symptom) OR INJURY (Accident) OR PREGNANCY(LMP)

15. IF PATIENT HAS HAD SAME OR SIMILAR ILLNESS. GIVE FIRST DATE MM | DD | YY

16. DATES PATIENT UNABLE TO WORK IN CURRENT OCCUPATION MM | DD | YY FROM   MM | DD | YY TO

17. NAME OF REFERRING PHYSICIAN OR OTHER SOURCE

17a.
17b. NPI

18. HOSPITALIZATION DATES RELATED TO CURRENT SERVICES MM | DD | YY FROM   MM | DD | YY TO

19. RESERVED FOR LOCAL USE

20. OUTSIDE LAB? YES ☐ NO ☐ $ CHARGES

21. DIAGNOSIS OR NATURE OF ILLNESS OR INJURY. (Relate Items 1,2,3 or 4 to Item 24e by Line)

1. ⌊___.___⌋   3. ⌊___.___⌋
2. ⌊___.___⌋   4. ⌊___.___⌋

22. MEDICAID RESUBMISSION CODE   ORIGINAL REF. NO.

23. PRIOR AUTHORIZATION NUMBER

24. A. DATE(S) OF SERVICE						B. PLACE OF SERVICE	C. EMG	D. PROCEDURES, SERVICES, OR SUPPLIES (Explain Unusual Circumstances)		E. DIAGNOSIS POINTER	F. $ CHARGES	G. DAYS OR UNITS	H. EPSDT Family Plan	I. ID. QUAL.	J. RENDERING PROVIDER ID.#
From MM	DD	YY	To MM	DD	YY			CPT/HCPCS	MODIFIER						
1														NPI	
2														NPI	
3														NPI	
4														NPI	
5														NPI	
6														NPI	

25. FEDERAL TAX I.D. NUMBER SSN ☐ EIN ☐

26. PATIENT'S ACCOUNT NO.

27. ACCEPT ASSIGNMENT? (For govt. claims, see back) YES ☐ NO ☐

28. TOTAL CHARGE $

29. AMOUNT PAID $

30. BALANCE DUE $

31. SIGNATURE OF PHYSICIAN OR SUPPLIER INCLUDING DEGREES OR CREDENTIALS (I certify that the statements on the reverse apply to this bill and are made a part thereof.)

SIGNED _____ DATE _____

32. SERVICE FACILITY LOCATION INFORMATION

a. NPI   b.

33. BILLING PROVIDER INFO & PHONE # ( )

a. NPI   b.

NUCC Instruction Manual available at: www.nucc.org

BECAUSE THIS FORM IS USED BY VARIOUS GOVERNMENT AND PRIVATE HEALTH PROGRAMS, SEE SEPARATE INSTRUCTIONS ISSUED BY APPLICABLE PROGRAMS.

NOTICE: Any person who knowingly files a statement of claim containing any misrepresentation or any false, incomplete or misleading information may be guilty of a criminal act punishable under law and may be subject to civil penalties.

REFERS TO GOVERNMENT PROGRAMS ONLY

MEDICARE AND CHAMPUS PAYMENTS: A patient's signature requests that payment be made and authorizes release of any information necessary to process the claim and certifies that the information provided in Blocks 1 through 12 is true, accurate and complete. In the case of a Medicare claim, the patient's signature authorizes any entity to release to Medicare medical and nonmedical information, including employment status, and whether the person has employer group health insurance, liability, no-fault, worker's compensation or other insurance which is responsible to pay for the services for which the Medicare claim is made. See 42 CFR 411.24(a). If item 9 is completed, the patient's signature authorizes release of the information to the health plan or agency shown. In Medicare assigned or CHAMPUS participation cases, the physician agrees to accept the charge determination of the Medicare carrier or CHAMPUS fiscal intermediary as the full charge, and the patient is responsible only for the deductible, coinsurance and noncovered services. Coinsurance and the deductible are based upon the charge determination of the Medicare carrier or CHAMPUS fiscal intermediary if this is less than the charge submitted. CHAMPUS is not a health insurance program but makes payment for health benefits provided through certain affiliations with the Uniformed Services. Information on the patient's sponsor should be provided in those items captioned "Insured"; i.e., items 1a, 4, 6, 7, 9, and 11.

BLACK LUNG AND FECA CLAIMS

The provider agrees to accept the amount paid by the Government as payment in full. See Black Lung and FECA instructions regarding required procedure and diagnosis coding systems.

SIGNATURE OF PHYSICIAN OR SUPPLIER (MEDICARE, CHAMPUS, FECA AND BLACK LUNG)

I certify that the services shown on this form were medically indicated and necessary for the health of the patient and were personally furnished by me or were furnished incident to my professional service by my employee under my immediate personal supervision, except as otherwise expressly permitted by Medicare or CHAMPUS regulations.

For services to be considered as "incident" to a physician's professional service, 1) they must be rendered under the physician's immediate personal supervision by his/her employee, 2) they must be an integral, although incidental part of a covered physician's service, 3) they must be of kinds commonly furnished in physician's offices, and 4) the services of nonphysicians must be included on the physician's bills.

For CHAMPUS claims, I further certify that I (or any employee) who rendered services am not an active duty member of the Uniformed Services or a civilian employee of the United States Government or a contract employee of the United States Government, either civilian or military (refer to 5 USC 5536). For Black-Lung claims, I further certify that the services performed were for a Black Lung-related disorder.

No Part B Medicare benefits may be paid unless this form is received as required by existing law and regulations (42 CFR 424.32).

NOTICE: Any one who misrepresents or falsifies essential information to receive payment from Federal funds requested by this form may upon conviction be subject to fine and imprisonment under applicable Federal laws.

NOTICE TO PATIENT ABOUT THE COLLECTION AND USE OF MEDICARE, CHAMPUS, FECA, AND BLACK LUNG INFORMATION
(PRIVACY ACT STATEMENT)

We are authorized by CMS, CHAMPUS and OWCP to ask you for information needed in the administration of the Medicare, CHAMPUS, FECA, and Black Lung programs. Authority to collect information is in section 205(a), 1862, 1872 and 1874 of the Social Security Act as amended, 42 CFR 411.24(a) and 424.5(a) (6), and 44 USC 3101;41 CFR 101 et seq and 10 USC 1079 and 1086; 5 USC 8101 et seq; and 30 USC 901 et seq; 38 USC 613; E.O. 9397.

The information we obtain to complete claims under these programs is used to identify you and to determine your eligibility. It is also used to decide if the services and supplies you received are covered by these programs and to insure that proper payment is made.

The information may also be given to other providers of services, carriers, intermediaries, medical review boards, health plans, and other organizations or Federal agencies, for the effective administration of Federal provisions that require other third parties payers to pay primary to Federal program, and as otherwise necessary to administer these programs. For example, it may be necessary to disclose information about the benefits you have used to a hospital or doctor. Additional disclosures are made through routine uses for information contained in systems of records.

FOR MEDICARE CLAIMS: See the notice modifying system No. 09-70-0501, titled, 'Carrier Medicare Claims Record,' published in the Federal Register, Vol. 55 No. 177, page 37549, Wed. Sept. 12, 1990, or as updated and republished.

FOR OWCP CLAIMS: Department of Labor, Privacy Act of 1974, "Republication of Notice of Systems of Records," Federal Register Vol. 55 No. 40, Wed Feb. 28, 1990, See ESA-5, ESA-6, ESA-12, ESA-13, ESA-30, or as updated and republished.

FOR CHAMPUS CLAIMS: PRINCIPLE PURPOSE(S): To evaluate eligibility for medical care provided by civilian sources and to issue payment upon establishment of eligibility and determination that the services/supplies received are authorized by law.

ROUTINE USE(S): Information from claims and related documents may be given to the Dept. of Veterans Affairs, the Dept. of Health and Human Services and/or the Dept. of Transportation consistent with their statutory administrative responsibilities under CHAMPUS/CHAMPVA; to the Dept. of Justice for representation of the Secretary of Defense in civil actions; to the Internal Revenue Service, private collection agencies, and consumer reporting agencies in connection with recoupment claims; and to Congressional Offices in response to inquiries made at the request of the person to whom a record pertains. Appropriate disclosures may be made to other federal, state, local, foreign government agencies, private business entities, and individual providers of care, on matters relating to entitlement, claims adjudication, fraud, program abuse, utilization review, quality assurance, peer review, program integrity, third-party liability, coordination of benefits, and civil and criminal litigation related to the operation of CHAMPUS.

DISCLOSURES: Voluntary; however, failure to provide information will result in delay in payment or may result in denial of claim. With the one exception discussed below, there are no penalties under these programs for refusing to supply information. However, failure to furnish information regarding the medical services rendered or the amount charged would prevent payment of claims under these programs. Failure to furnish any other information, such as name or claim number, would delay payment of the claim. Failure to provide medical information under FECA could be deemed an obstruction.

It is mandatory that you tell us if you know that another party is responsible for paying for your treatment. Section 1128B of the Social Security Act and 31 USC 3801-3812 provide penalties for withholding this information.

You should be aware that P.L. 100-503, the "Computer Matching and Privacy Protection Act of 1988", permits the government to verify information by way of computer matches.

MEDICAID PAYMENTS (PROVIDER CERTIFICATION)

I hereby agree to keep such records as are necessary to disclose fully the extent of services provided to individuals under the State's Title XIX plan and to furnish information regarding any payments claimed for providing such services as the State Agency or Dept. of Health and Human Services may request.

I further agree to accept, as payment in full, the amount paid by the Medicaid program for those claims submitted for payment under that program, with the exception of authorized deductible, coinsurance, co-payment or similar cost-sharing charge.

SIGNATURE OF PHYSICIAN (OR SUPPLIER): I certify that the services listed above were medically indicated and necessary to the health of this patient and were personally furnished by me or my employee under my personal direction.

NOTICE: This is to certify that the foregoing information is true, accurate and complete. I understand that payment and satisfaction of this claim will be from Federal and State funds, and that any false claims, statements, or documents, or concealment of a material fact, may be prosecuted under applicable Federal or State laws.

349

BECAUSE THIS FORM IS USED BY VARIOUS GOVERNMENT AND PRIVATE HEALTH PROGRAMS, SEE SEPARATE INSTRUCTIONS ISSUED BY APPLICABLE PROGRAMS.

NOTICE: Any person who knowingly files a statement of claim containing any misrepresentation or any false, incomplete or misleading information may be guilty of a criminal act punishable under law and may be subject to civil penalties.

REFERS TO GOVERNMENT PROGRAMS ONLY

MEDICARE AND CHAMPUS PAYMENTS: A patient's signature requests that payment be made and authorizes release of any information necessary to process the claim and certifies that the information provided in Blocks 1 through 12 is true, accurate and complete. In the case of a Medicare claim, the patient's signature authorizes any entity to release to Medicare medical and nonmedical information, including employment status, and whether the person has employer group health insurance, liability, no-fault, worker's compensation or other insurance which is responsible to pay for the services for which the Medicare claim is made. See 42 CFR 411.24(a). If item 9 is completed, the patient's signature authorizes release of the information to the health plan or agency shown. In Medicare assigned or CHAMPUS participation cases, the physician agrees to accept the charge determination of the Medicare carrier or CHAMPUS fiscal intermediary as the full charge, and the patient is responsible only for the deductible, coinsurance and noncovered services. Coinsurance and the deductible are based upon the charge determination of the Medicare carrier or CHAMPUS fiscal intermediary if this is less than the charge submitted. CHAMPUS is not a health insurance program but makes payment for health benefits provided through certain affiliations with the Uniformed Services. Information on the patient's sponsor should be provided in those items captioned in "Insured"; i.e., items 1a, 4, 6, 7, 9, and 11.

BLACK LUNG AND FECA CLAIMS

The provider agrees to accept the amount paid by the Government as payment in full. See Black Lung and FECA instructions regarding required procedure and diagnosis coding systems.

SIGNATURE OF PHYSICIAN OR SUPPLIER (MEDICARE, CHAMPUS, FECA AND BLACK LUNG)

I certify that the services shown on this form were medically indicated and necessary for the health of the patient and were personally furnished by me or were furnished incident to my professional service by my employee under my immediate personal supervision, except as otherwise expressly permitted by Medicare or CHAMPUS regulations.

For services to be considered as "incident" to a physician's professional service, 1) they must be rendered under the physician's immediate personal supervision by his/her employee, 2) they must be an integral, although incidental part of a covered physician's service, 3) they must be of kinds commonly furnished in physician's offices, and 4) the services of nonphysicians must be included on the physician's bills.

For CHAMPUS claims, I further certify that I (or any employee) who rendered services am not an active duty member of the Uniformed Services or a civilian employee of the United States Government or a contract employee of the United States Government, either civilian or military (refer to 5 USC 5536). For Black-Lung claims, I further certify that the services performed were for a Black Lung-related disorder.

No Part B Medicare benefits may be paid unless this form is received as required by existing law and regulations (42 CFR 424.32).

NOTICE: Any one who misrepresents or falsifies essential information to receive payment from Federal funds requested by this form may upon conviction be subject to fine and imprisonment under applicable Federal laws.

NOTICE TO PATIENT ABOUT THE COLLECTION AND USE OF MEDICARE, CHAMPUS, FECA, AND BLACK LUNG INFORMATION
(PRIVACY ACT STATEMENT)

We are authorized by CMS, CHAMPUS and OWCP to ask you for information needed in the administration of the Medicare, CHAMPUS, FECA, and Black Lung programs. Authority to collect information is in section 205(a), 1862, 1872 and 1874 of the Social Security Act as amended, 42 CFR 411.24(a) and 424.5(a) (6), and 44 USC 3101;41 CFR 101 et seq and 10 USC 1079 and 1086; 5 USC 8101 et seq; and 30 USC 901 et seq; 38 USC 613; E.O. 9397.

The information we obtain to complete claims under these programs is used to identify you and to determine your eligibility. It is also used to decide if the services and supplies you received are covered by these programs and to insure that proper payment is made.

The information may also be given to other providers of services, carriers, intermediaries, medical review boards, health plans, and other organizations or Federal agencies, for the effective administration of Federal provisions that require other third parties payers to pay primary to Federal program, and as otherwise necessary to administer these programs. For example, it may be necessary to disclose information about the benefits you have used to a hospital or doctor. Additional disclosures are made through routine uses for information contained in systems of records.

FOR MEDICARE CLAIMS: See the notice modifying system No. 09-70-0501, titled, 'Carrier Medicare Claims Record,' published in the <u>Federal Register</u>, Vol. 55 No. 177, page 37549, Wed. Sept. 12, 1990, or as updated and republished.

FOR OWCP CLAIMS: Department of Labor, Privacy Act of 1974, "Republication of Notice of Systems of Records," <u>Federal Register</u> Vol. 55 No. 40, Wed Feb. 28, 1990, See ESA-5, ESA-6, ESA-12, ESA-13, ESA-30, or as updated and republished.

FOR CHAMPUS CLAIMS: <u>PRINCIPLE PURPOSE(S):</u> To evaluate eligibility for medical care provided by civilian sources and to issue payment upon establishment of eligibility and determination that the services/supplies received are authorized by law.

<u>ROUTINE USE(S):</u> Information from claims and related documents may be given to the Dept. of Veterans Affairs, the Dept. of Health and Human Services and/or the Dept. of Transportation consistent with their statutory administrative responsibilities under CHAMPUS/CHAMPVA; to the Dept. of Justice for representation of the Secretary of Defense in civil actions; to the Internal Revenue Service, private collection agencies, and consumer reporting agencies in connection with recoupment claims; and to Congressional Offices in response to inquiries made at the request of the person to whom a record pertains. Appropriate disclosures may be made to other federal, state, local, foreign government agencies, private business entities, and individual providers of care, on matters relating to entitlement, claims adjudication, fraud, program abuse, utilization review, quality assurance, peer review, program integrity, third-party liability, coordination of benefits, and civil and criminal litigation related to the operation of CHAMPUS.

<u>DISCLOSURES:</u> Voluntary; however, failure to provide information will result in delay in payment or may result in denial of claim. With the one exception discussed below, there are no penalties under these programs for refusing to supply information. However, failure to furnish information regarding the medical services rendered or the amount charged would prevent payment of claims under these programs. Failure to furnish any other information, such as name or claim number, would delay payment of the claim. Failure to provide medical information under FECA could be deemed an obstruction.

It is mandatory that you tell us if you know that another party is responsible for paying for your treatment. Section 1128B of the Social Security Act and 31 USC 3801-3812 provide penalties for withholding this information.

You should be aware that P.L. 100-503, the "Computer Matching and Privacy Protection Act of 1988", permits the government to verify information by way of computer matches.

MEDICAID PAYMENTS (PROVIDER CERTIFICATION)

I hereby agree to keep such records as are necessary to disclose fully the extent of services provided to individuals under the State's Title XIX plan and to furnish information regarding any payments claimed for providing such services as the State Agency or Dept. of Health and Human Services may request.

I further agree to accept, as payment in full, the amount paid by the Medicaid program for those claims submitted for payment under that program, with the exception of authorized deductible, coinsurance, co-payment or similar cost-sharing charge.

SIGNATURE OF PHYSICIAN (OR SUPPLIER): I certify that the services listed above were medically indicated and necessary to the health of this patient and were personally furnished by me or my employee under my personal direction.

NOTICE: This is to certify that the foregoing information is true, accurate and complete. I understand that payment and satisfaction of this claim will be from Federal and State funds, and that any false claims, statements, or documents, or concealment of a material fact, may be prosecuted under applicable Federal or State laws.

According to the Paperwork Reduction Act of 1995, no persons are required to respond to a collection of information unless it displays a valid OMB control number. The valid OMB control number for this information collection is 0938-0008. The time required to complete this information collection is estimated to average 10 minutes per response, including the time to review instructions, search existing data resources, gather the data needed, and complete and review the information collection. If you have any comments concerning the accuracy of the time estimate(s) or suggestions for improving this form, please write to: CMS, Attn: PRA Reports Clearance Officer, 7500 Security Boulevard, Baltimore, Maryland 21244-1850.